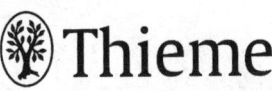

NANDA International, Inc.
Nursing Diagnoses

Definitions and Classification

2021–2023
Twelfth Edition

Edited by

T. Heather Herdman, PhD, RN, FNI, FAAN

Shigemi Kamitsuru, PhD, RN, FNI

Camila Takáo Lopes, PhD, RN, FNI

Thieme
New York • Stuttgart • Delhi • Rio de Janeiro

Library of Congress Cataloging-in-Publication Data is available from the publisher.

For information on licensing the NANDA International (NANDA-I) nursing diagnostic system or permission to use it in other works, please e-mail: nanda-i@thieme.com; additional product information can be found by visiting: www.thieme.com/nanda-i.

Thieme Medical Publishers, Inc.
333 Seventh Avenue, 18th Floor
New York, NY 10001, USA
www.thieme.com
+1-800-782-3488
customerservice@thieme.com

Cover design: © Thieme
Cover image source: © Gorodenkoff/stock.adobe.com – stock photo. Posed by models
Typesetting by DiTech Process Solutions, India; typeset using Arbortext.
Printed by King Printing Co., Inc.

Printed in the United States of America.

DOI 10.1055/b000000515

ISBN 978-1-68420-454-0
ISSN 1943-0728

6 5 4 3 2

Also available as an e-book:
eISBN 978-1-68420-455-7

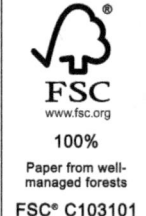

FSC
www.fsc.org
100%
Paper from well-managed forests
FSC® C103101

Dedication

The Board of Directors of NANDA International, Inc., would like to dedicate this book to nurses working on the front lines of the COVID-19 pandemic. We honor your courage and dedication during this time. We especially wish to recognize those nurses who lost their lives while caring for patients and families.

Preface

The International Year of the Nurse and Midwife began with a battle with COVID-19. I cannot thank healthcare professionals enough who are caring for patients despite, at times, the lack of protective equipment. I am writing this as the impact of COVID-19 is continuing around the world. I hope that by the time you read this text, effective treatments and preventive measures have been developed and are available to everyone.

A while back, a nurse fighting on the frontline asked me, "Which nursing diagnosis should I use for COVID-19 patients?" This question reminded me of the need to repeatedly emphasize the meaning of nursing diagnosis. Most importantly, patients with the same medical diagnosis do not necessarily have the same human responses (nursing diagnoses). Likewise, patients with the same genotype of coronavirus infection do not necessarily have the same human responses. That is why, prior to providing proper care for each patient, nurses must conduct a nursing assessment and identify his/her unique responses (nursing diagnoses). Even at times like those we are facing today, nurses need to identify what we independently diagnose and treat related to patients and their families, which are different from medical diagnoses. If nurses have properly documented the nursing diagnoses of patients with COVID-19 and their families, then in the near future, we will be able to identify commonalities and differences in their human responses, from an international perspective.

In this 2021–2023 version, the Twelfth Edition, the classification provides 267 diagnoses, with the addition of new diagnoses. Each nursing diagnosis has been the product of one or more of our many NANDA International (NANDA-I) volunteers, and most have a defined evidence base. Each new diagnosis has been reviewed and refined by our Diagnosis Development Committee (DDC) members assigned as primary reviewers, and by content experts, prior to receiving DDC approval. This DDC approval does not mean the diagnosis is "completed" or "ready to be used" across all countries or practice areas. We all know that practice and regulation of nursing varies from region to region. It is our hope that publication of these new diagnoses will facilitate further validation studies in different parts of the world, to achieve a higher level of evidence.

We always welcome submissions for new nursing diagnoses. At the same time, we have a serious need for revision of existing diagnoses to reflect the most recent evidence. In the eleventh edition, we identified approximately

90 diagnoses without an assigned level of evidence (LOE), or which required major updates. Thanks to the cooperation of many volunteers, most of whom were published in the focus area of the diagnosis, the majority of these diagnoses are now revised and have met requirements for our LOE criteria. However, we were not able to complete all revisions, so 32 diagnoses remain without an identified LOE. The intention is to revise or retire these remaining diagnoses by the next edition. I want to strongly encourage all students and researchers to submit their nursing diagnosis-related research results to NANDA-I, to improve the evidence base of the terminology.

The NANDA-I terminology is translated into more than 20 distinct languages. Translating abstract English terms into other languages can often be frustrating. During this cycle, a decision was made to incorporate standardized terms from the United States National Library of Medicine, the Medical Subject Headings (MeSH), to facilitate translation. Identifying the MeSH terms, where appropriate, that are found within our diagnostic indicators provides standardized definitions for terms, which we believe will support translators in their work.

The years since the past edition have also been the first in what we hope will be a lasting partnership with our academic partner, Boston College (BC) and the Connell School of Nursing. Under the direction of Dr. Dorothy Jones, the Marjory Gordon Program for Knowledge Development and Clinical Reasoning has been established. We held our first conference at BC in 2018, and had planned our second conference for 2020, which unfortunately was cancelled due to the impact of COVID-19. However, work on an online educational module has been completed as a joint venture between BC and NANDA-I, several postdoctoral scholars have been welcomed into the program from around the world (Brazil, Italy, Spain, Nigeria), and our collaboration continues. We look forward to additional conferences, educational opportunities, postdoctoral scholarships, and future opportunities that this partnership with BC will bring. I wish to extend my sincere gratitude to Dr. Jones, Dean Susan Gennaro, and Associate Dean Christopher Grillo for their collaboration, collegiality, and dedication to making this partnership a reality.

I want to acknowledge the work of all NANDA-I volunteers, committee members, chairpersons, and members of the Board of Directors for their time, commitment, devotion, and ongoing support. I would also like to thank the various content experts who, although not members of NANDA International, contributed countless hours to reviewing and revising diagnoses in their area of expertise. The NANDA-I staff, led by our Chief Executive Officer, Dr. T. Heather Herdman, is to be commended for its efforts and support.

My special thanks to the members of the DDC and the Expert Clinical Advisory Panel for their outstanding and timely efforts to review and edit the terminology represented within this book, and especially for the leadership of our new DDC Chair, Dr. Camila Takáo Lopes, who began her term in 2019. This remarkable committee, with representation from North and South America and Europe, is the true "powerhouse" of the NANDA-I knowledge content. I am deeply impressed and pleased by the astonishing, comprehensive work of these volunteers during this cycle, and I am confident that you will be, as well.

It has been my honor and privilege to serve as President of this dedicated association of international nurses, and I look forward to where the future will continue to take our work.

Shigemi Kamitsuru, PhD, RN, FNI
President, NANDA International, Inc.

Acknowledgments

Substantial changes have been made in this edition. That would not be possible without a significant amount of voluntary time and effort donated by many nurses around the world. We would especially like to show appreciation to the following:

Chapter Contributors.
Revised Level of Evidence Criteria for Diagnosis Submission
- Marcos Venícios de Oliveira Lopes, PhD, RN, FNI. *Universidade Federal do Ceará* (Federal University of Ceará), Brazil
- Viviane Martins da Silva, PhD, RN, FNI. *Universidade Federal do Ceará* (Federal University of Ceará), Brazil
- Diná Monteiro da Cruz, PhD, RN, FNI. *Universidade de São Paulo* (São Paulo University), Brazil

Nursing Diagnosis Basics, and Nursing Diagnosis: An International Terminology
- Susan Gallagher-Lepak, PhD, RN. University of Wisconsin – Green Bay, USA

Clinical Reasoning: From Assessment to Diagnosis Generation
- Dorothy A. Jones, EdD, RNC, ANP, FNI, FAAN. Boston College, USA
- Rita de Cássia Gengo e Silva Butcher, PhD, RN. The Marjory Gordon Program for Clinical Reasoning and Knowledge Development, Boston College, USA

Specifications and Definitions Within the NANDA International Taxonomy of Nursing Diagnoses
- Sílvia Caldeira, PhD, RN. *Universidade Católica Portuguesa* (Catholic Portuguese University), Portugal

Consultants.
Indication of content experts for the DDC Task Force 2019
- Emilia Campos de Carvalho, PhD, RN, FNI. *Universidade de São Paulo* (São Paulo University) Brazil

Mental health diagnostic content
- Jacqueline K. Cantor, MSN, RN, PMHCNS-BC, APRN. West Hartford, USA

Primary healthcare diagnostic content
- Ángel Martín García, RN. *Centro de Salud San Blas* (Sal Blas Healthcare Center), Spain
- Martín Rodríguez Álvaro, PhD, RN. *Universidad de la Laguna* (Laguna University), Spain

Critical care diagnostic content
- Fabio D'Agostino, PhD, RN. Saint Camillus International University of Health and Medical Sciences, Italy
- Gianfranco Sanson, PhD, RN. *Università degli studi di Trieste* (University of Trieste), Italy

Technical support.
The editors would like to extend a special acknowledgment to Mary Kalinosky, Senior Technical Developer, from Thieme Publishers. Her work to create and adapt the NANDA-I terminology database has significantly improved our ability to evaluate and revise the terms within the classification. We are in her debt for her dedication to this enormous project.

Please contact us at admin@nanda.org if you have questions on any of the content or if you find errors, so that these may be corrected for future publication and translation.

Sincerely,

T. Heather Herdman, PhD, RN, FNI, FAAN
Shigemi Kamitsuru, PhD, RN, FNI
Camila Takáo Lopes, PhD, RN, FNI
NANDA International, Inc.

Contents

Domain 2. Nutrition

Domain 3. Elimination and exchange

Domain 5. Perception/cognition

Domain 6. Self-perception

Domain 7. Role relationship

Domain 10. Life principles 447

Domain 11. Safety/protection 463

Class 3. Violence

Class 4. Environmental hazards

Class 5. Defensive processes

Part 1
The NANDA International Terminology: General Information

1 What's New in the NANDA-I 2021–2023 Edition

T. Heather Herdman, Shigemi Kamitsuru, Camila Takáo Lopes

1.1 Overview on Changes and Revisions in the NANDA-I 2021–2023 Edition

Part 1 presents an overview of major changes to this edition: new and revised diagnoses, retired diagnoses, continued revision to standardize diagnostic indicator terms, new level of evidence criteria for diagnosis submission, a proposed refinement to the terminology, and introductory recommendations on nursing diagnoses that require development.

It is our hope that the organization of this 12th edition will make it efficient and effective to use. We welcome your feedback. If you have suggestions, please send them by email to: admin@nanda.org.

Changes have been made in this edition based on feedback from users, to address both the needs of students, clinicians, and researchers, as well as to provide additional support to educators. New information has been added to assessment. Many diagnoses were revised by international collaborators of the Diagnosis Development Committee Task Force, in order to strengthen their level of evidence. The diagnostic indicators of each diagnosis were revised to decrease ambiguity and improve clarity. Editors referred to the Medical Subject Headings (MeSH, https://www.ncbi.nlm.nih.gov/mesh) whenever possible, to provide standardized definitions, which are available to translators to ensure consistency across languages. Revised level of evidence criteria are presented to ensure that all future diagnoses submitted for inclusion in the classification are at an appropriate level of evidence to represent the current strength of nursing knowledge.

Users who are familiar with previous editions of this text may note that the diagnostic focus is no longer highlighted in the diagnosis label. Instead, the diagnostic focus will be found below the label for each diagnosis in the classification. This was done to facilitate ease of identification of diagnostic foci across languages.

1.2 New Nursing Diagnoses

A significant body of work representing new and revised nursing diagnoses was submitted to the NANDA-I Diagnosis Development Committee. The editors would like to take this opportunity to congratulate those submitters who successfully met the level of evidence criteria with their submissions and/or revisions. Forty-six new diagnoses were approved by the Diagnosis Development Committee and were presented to the NANDA-I Board of Directors (▶ Table 1.1), and are now included here for members and users of the terminology. The submitters of each diagnosis are presented following the table.

Submitters of nursing diagnoses. Included here are those contributors who submitted new diagnoses or completed reviews of diagnoses including both label and definition change, or significant content change. Individuals who

Table 1.1 New NANDA-I Nursing Diagnoses, 2021–2023*

Domain	Diagnosis
1. Health Promotion	Risk for elopement attempt (00290)
	Readiness for enhanced exercise engagement (00307)
	Ineffective health maintenance behaviors (00292)*
	Ineffective health self-management (00276)*
	Readiness for enhanced health self-management (00293)*
	Ineffective family health self-management (00294)*
	Ineffective home maintenance behaviors (00300)*
	Risk for ineffective home maintenance behaviors (00308)
	Readiness for enhanced home maintenance behaviors (00309)
2. Nutrition	Ineffective infant suck-swallow response (00295)*
	Risk for metabolic syndrome (00296)*
3. Elimination and Exchange	Disability-associated urinary incontinence (00297)*
	Mixed urinary incontinence (00310)
	Risk for urinary retention (00322)
	Impaired bowel continence (00319)*
4. Activity/rest	Decreased activity tolerance (00298)*
	Risk for decreased activity tolerance (00299)*
	Risk for impaired cardiovascular function (00311)
	Ineffective lymphedema self-management (00278)
	Risk for ineffective lymphedema self-management (00281)
	Risk for thrombosis (00291)
	Dysfunctional adult ventilatory weaning response (00318)
5. Perception/cognition	Disturbed thought process (00279)
7. Role relationship	Disturbed family identity syndrome (00283)
	Risk for disturbed family identity syndrome (00284)
9. Coping/stress tolerance	Maladaptive grieving (00301)*
	Risk for maladaptive grieving (00302)*
	Readiness for enhanced grieving (00285)

Table 1.1 *(Continued)*

Domain	Diagnosis
11. Safety/protection	Ineffective dry eye self-management (00277)
	Risk for adult falls (00303)*
	Risk for child falls (00306)
	Nipple-areolar complex injury (00320)
	Risk for nipple-areolar complex injury (00321)
	Adult pressure injury (00312)
	Risk for adult pressure injury (00304)*
	Child pressure injury (00313)
	Risk for child pressure injury (00286)
	Neonatal pressure injury (00287)
	Risk for neonatal pressure injury (00288)
	Risk for suicidal behavior (00289)*
	Neonatal hypothermia (00280)
	Risk for neonatal hypothermia (00282)
13. Growth/ development	Delayed child development (00314)
	Risk for delayed child development (00305)*
	Delayed infant motor development (00315)
	Risk for delayed infant motor development (00316)

*For taxonomic purposes, when a diagnosis label and definition are revised, the original code is retired and a new code is assigned

worked as a group are listed together; in cases where more than one individual or group submitted content, they are listed separately.

Countries of submitters: 1. Brazil, 2. Germany, 3. Iran, 4. Mexico, 5. Spain, 6. Turkey, 7. USA

Domain 1. Health promotion

- Risk for elopement attempt
  - Amália F. Lucena, Ester M. Borba, Betina Franco, Gláucia S. Policarpo, Deborah B. Melo, Simone Pasin, Luciana R. Pinto, Michele Schmid[1]
- Readiness for enhanced exercise engagement
  - Raúl Fernando G. Castañeda[4]
- Ineffective health maintenance behaviors
  - Rafaela S. Pedrosa, Andressa T. Nunciaroni[1]
  - Camila T. Lopes[1]
- Ineffective health self-management
  - Camila S. Carneiro, Agueda Maria R. Z. Cavalcante, Gisele S. Bispo, Viviane M. Silva, Alba Lucia B.L. Barros[1]

- – Maria G.M.N. Paiva, Jéssica D.S. Tinôco, Fernanda Beatriz B.L. Silva, Juliane R. Dantas, Maria Isabel C.D. Fernandes, Isadora L.A. Nogueira, Ana B.A. Medeiros Marcos Venícios O. Lopes, Ana L.B.C. Lira[1]
- – Richardson Augusto R. Silva, Wenysson N. Santos, Francisca M.L.C. Souza, Rebecca Stefany C. Santos, Izaque C. Oliveira, Hallyson L.L. Silva, Dhyanine M. Lima[1]
- – Camila T. Lopes[1]
- – Readiness for enhanced health self-management
  - – DDC
- – Ineffective family health self-management
  - – Andressa T. Nunciaroni, Rafaela S. Pedrosa[1]
  - – Camila T. Lopes[1]
- – Ineffective home maintenance behaviors, Risk for ineffective home maintenance behaviors, Readiness for enhanced home maintenance behaviors
  - – Ángel Martín-García[5]
  - – Diagnosis Development Committee (DDC)

Domain 2. Nutrition
- – Ineffective infant suck-swallow response
  - – T. Heather Herdman[7]
- – Risk for metabolic syndrome
  - – DDC

Domain 3. Elimination and exchange
- – Disability-associated urinary incontinence, Mixed urinary incontinence
  - – Juliana N. Costa, Maria Helena B.M. Lopes, Marcos Venícios O. Lopes[1]
- – Risk for urinary retention
  - – Aline S. Meira, Gabriella S. Lima, Luana B. Storti, Maria Angélica A. Diniz, Renato M. Ribeiro, Samantha S. Cruz, Luciana Kusumota[2]
  - – Juliana N. Costa, Micnéias L. Botelho, Erika C.M. Duran, Elenice V. Carmona, Ana Railka S. Oliveira-Kumakura, Maria Helena B.M. Lopes[2]
- – Impaired bowel continence
  - – DDC
  - – Barbara G. Anderson[7]

Domain 4. Activity/rest
- – Decreased activity tolerance, Risk for decreased activity tolerance
  - – Jana Kolb, Steve Strupeit[2]

- Risk for impaired cardiovascular function
  - María B.S. Gómez[5], Gonzalo D. Clíments[5], Tibelle F. Mauricio[1], Rafaela P. Moreira[1], Edmara C. Costa[1]
  - Gabrielle P. da Silva, Francisca Márcia P. Linhares, Suzana O. Mangueira, Marcos Venícius O. Lopes, Jaqueline G.A. Perrelli, Tatiane G. Guedes[1]
- Ineffective lymphedema self-management, Risk for ineffective lymphedema self-management
  - Gülengün Türk, Elem K. Güler, İzmir Demokrasi[6]
  - DDC
- Risk for thrombosis
  - Eneida R.R. Silva, Thamires S. Hilário, Graziela B. Aliti, Vanessa M. Mantovani, Amália F. Lucena[1]
  - DDC
- Dysfunctional adult ventilatory weaning response
  - Ludmila Christiane R. Silva, Tânia C.M. Chianca[1]

Domain 5. Perception/cognition
- Disturbed thought process
  - Paula Escalada-Hernández, Blanca Marín-Fernández[5]

Domain 7. Role relationship
- Disturbed family identity syndrome, Risk for disturbed family identity syndrome
  - Mitra Zandi, Eesa Mohammadi[3]
  - DDC

Domain 9. Coping/stress tolerance
- Maladaptive grieving, Risk for maladaptive grieving, Readiness for enhanced grieving
  - Martín Rodríguez-Álvaro, Alfonso M. García-Hernández, Ruymán Brito-Brito[5]
  - DDC

Domain 11. Safety/protection
- Ineffective dry eye self-management
  - Elem K. Güler, İsmet Eşer[6], Diego D. Araujo, Andreza Werli-Alvarenga, Tânia C.M. Chianca[1]

- Jéssica N. M. Araújo, Allyne F. Vitor[1]
- DDC
- Risk for adult falls
  - Flávia O.M. Maia[1]
  - Danielle Garbuio, Emilia C. Carvalho[1]
  - Dolores E. Hernández[1]
  - Camila T. Lopes[1]
  - Silvana B. Pena, Heloísa C.Q.C.P. Guimarães, Lidia S. Guandalini, Mônica Taminato, Dulce A. Barbosa, Juliana L. Lopes, Alba Lucia B.L. Barros[1]
- Risk for child falls
  - Camila T. Lopes, Ana Paula D.F. Guareschi[1]
- Neonatal hypothermia, Risk for neonatal hypothermia
  - T. Heather Herdman[7]
- Nipple-areolar complex injury, Risk for nipple-areolar complex injury
  - Flaviana Vely Mendonca Vieira[1]
  - Agueda Maria Ruiz Zimmer Cavalcante[1]
  - Janaina Valadares Guimarães[1]
- Adult pressure injury, Risk for adult pressure injury
  - Amália F. Lucena, Cássia T. Santos, Taline Bavaresco, Miriam A. Almeida[1]
  - T. Heather Herdman[7]
- Child pressure injury, Risk for child pressure injury, Neonatal pressure injury, Risk for neonatal pressure injury
  - T. Heather Herdman[7]
  - Amália F. Lucena, Cássia T. Santos, Taline Bavaresco, Miriam A. Almeida[1]
- Risk for suicidal behavior
  - Girliani S. Sousa, Jaqueline G.A. Perrelli, Suzana O. Mangueira, Marcos Venícios O. Lopes, Everton B. Sougey[1]

Domain 13. Growth/development
- Delayed child development
  - Juliana M. Souza, Maria L.O.R. Veríssimo[1]
  - T. Heather Herdman[7]
- Risk for delayed child development, Delayed infant motor development, Risk for delayed infant motor development
  - T. Heather Herdman[7]

1.3 Revised Nursing Diagnoses

Sixty-seven diagnoses were revised during this cycle as part of the Diagnosis Development Committee Task Force. ▸ Table 1.2 shows those diagnoses. The contributors to revisions of each diagnosis are presented following the table. Not shown in this table are those diagnoses that have revisions strictly due to phrase refinement or minor editorial changes; only those diagnoses with content changes (label revision, diagnosis definition revision, or changes to diagnostic indicators) are shown here.

Contributors to revision of diagnoses. Included here are those contributors who completed reviews of diagnoses.

Countries of revisors: 1. Austria, 2. Brazil, 3. Germany, 4. Italy, 5. Japan, 6. Mexico, 7. Portugal, 8. Spain, 9. Switzerland, 10. Turkey, 11. USA

Domain 1. Health promotion
- Sedentary lifestyle
    - Marcos Venicios O. Lopes, Viviane Martins da Silva, Nirla G. Guedes, Larissa C.G. Martins, Marcos R. Oliveira[2]
    - Laís S.Costa, Juliana L. Lopes, Camila T. Lopes, Vinicius B. Santos, Alba Lúcia B.L. Barros[2]
- Ineffective protection
    - Livia M. Garbim, Fernanda T.M.M. Braga, Renata C.C.P. Silveira[2]

Domain 2. Nutrition
- Imbalanced nutrition: less than body requirements
    - Renata K. Reis, Fernanda R.E.G. Souza[2]
- Impaired swallowing
    - Renan A. Silva, Viviane M. Silva[2]
- Risk for unstable blood glucose level
    - Grasiela M. Barros, Ana Carla D. Cavalcanti, Helen C. Ferreira, Marcos Venícios O. Lopes, Priscilla A. Souza[2]
- Risk for imbalanced fluid volume, Deficient fluid volume, Risk for deficient fluid volume, Excess fluid volume
    - Mariana Grassi, Rodrigo Jensen, Camila T. Lopes[2]

Domain 3. Elimination and exchange
- Impaired urinary elimination, Urinary retention
    - Aline S. Meira, Gabriella S. Lima, Luana B. Storti, Maria Angélica A. Diniz, Renato M. Ribeiro, Samantha S. Cruz, Luciana Kusumota[2]

Table 1.2 Revised NANDA-I Nursing Diagnoses, 2021–2023

Diagnosis	Revision				
	Definition	DC added	DC removed	ReF/RiF added	ReF/RiF removed
Domain 1. Health promotion					
Sedentary lifestyle	X	X	X	X	
Ineffective protection		X		X	
Domain 2. Nutrition					
Imbalanced nutrition: less than body requirements		X	X	X	X
Impaired swallowing		X			
Risk for unstable blood glucose level				X	
Risk for imbalanced fluid volume				X	
Deficient fluid volume				X	
Risk for deficient fluid volume				X	
Excess fluid volume		X		X	
Domain 3. Elimination and exchange					
Impaired urinary elimination					X
Stress urinary incontinence	X	X		X	
Urge urinary incontinence	X			X	
Risk for urge urinary incontinence				X	
Urinary retention	X	X		X	
Constipation	X	X	X	X	X
Risk for constipation				X	
Perceived constipation				X	
Diarrhea	X			X	
Impaired gas exchange		X	X	X	
Domain 4. Activity/rest					
Insomnia	X	X	X	X	X
Impaired bed mobility		X		X	
Impaired wheelchair mobility		X		X	
Fatigue		X	X	X	X
Ineffective breathing pattern		X	X	X	X
Domain 5. Perception/cognition					
Chronic confusion				X	
Deficient knowledge	X	X		X	
Impaired memory				X	
Impaired verbal communication		X		X	

Table 1.2 *(Continued)*

Diagnosis	Revision				
	Definition	DC added	DC removed	ReF/RiF added	ReF/RiF removed
Domain 6. Self-perception					
Hopelessness	X	X	X	X	
Readiness for enhanced hope	X	X			
Chronic low self-esteem	X		X	X	
Risk for chronic low self-esteem	X				
Situational low self-esteem	X		X	X	
Risk for situational low self-esteem	X				
Disturbed body image	X	X	X	X	X
Domain 7. Role relationship					
Impaired parenting	X	X		X	
Risk for impaired parenting	X			X	
Readiness for enhanced parenting	X	X			
Impaired social interaction		X		X	
Domain 9. Coping/stress tolerance					
Anxiety	X	X	X	X	X
Death anxiety	X	X		X	
Fear	X	X	X	X	X
Powerlessness	X	X	X	X	
Risk for powerlessness	X			X	
Domain 10. Life principles					
Readiness for enhanced spiritual well-being	X	X			
Spiritual distress	X	X	X	X	X
Risk for spiritual distress				X	X
Domain 11. Safety/protection					
Risk for infection				X	
Ineffective airway clearance	X	X	X	X	X
Risk for aspiration				X	X
Risk for dry eye	X				X
Risk for urinary tract injury				X	
Risk for perioperative positioning injury				X	
Risk for shock	X			X	

Table 1.2 *(Continued)*

Diagnosis	Revision				
	Definition	DC added	DC removed	ReF/RiF added	ReF/RiF removed
Impaired skin integrity		X	X	X	
Risk for impaired skin integrity				X	
Delayed surgical recovery		X		X	
Risk for delayed surgical recovery				X	
Impaired tissue integrity		X	X	X	
Risk for impaired tissue integrity				X	
Risk for latex allergy reaction	X			X	
Hypothermia	X		X		
Risk for hypothermia					X
Risk for perioperative hypothermia				X	X
Domain 12. Comfort					
Chronic pain syndrome			X	X	
Labor pain				X	
Social isolation	X	X		X	

- Juliana N. Costa, Micnéias L. Botelho, Erika C.M. Duran, Elenice V. Carmona, Ana Railka S. Oliveira-Kumakura, Maria Helena B.M. Lopes[2]
- Stress urinary incontinence, Urge urinary incontinence, Risk for urge urinary incontinence
  - Juliana N. Costa, Maria Helena B.M. Lopes, Marcos Venícios O. Lopes[2]
  - Aline S. Meira, Gabriella S. Lima, Luana B. Storti, Maria Angélica A. Diniz, Renato M. Ribeiro, Samantha S. Cruz, Luciana Kusumota[2]
- Constipation, Risk for constipation
  - Barbara G. Anderson[11]
  - Cibele C. Souza, Emilia C. Carvalho, Marta C.A. Pereira[2]
  - Shigemi Kamitsuru[5]
- Perceived constipation
  - DDC

- Diarrhea
  - Barbara G. Anderson[11]
- Impaired gas exchange
  - Marcos Venícios O. Lopes, Viviane M. Silva, Lívia Maia Pascoal, Beatriz A. Beltrão, Daniel Bruno R. Chaves, Vanessa Emile C. Sousa, Camila M. Dini, Marília M. Nunes, Natália B. Castro, Reinaldo G. Barreiro, Layana P. Cavalcante, Gabriele L. Ferreira, Larissa C.G. Martins[2]

Domain 4. Activity/rest

- Insomnia
  - Lidia S. Guandalini, Vinicius B. Santos, Eduarda F. Silva, Juliana L. Lopes, Camila T. Lopes, Alba Lucia B. L. Barros[2]
- Impaired bed mobility
  - Allyne F. Vitor, Jéssica Naiara M. Araújo, Ana Paula N.L. Fernandes, Amanda B. Silva, Hanna Priscilla da Silva [2]
- Impaired wheelchair mobility
  - Allyne F. Vitor, Jéssica Naiara M. Araújo, Ana Paula N.L. Fernandes, Amanda B. Silva, Hanna Priscilla da Silva [2]
  - Camila T. Lopes[2]
- Fatigue
  - Rita C.G.S. Butcher, Amanda G. Muller, Leticia C. Batista, Mara N. Araújo[2]
  - Vinicius B. Santos, Rita Simone L. Moreira[2]
- Ineffective breathing pattern
  - Viviane M. Silva, Marcos Venícios O. Lopes, Beatriz A. Beltrão, Lívia Maia Pascoal, Daniel Bruno R. Chaves, Livia Zulmyra C. Andrade, Vanessa Emile C. Sousa[2]
  - Patricia R. Prado, Ana Rita C. Bettencourt, Juliana. L. Lopes[2]

Domain 5. Perception/cognition

- Chronic confusion, Impaired memory
  - Priscilla A. Souza[2], Kay Avant[11]
- Deficient knowledge
  - Cláudia C. Silva, Sheila C.R.V. Morais e Cecilia Maria F.Q. Frazão[2]
  - Camila T. Lopes[2]
- Impaired verbal communication
  - Amanda H. Severo, Zuila Maria F. Carvalho, Marcos Venícios O. Lopes, Renata S.F. Brasileiro, Deyse C.O. Braga[2]
  - Vanessa S. Ribeiro, Emilia C. Carvalho[2]

Domain 6. Self-perception
- Hopelessness
  - Ana Carolina A.B. Leite, Willyane A. Alvarenga, Lucila C. Nascimento, Emilia C. Carvalho[2]
  - Ramon A., Cibele Souza, Marta C.A. Pereira[2]
  - Camila T. Lopes[2]
- Readiness for enhanced hope
  - Renan A. Silva[2], Geórgia A.A. Melo[2], Joselany A. Caetano[2], Marcos Venícios O. Lopes[2], Howard K. Butcher[11], Viviane M. Silva[2]
- Chronic low self-esteem and Risk for chronic low self-esteem
  - Natalia B. Castro, Marcos Venícios O. Lopes, Ana Ruth M. Monteiro[2]
  - Camila T. Lopes[2]
- Situational low self-esteem
  - Natalia B. Castro, Marcos Venícios O. Lopes, Ana Ruth M. Monteiro[2]
  - Francisca Marcia P. Linhares, Gabriella P. da Silva, Thais A.O. Moura[2]
  - Camila T. Lopes[2]
- Risk for situational low self-esteem
  - Natalia B. Castro, Marcos Venícios O. Lopes, Ana Ruth M. Monteiro[2]
  - Francisca Marcia P. Linhares, Ryanne Carolynne M. Gomes, Suzana O. Mangueira[2]
  - Camila T. Lopes[2]
- Disturbed body image
  - Julie Varns[11]

Domain 7. Role relationships
- Impaired parenting, Risk for impaired parenting, Readiness for enhanced parenting
  - T. Heather Herdman[10]
- Impaired social interaction
  - Hortensia Castañedo-Hidalgo[6]

Domain 9. Coping/stress tolerance
- Anxiety, Fear
  - Aline A. Eduardo[2]
- Death anxiety
  - Claudia Angélica M.F. Mercês, Jaqueline S.S. Souto, Kênia R.L. Zaccaro, Jackeline F. Souza, Cândida C. Primo, Marcos Antônio G. Brandão[2]
- Powerlessness, Risk for Powerlessness

- Renan A. Silva[2], Álissan Karine L. Martins[2], Natália B. Castro[2], Anna Virgínia Viana[2], Howard K. Butcher[11], Viviane M. Silva[2]

Domain 10. Life principles
- Readiness for enhanced spiritual wellbeing
  - Chontay D. Glenn[11]
  - Silvia Caldeira, Joana Romeiro, Helga Martins[7]
  - Camila T. Lopes[2]
- Spiritual distress and Risk for spiritual distress
  - Silvia Caldeira, Joana Romeiro, Helga Martins[7]
  - Chontay D. Glenn[11]

Domain 11. Safety/protection
- Risk for infection
  - Camila T. Lopes, Vinicius B. Santos, Daniele Cristina B. Aprile, Juliana L. Lopes, Tania A. M. Domingues, Karina Costa[2]
- Ineffective airway clearance
  - Viviane M. Silva, Marcos Venícios O. Lopes, Daniel Bruno R. Chaves, Livia M. Pascoal, Livia Zulmyra C. Andrade, Beatriz A. Beltrão, Vanessa Emile C. Sousa[2]
  - Silvia A. Alonso, Susana A. López, Almudena B. Rodríguez, Luisa P. Hernandez, Paz V. Lozano, Lidia P. López, Ana Campillo, Ana Frías María E. Jiménez, David P. Otero, Respiratory Nursing Group Neumomadrid[8]
  - Gianfranco Sanson[4]
- Risk for aspiration
  - Fernanda R.E.G. Souza, Renata K. Reis[2]
  - Nirla G. Guedes, Viviane M. Silva, Marcos Venícios O. Lopes[2]
- Risk for dry eye
  - Elem K. Güler, İsmet Eşer[10]
  - Diego D. Araujo, Andreza Werli-Alvarenga, Tânia C.M. Chianca[2]
  - Jéssica N. M. Araújo, Allyne F. Vitor[2]
- Risk for urinary tract injury
  - Danielle Garbuio, Emilia C. Carvalho, Anamaria A. Napoleão[2]
- Risk for perioperative positioning injury
  - Danielle Garbuio, Emilia C. Carvalho[2]
  - Camila Mendonça de Moraes, Namie Okino Sawada[2]
- Risk for shock
  - Luciana Ramos Corrêa Pinto, Karina O. Azzolin, Amália de Fátima Lucena[2]

- Impaired skin integrity, Risk for impaired skin integrity, Impaired tissue integrity and Risk for impaired tissue integrity
  - Edgar Noé M. García[6]
  - Camila T. Lopes[2]
- Delayed surgical recovery and Risk for delayed surgical recovery
  - Thalita G. Carmo, Rosimere F. Santana, Marcos Venícios O. Lopes, Simone Rembold[2]
- Risk for latex allergy reaction
  - Sharon E. Hohler[11]
  - Camila T. Lopes[2]
- Hypothermia and Risk for hypothermia
  - T. Heather Herdman[11]
- Risk for perioperative hypothermia
  - Manuel Schwanda[1], Maria Müller-Staub[9], André Ewers[1]

Domain 12. Comfort
- Chronic pain syndrome
  - Thainá L. Silva, Cibele A.M. Pimenta, Marina G. Salvetti[2]
- Labor pain
  - Luisa Eggenschwiler, Monika Linhart, Eva Cignacco[9]
- Social isolation
  - Hortensia Castañeda-Hidalgo[6]
  - Amália de Fátima Lucena[2]

1.4 Changes to Nursing Diagnosis Labels

Changes were made to 17 nursing diagnosis labels to ensure that the diagnostic label was consistent with current literature, and reflected a human response. The diagnostic label changes are shown in ► Table 1.3. Because major changes also occurred to definitions and diagnostic indicators, the original diagnoses were retired from the classification, new diagnoses replaced the originals, and new codes were assigned.

1.5 Retired Nursing Diagnoses

In the previous edition of the NANDA-I classification, 92 diagnoses were slotted for removal from this edition, unless additional work was completed to bring them to an adequate level of evidence, or to identify appropriate diagnostic indicators. Among those, 52 were successfully revised and submitted to NANDA-I as part of the DDC Task Force, or by individuals who

Table 1.3 Changes to nursing diagnosis labels of NANDA-I nursing diagnoses, 2021–2023

Domain	Previous diagnosis label	New diagnosis label
1. Health promotion	Ineffective health maintenance (00099)	Ineffective health maintenance behaviors (00292)
	Ineffective health management (00078)	Ineffective health self-management (00276)
	Readiness for enhanced health management (00162)	Readiness for enhanced health self-management (00293)
	Ineffective family health management (00080)	Ineffective family health self-management (00294)
	Impaired home maintenance (00098)*	Ineffective home maintenance behaviors (00300)
2. Nutrition	Ineffective infant feeding pattern (00107)	Ineffective infant suck-swallow response (00295)
	Risk for metabolic imbalance syndrome (00263)	Risk for metabolic syndrome (00296)
3. Elimination and exchange	Functional urinary incontinence (00020)	Disability-associated urinary incontinence (00297)
	Bowel incontinence (00014)	Impaired bowel continence (00319)
4. Activity/rest	Activity intolerance (00092)	Decreased activity tolerance (00298)
	Risk for activity intolerance (00094)	Risk for decreased activity tolerance (00299)
9. Coping/stress tolerance	Complicated grieving (00135)	Maladaptive grieving (00301)
	Risk for complicated grieving (00172)	Risk for maladaptive grieving (00302)
11. Safety/ protection	Risk for falls (00155)	Risk for adult falls (00303)
	Risk for pressure ulcer (00249)	Risk for adult pressure injury (00304)
	Risk for suicide (00150)	Risk for suicidal behavior (00289)
13. Growth/ development	Risk for delayed development (00112)	Risk for delayed child development (00305)

*Previously this diagnosis was slotted under Domain 4. With the new conceptualization, it is now slotted under Domain 1.

independently provided revisions. However, we did not receive any revisions on 40 diagnoses. Because of delays between the release in English and translated releases in other countries, we have postponed the removal of these remaining diagnoses, in order to give researchers more time to address their revisions. If additional work is not completed, they will be removed from the 2024–2026 edition. It should be noted that the revision of these diagnoses is considered a priority for NANDA-I in the next cycle of the DDC.

Table 1.4 Diagnoses removed from NANDA-I nursing diagnoses, 2021–2023

Domain	Class	Diagnosis label	Code
1	2	Ineffective health maintenance	00099
	2	Ineffective health management	00078
	2	Readiness for enhanced health management	00162
	2	Ineffective family health management	00080
2	1	Ineffective infant feeding pattern	00107
	4	Risk for metabolic imbalance syndrome	00263
3	1	Functional urinary incontinence	00020
	1	Overflow urinary incontinence	00176
	1	Reflex urinary incontinence	00018
	2	Bowel incontinence	00014
4	4	Activity intolerance	00092
	4	Risk for activity intolerance	00094
	5	Impaired home maintenance	00098
9	2	Grieving	00136
	2	Complicated grieving	00135
	2	Risk for complicated grieving	00172
	3	Decreased intracranial adaptive capacity	00049
11	2	Risk for falls	00155
	2	Risk for pressure ulcer	00249
	2	Risk for venous thromboembolism	00268
	3	Risk for suicide	00150
	5	Latex allergy reaction	00041
13	2	Risk for delayed development	00112

Twenty-three of the 52 diagnoses that were reviewed by context experts were removed from the classification, based on evidence presented to support removal. The diagnoses that have been removed from the classification are listed in ▶ Table 1.4.

The rationale for retirement of these diagnoses clustered into a few categories: (1) new research is available suggesting previous terms are outdated or have been replaced in the nursing literature, (2) lack of related factors modifiable by independent nursing interventions, (3) diagnosis does not meet the definition of a problem-focused diagnosis.

Ineffective health maintenance, impaired home maintenance, ineffective health management, readiness for enhanced health management, ineffective family health management, risk for metabolic imbalance syndrome, bowel incontinence and *functional urinary incontinence* were removed because content experts, in the course of literature review, found more appropriate terms to describe the diagnostic focus. Additionally, clarity to definitions and related factors were provided from these literature reviews. It was indicated that NANDA-I needed to retire old terms, which could be confusing to clinicians, and adopt those with support from current research literature. Refer to ▶ Table 1.3.

Overflow urinary incontinence was removed because it is a defining characteristic of *urinary retention*, which should be the actual focus of nursing interventions.

The absence of related factors modifiable by independent nursing interventions in the literature led to the removal of *reflex urinary incontinence and decreased intracranial adaptive capacity.*

Ineffective infant feeding pattern was removed because the phrase "feeding pattern", when translated from English to other languages, might be misleading and inadequately interpreted as *the act of being fed*, as opposed to the ability of an infant to suck or to coordinate the suck-swallow response. This diagnosis is now represented by the label, *ineffective infant suck-swallow response (00295).*

Activity intolerance and *risk for activity intolerance* were removed to enable the creation of diagnostic labels that incorporate a judgment term. These diagnoses were replaced by *decreased activity tolerance (00298)* and *risk for decreased activity tolerance (00299).*

No related factors were found by reviewers for *latex allergy reaction* that were modifiable by independent nursing interventions. However, nurses do assess for, and can independently intervene on, *risk for latex allergy reaction (00217),* which remains in the classification.

Grieving is a normal human response and therefore does not meet the definition of a problem-focused nursing diagnosis. This does not suggest that nurses do not support patients who are grieving. Nurses should assess for *risk for maladaptive grieving* (00302) and *maladaptive grieving* (00301). Additionally, patients may indicate a desire to enhance their grief experience (*readiness for enhanced grieving*, 00285)

Risk for falls and *risk for pressure ulcer* were removed because literature reviews performed by content experts provided evidence that there are sufficiently different risk factors for falls and pressure injury among adults, children and/or neonates. Therefore, these diagnoses were replaced by more granular, specific terms. In addition, the diagnostic focus *pressure ulcer* was updated to *pressure injury*, according to the most updated specialized literature.

Risk for venous thromboembolism was removed because no sufficiently distinct risk factors for venous thromboembolism and arterial thromboembolism were found that are modifiable by independent nursing interventions. The new diagnosis, *risk for thrombosis (00291),* includes risk factors for both types of thromboses.

Risk for suicide was removed because the new diagnostic focus, *suicidal behavior,* represents more accurately the phenomenon of concern to nurses. *Suicide* – the act of killing oneself – would be an undesirable outcome following suicidal behaviors. This diagnosis was replaced by *risk for suicidal behavior* (00289).

Risk for delayed development was retired because its definition was more accurately represented by the addition of the age axis, *child,* to the label. Therefore, this diagnosis was replaced by *risk for delayed child development* (00305).

1.6 NANDA-I Nursing Diagnoses: Indicator Term Standardization

Our work to decrease variation in terms used for defining characteristics, related factors, and risk factors continued during this twelfth edition of the classification. It involved literature searches, discussion, and consultation with clinical experts in different nursing specialties around the world. Although development of technology made it easier to find similar terms/phrases or those which had difficulties for translation, for example, this was not a simple task and took dozens of hours to complete. Despite this, we know it will not be perfect, and that work will continue into the next edition.

Readers will notice that many diagnoses have minor edits to terms (e.g., *alteration in metabolism* in the 11th edition will be *impaired metabolism* in the current edition). Work was also completed on all *associated conditions* and *at risk populations,* as it was noted in the previous edition that this work would occur during this cycle. This work focused on clarity of terms, and standardizing the way in which terms were stated. These changes are not considered to be content edits, but rather they are editorial changes. Those diagnoses with terms that had editorial changes *only* do not appear in ▸ Table 1.2.

The benefits of this revision work are many, but the following three are perhaps the most notable:

1.6.1 Improving Translation

There have been multiple questions and comments from translators regarding previous terms, which reminded us of the need for this work. For example:

- *There are many similar terms/phrases and the way I would translate these terms is exactly the same in my language. Can I use the same term/phrase, or must I translate these terms differently, even if we would not do so in daily practice?* To date, we have not required submitters of nursing diagnoses to search the terminology for terms/phrases that already exist to standardize their terms. As a result, the number of diagnostic indicator terms/phrases in the terminology have increased substantially over the years.
- It is important for translators to ensure conceptual clarity when translating the term/phrase. If there is a conceptual difference in two terms in the original English (e.g., helplessness and hopelessness), then they cannot use the same term to represent these two separate concepts. However, translators' struggles often result from a lack of standardization of the original English terms/phrases. Here is one of the examples in the 11th edition: the term, *anorexia*, was used in eight diagnoses, *poor appetite* appeared in three diagnoses, *decrease in appetite* in two diagnoses, and *loss of appetite* in one diagnosis! It would be difficult, if not impossible to translate these terms in some languages in a way that clearly differentiates the terms.

Decreasing the variation in these terms/phrases should facilitate the translation process, as one term/phrase will now be used throughout the terminology for similar diagnostic indicators. In this edition, we initiated the incorporation of Medical Subject Headings (MeSH) terms whenever possible. The MeSH make up the USA National Library of Medicine's controlled vocabulary thesaurus, used for indexing articles for the MEDLINE®/PubMED® database. The MeSH terms are defined and serve as a thesaurus that facilitates searching. Although the MeSH terms are not viewable in this text, our translators were provided access to the MeSH terms, whenever they were adopted, along with their definitions. These MeSH terms and their definitions should assist translators in creating more precise translation. For the example we discussed above, related to appetite, we have adopted the MeSH term, *anorexia*, which is defined as "the lack or loss of appetite accompanied by an aversion to food and the inability to eat". This means that this one term replaces the previous four terms.

We have also done our best to condense terms and standardize them, whenever possible.

1.6.2 Improving Terminological Consistency

We have received other questions that were difficult to answer. For instance: *When you say "inadequate" in English, does that mean a lack of quality, or is it the quantity that is lacking?* The answer is often, "Both!" Although the duality of this word is well accepted in English, the lack of clarity does not support the clinician in any language, and it makes it very difficult to translate into languages in which a different word would be used depending on the intended meaning. Unfortunately, other similar words, such as *insufficient*, *inadequate*, and *deficient*, have been also used in the terminology. In this edition, we decided to use the term, *inadequate*, consistently to point a lack of quality and/or lack of quantity, whereas the term, *insufficient*, is used solely to indicate lack of quantity. Moreover, the word, *deficient*, is used to mean lacking some elements or characteristics. For example, the phrases, *insufficient access to resources* and *deficient immunity*, in the eleventh edition, are revised to *inadequate access to resources* and *altered immune functioning*, respectively, in this edition.

Another question identified the need for clear differentiation between commonly used terms: *What are the differences, if any, between disease and illness?* These terms are not completely exclusive, and the English definitions can be confusing. However, some rules need to be set for consistent use of these terms in the terminology. The MeSH term, *disease*, is defined as "a definite pathologic process with a characteristic set of signs and symptoms". That is, *disease* is used for a specific medical condition with a clear name and symptoms, which needs to be treated, such as *cardiovascular disease* or *inflammatory bowel disease*. Meanwhile, *illness* is used for the patient's subjective experience of symptoms and unhealthy conditions, which needs to be managed, such as *chronic illness* or *physical illness*.

1.6.3 Facilitating Diagnostic Indicator Coding

We often hear voices from nurses and students confused by the long list of diagnostic indicators. *I really do not know if this diagnosis is right for my patient. Do I have to find all defining characteristics and related factors of the diagnosis with my patient?* At the current developmental stage of nursing diagnoses, the diagnostic criteria are not as clear as in most medical diagnoses. Identification of nursing diagnostic criteria based on research is an urgent task for the nursing community. Without diagnostic criteria, it is difficult for us to make an accurate nursing diagnosis. Additionally, there is no guarantee that nurses around the world use the same nursing diagnosis for a similar human response.

This work facilitates the coding of the diagnostic indicators, which should facilitate their use for populating assessment databases within electronic health records (EHR). All terms are now coded for use in EHR systems, which is something we have been frequently asked to do by many organizations and vendors alike. In near future, it is possible to find out which defining characteristics most often occur within the assessment data when a nursing diagnosis is documented, which could lead to the identification of critical diagnostic criteria. Additionally, identification of the most common related (causative) factors found for each diagnosis will also facilitate appropriate nursing interventions. This all facilitates the development of decision-support tools regarding accuracy in diagnosis, as well as linking diagnosis to assessment, and linking related/risk factors to appropriate treatment plans.

2 International Considerations on the Use of the NANDA-I Nursing Diagnoses

T. Heather Herdman

As we noted earlier, NANDA International, Inc. initially began as a North American organization and, therefore, the earliest nursing diagnoses were primarily developed by nurses from the United States and Canada. However, over the past 20 to 30 years, there has been an increasing involvement by nurses from around the world, and membership in NANDA International, Inc. now includes nurses from nearly 40 countries, with nearly two-thirds of its members coming from countries outside North America. Work is occurring across all continents using NANDA-I nursing diagnoses in curricula, clinical practice, research, and informatics applications. Development and refinement of diagnoses is ongoing across multiple countries, and the majority of research related to the NANDA-I nursing diagnoses is occurring outside North America.

As a reflection of this increased international activity, contribution, and utilization, the North American Nursing Diagnosis Association changed its scope to an international organization in 2002, changing its name to **NANDA International, Inc.** So, please, we ask that you **do not refer to the organization as the *North American Nursing Diagnosis Association (or as the North American Nursing Diagnosis Association International)*,** unless referring to something that happened prior to 2002 – it simply does not reflect our international scope, and **it is not the legal name of the organization.** We retained "NANDA" within our name because of its status in the nursing profession, so think of it more as a trademark or brand name than as an acronym, since it no longer "stands for" the original name of the association.

As NANDA-I experiences increased worldwide adoption, issues related to differences in the scope of nursing practice, diversity of nurse practice models, divergent laws and regulations, nurse competency, and educational differences must be addressed. In 2009, NANDA-I held an International Think Tank Meeting, which included 86 individuals representing 16 countries. During that meeting, significant discussions occurred as to how best to handle these and other issues. Nurses in some countries are not able to utilize nursing diagnoses of a more physiologic nature because they are in conflict with their current scope of nursing practice. Nurses in other nations are facing regulations aimed to ensure that everything done within nursing practice can be demonstrated to be evidence-based, and therefore face difficulties with some of the older nursing diagnoses and/or those linked interventions that are not supported by a strong level of research literature. Discussions were therefore held with international leaders in nursing diagnosis use and research, looking for direction that would meet the needs of the worldwide community.

These discussions resulted in a unanimous decision to maintain the taxonomy as an intact body of knowledge in all languages, in order to enable nurses around the world to view, discuss, and consider diagnostic concepts being used by nurses within and outside of their countries, and to engage in discussions, research, and debate regarding the appropriateness of all of the diagnoses. A critical statement agreed upon in that Summit is noted here prior to introducing the nursing diagnoses themselves:

> Not every nursing diagnosis within the NANDA-I taxonomy is appropriate for every nurse in practice – nor has it ever been. Some of the diagnoses are specialty-specific, and would not necessarily be used by all nurses in clinical practice ... There are diagnoses within the taxonomy that may be outside the scope or standards of nursing practice governing a particular geographic area in which a nurse practices.

Those diagnoses and/or related/risk factors would, in these instances, not be appropriate for practice, and should not be used if they lie outside the scope or standards of nursing practice for a particular geographic region. However, it is appropriate for these diagnoses to remain visible in the classification, because the classification represents clinical judgments made by nurses *around the world*, not just those made in one region or country. Every nurse should be aware of, and work within, the standards and scope of practice and any laws or regulations within which he/she is licensed to practice. However, it is also important for all nurses to be aware of the areas of nursing practice that exist globally, as this informs discussion and may over time support the broadening of nursing practice across other countries. Conversely, these individuals may be able to provide evidence that would support the removal of diagnoses from the current classification, which, if they were not shown in their translations, would be unlikely to occur.

That said, it is important that you are not avoiding the use of a diagnosis because, in the opinion of one local expert or published textbook, it is not appropriate. I have met nurse authors who indicate that operating room nurses "cannot diagnose because they don't assess", or that intensive care unit nurses "have to practice under strict physician protocol that doesn't include nursing diagnosis". Neither of these statements is factual, but rather represents the personal opinions of those nurses. It is, therefore, important to truly educate oneself on regulation, law, and professional standards of practice in one's own country and area of practice, rather than relying on the word of one person, or group of people, who may be inaccurately defining or describing nursing diagnosis.

Ultimately, nurses must identify those diagnoses that are appropriate for their area of practice, that fit within their scope of practice or legal regulations, and for which they have competency. Nurse educators, clinical experts, and nurse administrators are critical to ensuring that nurses are aware of diagnoses that are truly outside the scope of nursing practice in a certain geographic region. Multiple textbooks in many languages are available that include the entire NANDA-I terminology, so for the NANDA-I text to remove diagnoses from country to country would no doubt lead to a great level of confusion worldwide. Publication of the classification in no way requires that a nurse utilize every diagnosis within it, nor does it justify practicing outside the scope of an individual's nursing license or regulations to practice.

Part 2
Recommendations for Research to Improve the Terminology

3 Future Improvement of the NANDA-I Terminology

Shigemi Kamitsuru, T. Heather Herdman, Camila Takáo Lopes

3.1 Research Priorities

As noted previously, one of the major priorities for the upcoming cycle is the revision or retirement of the 41 diagnoses that were not revised for this 12th edition. Secondly, we encourage clinical validation studies of diagnoses, with large sample sizes and preferably across sites and patient population. Many studies are conducted with patient populations who have a particular medical diagnosis (associated condition), for example the study by Ferreira et al. (2020) on *sexual dysfunction (00059)* in patients with breast cancer. In other cases, validation studies occur in at risk populations, such as *impaired walking (00088)* in the elderly (Marques-Vieria et al., 2018). While these studies are helpful for those working in specialty areas, they do not provide the breadth of understanding of a diagnosis that could occur if an approach looked at all patients admitted to hospital, or receiving in-home care, or being seen in an ambulatory clinic, for example. It is likely that there are core clinical indicators that cross all patients, in addition to those that may only occur within specific patient populations.

Further research is critical that provides information on which assessment indicators are most predictive of a patient developing a condition which is represented by a nursing diagnosis. This will allow us to narrow the list of clinical indicators, or separate the lists into critical defining characteristics (DCs), or those that must be present to make a diagnosis, and supportive DCs. Likewise, there has been little focus on related risk factors for nursing diagnoses in research studies, yet it is the related/risk factors that should primarily drive intervention. Thus, we strongly support studies which provide nurses with information on which related factors are most critical for diagnoses, so that intervention studies can be undertaken to remove or minimize the effects of the causes of diagnoses, or risk factors for a diagnosis.

Since at risk populations and associated conditions are supportive information for diagnostic reasoning, but not core elements of a diagnosis, research focusing solely on these elements is not encouraged.

3.2 Refinement and Diagnoses to be Developed

The evolution of our scientific language is an ongoing process; there is no end point at which the terminology will be complete. Rather, there will be continuous revisions and additions to the terminology, along with retirements from it, as knowledge evolves. Some of these evolutions are more editorial in nature, such as developing a specific schema for definitions and phrases of diagnostic indicator terms. Others are more complex and require extensive discussions and research to better position the NANDA-I terminology to be the strongest, most evidence-based, standardized nursing diagnosis language. The following issues represent some of the critical issues to which we hope to draw researchers' immediate attention.

Symptoms or nursing diagnoses? The NANDA-I nursing diagnoses are concepts constructed by means of a multi-axial system; however, some of the current diagnosis labels do not meet the specification of this model. Some labels are constructed with just one term from axis 1 (the focus of diagnosis), and are often considered symptoms: for example, *constipation* (00011), *insomnia* (00095), *wandering* (00154), *hopelessness* (00124), *fear* (00148), and *hyperthermia* (00007). Although some others are constructed with two terms, one from axis 1 and another from axis 6 (time), they also can be symptoms: for example, *acute confusion* (00128), *chronic sorrow* (00137), and *acute pain* (00132). None of these diagnosis labels have explicit terms from axis 3 (judgment), which are supposed to be included in the focus of diagnosis. What exactly do nurses assess, and what is their judgment about these symptoms? Is it the presence, severity, or self-management of the symptom, for example?

There is another issue with these diagnosis labels. Currently, *anxiety* (00146) and *fatigue* (00093) are classified as diagnoses within the NANDA-I nursing diagnosis classification. However, these terms are also found as defining characteristics of many other nursing diagnoses. It is difficult to comprehend that they can be both nursing diagnoses and defining characteristics. This is confusing for many users, so we often hear: "Am I supposed to diagnose *anxiety* itself, or should I consider anxiety as a defining characteristic of other nursing diagnoses?" "I think my patient's problems are *fatigue* and *ineffective coping* (00069). Should I document both diagnoses, or just *ineffective coping, since it* includes fatigue within its defining characteristics?"

We recommend a review of these issues to determine whether symptoms should belong within the current NANDA-I nursing diagnosis classification. We may need to create a secondary classification of symptoms, or we may need to remove them from the classification altogether because these symptoms do not fit within the multiaxial structure. Recently, the concepts of "symptom control" and "symptom self-management" are receiving a great deal of attention in the nursing literature. We may need to reconceptualize symptom diagnoses within the NANDA-I classification to reflect the most recent evidence. For example, rather than simply naming the symptom of *nausea* (00134), a clinically useful diagnosis label may be *"ineffective nausea control"* and/or *"ineffective nausea self-management"*. Likewise, rather than the symptom diagnosis of chronic pain (00133), "ineffective chronic pain control" and/or "ineffective chronic pain self-management" may be more clinically useful. However, it is important that these diagnosis labels represent the patient's human responses, and not indicate a nursing care issue.

Appropriate level of diagnosis granularity. Another frequent topic of discussion is what level of granularity should be used for nursing diagnoses in the terminology. Should the diagnoses be broad (abstract), specific (concrete), or both? For example, there are two problem-focused diagnoses that address issues with body weight: *overweight* (00233) and *obesity* (00232). These are specifically diagnosed based on body mass index (BMI). However, there is no broader diagnosis that would address the continuum of body weight management, such as *ineffective weight control* or *ineffective weight self-management*. Another example is three diagnoses focusing issues on eating (feeding) dynamics: *ineffective adolescent eating dynamics* (00269), *ineffective child eating dynamics* (00270), and *ineffective infant feeding dynamics* (00271). These are three specific diagnoses based on the age/developmental stage of the subject. However, there is no broader diagnosis that would address the problem of eating dynamics across all age groups, such as *ineffective eating dynamics*.

The current NANDA-I classification includes nursing diagnoses with various level of granularity. For example, the diagnosis, *impaired tissue integrity* (00044) is broader than *impaired skin integrity* (00046) and *impaired oral mucous membrane integrity* (00045). Some nurses would argue that *impaired tissue integrity* is all that is required, because problems related to skin and mucous membranes could all be treated using this diagnosis; other nurses prefer the more specific diagnoses. In general, however, more granular, or more specific diagnoses may better direct precise patient care.

Having both broad and specific nursing diagnoses will help us to develop a taxonomy which is more organized and hierarchical. Moreover, our classification of nursing diagnoses, with various level of granularity, may support nurses' clinical reasoning by guiding the categorization of clinical data from the abstract to more concrete. For example, when assessing a patient who is complaining of incontinence, you may first consider a broad, or more general diagnosis such as, *impaired urinary elimination* (00085). Then, upon further assessment and/or reflection, you may be able to narrow down the focus to a more specific diagnosis, *urge urinary incontinence* (00238).

We are not opposed to developing granular diagnoses, because these can direct specific nursing care. However, there is a great need to determine what level of granularity would be considered sufficient. Is there a level of granularity that might be considered too specific? For example, do we really want to have a diagnosis, *impaired left thumb mobility*?

What is needed to improve translation? The issue of granularity is also important in translation, in the understanding of the focus of the diagnosis in different languages, and in the applicability of diagnoses in clinical practice internationally. An example of this might be the diagnosis, *risk for adult falls* (00303). A person can fall down the stairs, fall out of bed, or fall down while walking across the room. However, in the original English language, there is just one term – fall – that is used to express any unintended drop from higher surfaces to lower ones, or from a standing position to a lower position on the same surface. In some languages, these are different concepts, and the terms used are therefore different. As a result, nurses take different precautions for each type of fall, and report on these incidents separately. It might even be considered dangerous to combine two different nursing problems into a single nursing diagnosis. It may be necessary to consider that some languages would be better served to have different nursing diagnoses to address those phenomena which cannot accurately be translated as one term from the original English language.

In this edition, the diagnosis label, *activity intolerance* (00092) has been revised to *decreased activity tolerance* (00298). This revision was based on the discussion regarding axes, especially axis 1 (the focus of the diagnosis) and axis 3 (judgment). It has been previously explained that the focus of *activity intolerance* is activity tolerance, and the diagnosis label contained the judgment "in-". The English, the prefix "in-" generally means "not" or "impossible". However, simply negating the human response of "activity tolerance" does not make sense as a diagnosis label, and it has proven to be difficult to translate this term in some languages. Therefore, the definition was carefully examined, and the judgment term reflected in that definition was determined to be "decreased". This modification will facilitate accurate translation as well as the consistent use of diagnosis labels internationally. Similarly, there are some other diagnosis labels to be considered: for example, *imbalanced nutrition: less than body requirements* (00002) and *sexual dysfunction* (00059) also cause difficulties with translation.

Does the focus of the diagnosis capture the appropriate human response? The focus of a diagnosis (axis 1) describes the human response that is the core of the diagnosis. However, a careful examination of axis 1 of diagnosis labels in the NANDA-I classification revealed questionable labels: *deficient knowledge* (00126) and *readiness for enhanced knowledge* (00161). The focus of these diagnoses is obviously "knowledge". However, does knowledge reflect a human response?

The National Library of Medicine's MeSH database defines knowledge as "the body of truths or facts accumulated in the course of time, the cumulated sum of information, its volume and nature, in any civilization, period, or country". The term, knowledge, therefore, does not contain a human response to internal or external stimulus. In some languages, a literal translation of *readiness for enhanced knowledge* did not make sense, so a local term which means "acquisition" has been added after the term "knowledge". It is possible that, in the original English, the focus of the diagnosis could also be changed to knowledge acquisition, knowledge attainment, or knowledge acquirement.

At the same time, the judgment term should probably be revised from "deficit" to, for example, "impaired" or "insufficient". Thus, we might have a diagnosis label, *insufficient knowledge attainment*, or *impaired knowledge acquisition*. Although this term might seem awkward in everyday vernacular in English, and in other languages as well, it is important to remember that we need labels that truly reflect human responses, and that adhere to a multiaxial structure. In practice, nurses may talk about *a patient's misunderstanding or lack of knowledge* of a patient when speaking with one another or with other health professionals, but the term in the patient record may be different (for example, *deficient knowledge*, 00126). This is true in medicine, as well, when we talk with patients about their "heart attack", but chart the term, *acute myocardial infarction*.

Is NANDA-I taxonomy user-friendly? Six new nursing diagnoses appear in this edition of the classification that incorporate a term, "self-management" in the focus of the diagnosis (axis 1). We spent a considerable time discussing where - in which domain - each of these diagnoses should be classified. The problem is that the human response of these diagnoses is not only *self-management*, but it is combined with specific terms that describe the target of self-management: *health, lymphedema,* and *dry eye.* Everyone will agree that *health self-management* is definitely a human response in Domain 1 (health promotion). However, where would you look to find *lymphedema self-management* or *dry eye self-management*? Nurses previously have addressed patients' responses related to lymphedema with the diagnosis, *ineffective peripheral tissue perfusion* (00204), which is found within Domain 4 (activity/rest). Another diagnosis focusing on dry eye, *risk for dry eye* (00219) has been slotted in Domain 11 (safety/protection) since 2012.

Although definitions of all of these new *self-management* diagnoses are similar to the definition of Domain 1-Class 2 (health management), we ultimately decided to classify each diagnosis based on user-friendliness. For example, would a nurse think to look in two different domains for a diagnosis to be used with patients having lymphedema? As a result, you will find the *lymphedema self-management* diagnosis in Domain 4, and the *dry eye self-management* diagnosis in Domain 11. The domain and class of these diagnoses may change in the future, depending on the advancement of the taxonomic structure, as well as possible changes in our perspectives. However, our goal was to ensure that diagnoses were classified within the taxonomic structure in a way that was clinically consistent.

In terms of clinical usability of the NANDA-I taxonomy, we will continue to examine its structure. Some nurses have struggled to locate diagnoses related to respiration, which are classified in three domains: Domain 3 (elimination and exchange), Domain 4 (activity/rest) and Domain 11 (safety/protection). Other nurses have had difficulty locating emotional response diagnoses, which are classified in three domains: Domain 6 (self-perception), Domain 9 (coping/stress tolerance), and Domain 12 (comfort). There are strong reasons for locating these diagnoses in different domains, when you review the definition of the diagnoses. However, it is critical that the taxonomy provides a structure that makes sense to those who are using it. Even if a perfect taxonomy is not possible, we should strive for it.

We are always faced with new challenges, new knowledge, and new ways of thinking about the human responses that nurses diagnose. We look forward to receiving your feedback and research findings on these and other issues for the further improvement of the NANDA-I terminology.

3.3 References

Ferreira IS, Fernandes AFC, Rodrigues AB, Santiago JCDS, de Sousa VEC, Lopes MVDO, Moreira CB. Accuracy of the Defining Characteristics of the Sexual Dysfunction Nursing Diagnosis in Women with Breast Cancer. International Journal of Nursing Knowledge 2020; 31(1): 37–43.

Marques-Vieira C, Sousa L, Costa D, Mendes C, Sousa L, Caldeira S. Validation of the nursing diagnosis of impaired walking in elderly. BMC Health Services Research 2018; 18 (Suppl 2): P176.

4 Revised Level of Evidence Criteria for Diagnosis Submission

Marcos Venícios de Oliveira Lopes, Viviane Martins da Silva, Diná de Almeida Lopes Monteiro da Cruz

4.1 Introduction

This chapter aims to present the new criteria for the evidence levels of validity of the NANDA International (NANDA-I) diagnoses, and how they should be used in the process of submitting new diagnoses. The text was organized starting with presentation and a brief discussion of the concepts of clinical evidence and validity theory, then describing and exemplifying the levels of evidence for nursing diagnoses.

The level of evidence (LOE) used in this edition does not reflect these new changes. Work is underway to convert all LOEs for current diagnoses, and this will be available in the 14th edition. However, we do require all submitters of new diagnoses to refer to these updated LOE criteria.

This section will be primarily of interest to researchers, graduate students, and others who are contemplating development of a new nursing diagnosis, or revision to improve the level of evidence of an existing diagnosis.

"Evidence" is a term that is difficult to define and has generated numerous debates in the health area (Pearson et al., 2005; Miller & Fredericks, 2003). In general, the term, evidence, refers to research results that test the effectiveness of interventions, presenting a central role for evidence-based practice which seeks to define the best option between different treatments. This notion has been expanded and organizations that are dedicated to the development of evidence-based practice have developed other types of approaches, including: proposals for evaluating evidence regarding the meaning that interventions have for the people who receive it; the feasibility of interventions in certain contexts (Pearson et al., 2007); or evidence of the accuracy of a particular diagnostic test (Pearson et al., 2005).

Evidence is a continuous phenomenon and is organized in hierarchies according to its robustness. This means that regardless of the type of evidence, it can be weaker or stronger. Very strong evidence would be a fact – or a set of facts – that, beyond any suspicion, confirms a statement. When it is said that evidence is very weak, it is because it is acknowledged that new facts may arise that contradict the fact that we have today. Several scholars and organizations have endeavored to create criteria to define hierarchies of evidence in health to assist professionals in making decisions in their practices, including the topic of interventions, among others (Merlin et al., 2009).

NANDA-I is the only association concerned with the criteria for the degrees of evidence of diagnostic validity, in this case, nursing diagnoses. In no other area that uses diagnostic language standardization do criteria exist for the degrees of evidence of their validity. As you will see later, the hierarchy of evidence for the validity of NANDA-I diagnoses is guided by criteria relating to the types of studies that generated them. But before that, it is necessary to relate "clinical evidence" and "theory of validity", since we are dealing with degrees of evidence of validity of nursing diagnoses.

4.2 Relationship Between Clinical Evidence and Validity Theory

The theory of validity has its origin in the development of instruments for assessing cognitive performance and skills, particularly aimed at the selection of candidates for public office or European and North American universities in the mid-19th century (Gregory, 2010). The first definitions of validity try to represent it as the characteristic of an instrument, meaning that it measures what it proposes to measure. If we transpose this definition to a nursing diagnosis, we would identify that a valid nursing diagnosis would be one whose defining characteristics measure the diagnosis that it is supposed to represent. For example, the *acute pain* (00132) diagnosis would not be valid in itself; what would be valid would be the set of defining characteristics that supposedly "measure" acute pain, regardless of the clinical context, population, environment, or the subject evaluated.

You might believe that such a definition seems obvious and relatively simple. And indeed it is! However, the simplicity of this initial definition has raised some doubts over time. How does one prove the measurement capacity of an instrument? If an instrument was proven to measure a phenomenon in a specific population, could it be used to measure the same phenomenon in another population if it is clinically distinct from the first? If the evaluation itself is developed to draw a conclusion based on the presence/absence of a phenomenon, is the instrument itself, or the interpretation that is obtained from it, considered to be valid?

To better understand, let's rewrite these same questions in context for nursing diagnoses: how do we prove that the defining characteristics represent a nursing diagnosis, if most human responses are not subject to direct observation (that is, there is no gold standard for most nursing diagnoses)? If a set of defining characteristics were proven to represent a nursing diagnosis in a specific population (for example, *hopelessness,* 00124, among adolescents), would they represent the same diagnosis in another population that is clinically distinct from the first (such as, *hopelessness* among adult cancer patients)? If the assessment itself is developed to conclude with a finding of the presence/absence of a nursing diagnosis, is the set of defining characteristics or the interpretation that is obtained from them (the diagnosis itself) considered to be valid?

These questions led to reformulations of the concept of validity, as well as of the methods that have been developed to identify such a concept, which are commonly called validation. After decades of discussions and developments, the concept of validity among scholars in the fields of psychology and education has evolved, and led to the understanding of validity as the degree to which accumulated evidence and theory support the specific interpretation of test scores (understood as an instrument of evaluation of a psychological attribute) for a given use of this test (American Educational Research Association; American Psychological Association; National Council on Measurement in Education, 2014).

Transporting this definition to the context of nursing diagnoses, we can assume that the validity of a diagnosis is the degree to which evidence and theory support that it (the diagnosis) is the appropriate interpretation, for a given clinical use, of a given set of manifestations (understood as the defining characteristics of the diagnosis). From this definition it can be extrapolated that the validity of a diagnosis: a) can be presented at several levels (degrees); b) depends on the available evidence; c) depends on the underlying theory; d) is a property of the diagnosis and not of its components (the diagnosis is valid, not its characteristics); and, e) depends on the intended clinical use. The process of generating evidence of the validity of a nursing diagnosis is continuous, cumulative, and involves several interrelated steps. These range from the statement of a label, a term or expression to designate a more or less clear idea of a human response pertinent to nursing, to the collection of empirical data that "the observations selected to represent or indicate a concept in fact do so. Assessment of the validity of an operationalization is an ongoing process that requires empirical investigation" (Waltz et al., 2017, p .54).

4.3 Evidence Levels of Validity for NANDA-I Diagnoses

As we have seen, the validity of a diagnosis is directly related to the evidence of such validity. Evidence of validity of a diagnosis can have different levels, depending on the methodology used to generate them and the clinical context in which the diagnosis will be used; that is, the validity of a diagnosis depends on a continuous investigation process that allows for expansion of its use for different populations as clinical evidence accumulates. In the NANDA-I terminology, the level of evidence of a diagnosis has been related to the strength of the evidence that supports its development or validation (Herdman & Kamitsuru, 2018). It is, therefore, evidence of validity. In this review, the evidence level of validity of a diagnosis refers to the degree to which accumulated evidence and theory support the interpretation of the human response, represented by the diagnostic label, is the correct interpretation of the set of attributes (defining characteristics, related factors, risk factors, associated conditions, and at risk populations) for established clinical purposes (i.e., for the context and/or population from which the respective evidence was extracted). Thus, NANDA-I revised its structure of evidence levels of validity of its diagnoses in order to better reflect the state of science related to evidence-based practice, associating them with the types of studies capable of producing results compatible with the interpretations and their expected uses.

This new classification of the evidence level of validity for nursing diagnoses in NANDA-I is organized into two major levels: Level 1 represents the initial stages of development that precede the inclusion of the diagnosis in the terminology, and Level 2 refers to the various stages of clinical development of the diagnosis, according to the strength of the best available evidence, including those produced by expert opinion studies or with populations susceptible to it. Each level consists of sub-levels structured according to the study methods. A diagnosis will have higher levels of evidence the more robust the evidence is, according to the type of research that produced it, from studies of operationalization of concepts, culminating in high quality systematic reviews.

Evidence levels of diagnostic validity are used by the NANDA-I Diagnosis Development Committee (DDC) to make decisions about including new diagnoses in the terminology. Level 1 is assigned to diagnoses that are presented to the DDC to be included in the terminology. This first level deals with the presentation of the initial diagnosis structure to the DDC until the presentation of a theoretical review that proves the structural and conceptual consistency of the diagnostic proposal. After reaching a level of evidence of 1.3., the proposal is recommended for the development of theoretical and clinical studies, starting with conceptual validation, then moving on to content validation by experts and by qualitative analysis of the population supposedly exposed to the diagnosis. Level 2 includes gradually more robust methods of validation, strongly based on epidemiological approaches that aim to establish the accuracy of clinical indicators, the capacity for diagnostic screening, the potential for prognosis, the ability to differentiate between groups of diagnoses with similar concepts, relationships of causality (including causal interrelationships that can determine diagnostic syndromes), systematic reviews that make it possible to establish relationships between diagnostic components in multiple populations or multiple studies in similar populations, and studies of etiological factors based on case-control and/or cohort approaches. The interpretation of the evidence levels of the diagnoses will always be relative and gradual, that is, higher sub-levels in the classification indicate diagnoses with more robust evidence than diagnoses in lower sub-levels. A summary of the evidence levels of nursing diagnoses can be seen in ▸ Table 4.1.

4.3.1 Level 1. Proposal Received by the DDC for Development

If the reader identifies a human response that is not found within NANDA-I's terminology, the first step will be to develop a diagnostic proposal comprising a label, a definition, possible components (defining characteristics/related or risk factors/associated conditions/at risk population), and the relationship of the alleged diagnosis with possible nursing interventions and outcomes. The diagnostic development processes in this first level include direct monitoring by the DDC and execution by the submitter. Level 1 is divided into three sub-levels. The diagnostic proposal can present a structure resulting from the three levels to the DDC, sequentially, or it can consider two or even three sub-levels concurrently.

Level 1.1. Label only. The first task will be to develop a title (label) using the multiaxial system that represents a human response which could be identified as a nursing diagnosis. The level of evidence criterion is defined by a diagnostic label that is considered clear and is supported by a previously conducted literature review, and presented in a report format. The DDC will consult with the submitter, and provide guidance related to diagnostic development through guidelines, written consultation, and workshops. At this stage, the label is categorized as "Received for Development", and identified as such on the NANDA-I website.

Level 1.2. Label and definition. This level of evidence criterion is defined by the presentation of the diagnostic label and a clear and distinct definition from other NANDA-I diagnoses and definitions. The definition should differ from the defining characteristics, and the label and its components should not be included in the definition. A diagnosis must be consistent with the current NANDA-I definition of nursing diagnoses; that is, its proposal must represent

Table 4.1 Levels of evidence for nursing diagnoses

Level of diagnosis development	Criteria for classification
Concept generation	**Level 1. Proposal received by the DDC for development**
	1.1. Label only
	1.2. Label and definition
	1.3. Diagnostic components and relationship with outcomes and interventions
Theoretical support	**Level 2. Inclusion in terminology and clinical testing**
	2.1. Conceptual validity
	2.1.1. Conceptual validity of the elements
	2.1.2. Theoretical-causal validity
	2.1.3. Terminological validity
	2.2. Diagnostic content validity
	2.2.1. Initial validity of diagnostic content
	2.2.2. Potential validity of diagnostic content
	2.2.3. Advanced validity of diagnostic content
	2.2.4. Consolidated validity of diagnostic content
Clinical support	2.3. Clinical validity
Block 1 *Identification of populations in which a diagnosis may be applicable*	
	2.3.1. Qualitative validity
	2.3.2. Demographic validity
Block 2 *Utility of defining characteristics for clinical purposes*	
	2.3.3. Clinical construct validity
	2.3.4. Selective validity
	2.3.5. Discriminant validity
	2.3.6. Prognostic validity
	2.3.7. Generalizable validity of defining characteristics
Block 3 *Identification of related/risk factors, at risk populations, and associated conditions*	
	2.3.8. Diagnosis-specific causal validity
	2.3.9. Causal validity of exposure variable
	2.3.10. Generalized validity of related / risk factors

a human response for which the nurse can implement independent nursing interventions. The label and definition must be based on a literature review, which must be presented and evaluated by the DDC. At this stage, the label and its definition are categorized as "Received for Development", and identified as such on the NANDA-I website.

Level 1.3. Diagnostic components, and relationship with outcomes and interventions. A proposal at this level should include the label, definition, and other components of the diagnosis (defining characteristics, related/risk factors, and, when applicable, associated conditions, at risk populations), presented with the references obtained from a literature review. Although proposals at this level are not yet part of the terminology, they should support the discussion of the concept, the assessment of its clinical usefulness and applicability, and its validation through robust research methods. In addition, the proponent will be required to present the relationship of the diagnosis under development with interventions and outcomes as represented in other standardized terminologies (e.g., the Nursing Outcomes and Nursing Interventions Classifications). At this stage, the diagnostic proposal is categorized as "Received for clinical development and validation", and identified as such on the NANDA-I website and in a separate section of the book with the current terminology. It is worth mentioning that the submitter will be able to present a proposal beginning at level 1.3., without having to go sequentially through levels 1.1. and 1.2.

4.3.2 Level 2. Inclusion in Terminology and Clinical Testing

A new diagnosis is included in the NANDA-I terminology when evidence of second-level validity is generated. This level is subdivided into three sub-levels: 2.1. Conceptual validity; 2.2. Content validity; and 2.3. Clinical validity. To include a new diagnosis in the classification, the submitter must identify or develop theoretical studies that allow the construction of evidence of validity of at least the first sub-level, that is, conceptual validity. However, maintaining the diagnosis in the classification will depend on the continuity of studies that allow for the identification of evidence of validity of the third sub-level, that is, clinical validity. Note that each of these sub-levels has other subdivisions that will be characterized and exemplified below.

Level 2.1. Conceptual validity. Conceptual validity refers to the development of a conceptual framework and/or substantive theory that should support the interpretations obtained from the constituent elements of the nursing diagnosis. In the first sub-level, the elements initially developed are subjected to a concept analysis to demonstrate the existence of a body of knowledge underlying the diagnosis. Conceptual analysis provides support for the label and definition, includes a discussion and supports the defining characteristics and related factors (problem-focused diagnoses), risk factors (risk diagnoses), or defining characteristics (health promotion diagnoses). The components known as *associated conditions* and *at risk populations* may be included in this discussion, if applicable. This level should allow the construction of a substantive theory that, in addition to identifying the components of the diagnosis, leads to an understanding of the clinical and/or psychosocial relationships that underlie the diagnosis. This sub-level has three subdivisions, which are explained below.

Level 2.1.1. Conceptual validity of the elements. In this first level are diagnoses whose level of evidence criterion refers to the development of a concept analysis. This analysis can be developed for three purposes:

1. To explain the scope of the diagnosis, including identifying the appropriate domain and class, and the subject of the diagnosis (individual, caregiver, group, family, community). These studies could include those which develop the analysis within a group of patients who all experience the same clinical condition (associated condition), such as an analysis of impaired coping in patients with breast cancer, for example.
2. To clarify the definition of the diagnosis (and its components), the clinical indicators that will constitute the defining characteristics, and the etiological factors that will compose the set of related/risk factors, and any relevant associated conditions/at risk populations.
3. To differentiate the diagnosis from others existing in the taxonomy, identifying components that establish its clinical limits in relation to the others, characterizing it as a specific phenomenon. In the case of a syndrome diagnosis, the conceptual analysis should describe the relationships between the components of the diagnostic syndrome, differentiating it from clinical situations that represent only the individual diagnostic components.

The study by Cabaço et al. (2018) is an example of a concept analysis based on the evolutionary method, in which the authors present the structural elements for the development of three nursing diagnoses related to spiritual coping. Its analysis was developed from a literature review of qualitative studies and allowed the development of potential diagnoses, *spiritual coping, risk for impaired spiritual coping*, and *readiness for enhanced spiritual coping*.

Level 2.1.2. Theoretical-causal validity. In this second level, the submitter should identify or develop, as a criterion for the level of evidence, a broad theoretical study with the objective of establishing hypotheses for the clinical and causal relationships that justify the components (defining characteristics, related/risk factors, and when indicated, associated conditions/at risk populations) that make up the diagnosis. The preferred approach for this purpose is the development of middle-range theories, which represent theories composed of a limited number of concepts and which are aimed at describing, explaining, or predicting clinical practice situations (Lopes, Silva & Herdman, 2017). An example of the application of this approach is the study by Lemos et al. (2020) which presents a middle-range theory based on an integrative literature review for the nursing diagnosis, *dysfunctional ventilatory weaning response (00034)*, including the main concepts, pictorial diagrams, propositions, and causal relationships for use in clinical practice. In this study, the authors identified 13 clinical antecedent and 21 consequent results related to this nursing diagnosis that occurs when ventilatory weaning fails.

Level 2.1.3. Terminological validity. Terminological validity refers to the adequacy of interpretations obtained from health records of terms that are supposed to represent components of a nursing diagnosis. The level of evidence includes diagnoses submitted to validation processes based on secondary data, for the identification of diagnostic components and/or the diagnostic prevalence. Terminological validity of the diagnosis is verified from the documentation of components (defining characteristics, related/risk factors) in health records. These studies must be based on large samples of health records that allow sufficient data to be obtained to identify the diagnostic components. An important requirement with these studies is verification of the adequacy, precision, and accuracy of the records used. An example of this type of study can be found in the article by Ferreira et al. (2016), who cross-mapped 832 terms found in 256 health records with 52 NANDA-I diagnosis labels in an intensive care unit. It is important to note that terminological validity depends on the description of tools used to verify the quality of the information obtained. Simply having recorded terms in the health record *does not guarantee* that the interpretations obtained from them are valid.

Level 2.2. Diagnostic content validity. The criteria in any one of the previous levels (2.1.1., 2.1.2., 2.1.3.) must be fulfilled so that the submitter's proposal raises the evidence of validity of the diagnosis to a level of evidence of 2.2. The criterion for this level of evidence is a content analysis study by a group of experts with knowledge about the focus of the diagnosis. Content validity refers to how representative diagnostic components, identified at the previous level, are of the clinical content domain of the diagnosis. This level of evidence has four subdivisions, organized according to the sample size of experts and their respective level of expertise. Content validation is more strongly related to level of expertise than to the sample size of experts. In addition, it is important to consider the inclusion of both experts with clinical experience and researchers on the subject of diagnosis, in order to consider clinical experience and broader theoretical reflections on the diagnosis. A diagnosis is classified in the terminology based on the most advanced level achieved, according to evaluation led by the DDC and Research Directors. An example of a diagnostic content validation study is the article by Zeleníková, Žiaková, Čáp, & Jarošová (2014), who validated the nursing diagnosis, acute pain (00132), with Czech and Slovakian nurses, using the Fehring model. A total of 17 defining characteristics were validated.

Level 2.2.1. Initial validity of diagnostic content. Diagnoses whose validation process was developed with a small number of experts, with a predominantly beginner/advanced beginner profile, are found in this level. Group evaluation techniques are used at this level, such as the Delphi technique. The analysis follows a more qualitative approach and tends to confirm the structure built at sub-level 2.1. In addition, validation processes with these characteristics allow for verification of how comprehensive the diagnostic structure is for beginners, in order to glimpse its clarity and possible usefulness in clinical practice. Diagnoses at this level have moderate potential for content validity. A description of the use of the Delphi technique for content validation processes in nursing diagnoses can be found in the article by Grant & Kinney (1992). An example of this type of study can be found in the study by Melo et al. (2011), who used the Delphi technique with 25 experts in three rounds. In this study, the experts identified eight factors that represented a higher risk for the development of the diagnosis, *decreased cardiac output (00270)*.

Level 2.2.2. Potential validity of diagnostic content. The validation process at this level is developed with a large sample of experts who have a beginner/advanced beginner expertise profile. The research will generally include descriptive and inferential statistical analysis, with the possibility of verifying the adequacy of the diagnosis for use by nurses with little clinical experience. When evaluating diagnoses using this type of studies, the expert sample size must be sufficient to allow for the generalization of opinions. Often these opinions will be obtained from questionnaires, and their statistical analysis will include content validity indexes, proportions tests, and agreement coefficients, among other statistical measures. The previously mentioned study by Paloma-Castro et al. (2014) is an example, although their sample probably included experts with different levels of expertise. The data available in the article did not allow for the identification of the experts' level of expertise who participated in the study.

Level 2.2.3. Advanced validity of diagnostic content. This level requires analyses by participants with a high level of expertise. Most studies base their analysis of expertise on academic criteria, and often a critical analysis of the level of expertise is absent, making it difficult to identify these studies. The validation process is developed with a small number of individuals with predominantly proficient/expert levels of expertise. Diagnoses in this sub-level undergo a qualitative assessment by a group with greater knowledge and experience. The evaluation of these experts should be sufficient to confirm the relevance, adequacy, and clarity of the elements that make up the diagnosis.

Level 2.2.4. Consolidated validity of diagnostic content. The characteristic that differentiates this level from the previous one is the large sample of experts with predominantly proficient/expert levels of expertise. In addition to the difficulty of obtaining a sample of adequate size and quality, data analysis includes content validity indexes, tests of proportions, coefficients of agreement, and analysis of the internal consistency of the experts' assessments. The process can become more complex if the methods used include revisions of the structure, based on suggestions made by the experts. This is the most important subdivision of diagnostic content validation, and also the most difficult. Suggestions for strengthening this process include: obtain a larger sample than may be deemed initially necessary, use objective instruments, use electronic means of contact and data collection, seek experts in different countries, and organize a research schedule that takes into account a longer data collection period.

Level 2.3. Clinical validity. This is the highest and most desirable level for a diagnosis to remain in the classification. A content validation study must be completed prior to a clinical validity study. Prior to clinical validation, it should be established that the diagnosis has undergone content validation: is it classified as level 2.2.? This level has the largest number of subdivisions, and these are tied to the use of the diagnosis in clinical practice. The levels of evidence correspond to the type of clinical inference to be obtained from its clinical components, which may include the period beginning with the establishment of a clinical construct through to the development of causal processes. For better organization, this sublevel is divided into three blocks according to the purposes of the clinical validation process.

The first block includes the first two subdivisions (2.3.1. and 2.3.2.) and refers to descriptive studies that attempt to obtain initial profiles of the diagnostic components in populations that have supposedly experienced the phenomena; thus, this block represents evidence of clinical validity whose purpose is to identify in which populations a diagnosis may be applicable in practice. The second block includes the subsequent five sub-levels (2.3.3., 2.3.4., 2.3.5., 2.3.6. and 2.3.7.) and refers to validation processes that focus on the utility of defining characteristics for different clinical purposes, including diagnostic inference itself, screening capacity, prognosis establishment, differentiation capacity, and generalization across multiple populations. The third block includes the last three subdivisions (2.3.8. to 2.3.10.) and refers to validation processes that seek to identify related/risk factors, at risk populations, and associated conditions. The studies developed to reach the levels of evidence in this last block have the purpose of producing evidence regarding the factors that contribute to the occurrence of the nursing diagnosis.

The sublevels were organized considering that defining characteristics represent the main elements for the determination of a nursing diagnosis, and its validity for a specific purpose. Related factors, in turn, are causal elements that can only be identified if there is a certain degree of accuracy in the diagnostic inference process, which is based on defining characteristics. Thus, processes of clinical validation involving related factors (and other causal components) can only be properly designed and conducted for diagnoses with confirmed lower-level validity.

Level 2.3.1. Qualitative validity. Qualitative validity refers to the degree to which diagnostic interpretation is supported by clinical elements captured from individual subjective experiences. In this level, the level of evidence criterion relies on the development of qualitative studies to delimit the phenomenon based on the perception of those individuals believed to be experiencing it. These diagnoses must have been evaluated by a small group of subjects who possibly present with the diagnosis, in order to obtain information about the perception, beliefs, attitudes, and nuances of these individuals that can influence/characterize the phenomenon. Typically, intentional or convenience samples are used, and qualitative approaches are used for analysis. The study by Pinto et al. (2017) is an example of qualitative validation, in which the authors used interpretive content analysis to derive diagnoses related to patient comfort in palliative care. The authors derived 17 different diagnoses from the reported experiences of 15 patients from clinical-surgical units in a hospital in Portugal.

Level 2.3.2. Demographic validity. This is the last subdivision of the first block, and represents the degree to which demographic characteristics of a population can influence the interpretations obtained from the diagnostic components. This is a type of validity that has a strong relationship with causal components (related/risk factors, associated conditions, and at risk populations). The evidence level criteria consist of validation studies based on cross-sectional studies to identify elements associated with nursing diagnoses (defining characteristics/related/risk factors). These studies must be developed with large samples of subjects believed to be presenting with the diagnosis, whose selection of subjects can occur consecutively (as patients are admitted, for example) or by a random sampling process. The diagnostic inference process is based on a small group of nurse diagnosticians with proven experience with the diagnosis, and/or who have received specific training to identify it.

Data analysis must include verification of the association between socio-demographic variables, defining characteristics, and factors related to the diagnostic inference performed. In addition, some multivariate analysis techniques, such as logistic regressions, can be used to establish sets of defining characteristics, hierarchical models of related/risk factors, or models of joint association of human responses (for diagnoses that represent syndromes). For example, the study by Oliveira et al. (2016) analyzed the association between related factors and the presence of *sedentary lifestyle* (00168), adjusted for gender among Brazilian adolescents, to verify possible differences in the gender-influenced causality. The study included a total of 564 adolescents and identified four defining characteristics and six related factors strongly associated with a sedentary lifestyle. Some related factors showed differences by gender, being more strongly associated with men. In this case, the interpretations obtained from the defining characteristics identified among adolescents must be analyzed considering possible etiological differences by gender.

Level 2.3.3. Clinical construct validity. Unlike previous levels that focused on general exploratory approaches, this level is focused on specific components (defining characteristics) and represents the main category of evidence levels. Clinical construct validity is the degree to which a set of defining characteristics allows the correct interpretation (inference) of the nursing diagnosis from a defined clinical context. At this level, evidence level criteria include studies on the ability of defining characteristics to correctly classify subjects regarding the presence/absence of the diagnosis. Evidence of clinical construct validity should measure the accuracy (sensitivity and specificity) of each defining characteristic. It can also verify the importance of a group of defining characteristics and the influence of their clinical spectrum to modify the diagnostic inference.

The selection of patients included in these studies occurs in a naturalistic (consecutive) way, with a sufficient number of subjects to allow for the calculation of diagnostic accuracy. In general, diagnostic inference can be obtained by a panel of nurse diagnosticians, or through latent variable models for direct calculation of diagnostic accuracy. The study by Mangueira & Lopes (2016) is an example of this type of validation in which the authors evaluated 110 alcoholic patients and measured the diagnostic accuracy of 115 defining characteristics and, using four different latent class models, identified 24 characteristics with statistically significant measures of sensitivity or specificity for *dysfunctional family processes (00063)*.

Clinical construct validity seeks defining characteristics that allow for a more accurate diagnostic inference, representing the nursing diagnosis in its most complete form. The subsequent levels of clinical validity (2.3.4., 2.3.5., and 2.3.6.) differ from clinical construct validity in that they represent more specific uses and interpretations. These studies include those that aim to establish

- specific defining characteristics for screening and rapid decision making,
- defining characteristics which enable differentiation from similar diagnoses,
- and defining characteristics representing clinical deterioration.

The first two levels are applicable to few nursing diagnoses, while the last can be applicable to all diagnoses, and rely on the development of longitudinal studies.

Level 2.3.4. Selective validity (clinical screening). Selective validity refers to the degree to which a minimum set of characteristics can be used in a heuristic manner for a minimally acceptable interpretation of the presence of a nursing diagnosis. This enables rapid decision making in clinical settings such as urgent and emergency situations. The level of evidence criteria include studies that establish conditioned probabilities among small groups of defining characteristics, allowing for a rapid interpretation for use in risk classification protocols or clinical screening scenarios.

It must be taken into account that a clinical construct validation must have been conducted so that, based on these data, a minimum set of defining characteristics can be identified for use in diagnostic screening and rapid clinical decision making. Data analysis techniques for this type of validation, include the use of algorithms for the construction of classification trees. However, this technique requires large samples that allow for the calculation of conditioned probabilities for a pre-established minimum number of defining characteristics that should compose a decision-making model. For these studies, panels of nurse diagnosticians may be used for diagnostic inference, and the entire validation process of the classification tree must be reported.

The study by Chaves et al. (2018) is an example of the process used to establish this type of validity. The authors developed a classification tree for quick decision making for identifying *ineffective airway clearance* (00031) among children with acute respiratory infection. Its classification tree was based on comparing the results of three different algorithms in a sample of 249 children with acute respiratory infection. The best performing tree included the defining characteristics, *ineffective cough* and *adventitious breath sounds,* which were found to be suitable for screening children with *ineffective airway clearance* receiving care in the emergency department.

Level 2.3.5. Discriminant validity. Discriminant validity aims to determine the set of defining characteristics that allow for the differentiation between diagnoses that share similar signs and symptoms. This type of validity is defined as the degree to which a set of defining characteristics makes it possible to establish an interpretive boundary between diagnoses with similar clinical components. Thus, to consider investigating discriminant validity for two nursing diagnoses, both must have clinical construct validity: the level 2.3.3. criteria must be met. The level of evidence criteria may include studies with a different number of phases, ranging from a simultaneous concept analysis to an analysis with a population susceptible to the diagnoses to be differentiated. The samples must be large enough to calculate estimates, and the analysis is based on techniques such as multiple correspondence analysis or fuzzy sets (fuzzy logic).

An example of this type of validity can be found in the study by Pascoal et al. (2016a), who developed a discriminant validation study for the diagnoses, *ineffective airway clearance* (IAC, 00031), *ineffective breathing pattern* (IBP, 00032) *and impaired gas exchange* (IGE, 00030) among children with acute respiratory infection. The authors identified 27 defining characteristics that presented discriminating capacity among the three diagnoses.

Level 2.3.6. Prognostic validity. Prognostic validity refers to the degree to which a specific set of defining characteristics supports the interpretation of a patient's clinical deterioration, related to a nursing diagnosis in a specific context. This level of evidence criterion is based on the identification of lower survival/recovery rates of subjects with those defining characteristics. This criterion includes complex longitudinal studies whose objective is to identify a set of defining characteristics that allows for a prognostic assessment: to establish clinical signs that are markers of deterioration in the patient's clinical status. In order to achieve this type of validity, the diagnosis must have clinical construct validity (the 2.3.3. criteria must have been fulfilled).

This validation process is based on diagnostic cohort studies, in which the occurrence of defining characteristics must be evaluated and recorded at various points during follow-up. The length of patient follow-up will depend on each diagnosis, especially if its clinical trajectory tends to be acute or chronic, which can take anywhere from days to years of follow-up to establish reliable prognostic markers. Samples are typically obtained consecutively and/or by referral of subjects believed to be experiencing the diagnosis. The analysis of this type of study includes specific statistical techniques, such as measures of relative risk, incidence coefficients, and survival rates. Additionally, statistical models based on multivariate methods are used, such as generalized estimation equations and Cox proportional hazards models.

An example of prognostic validity can be found in the study by Pascoal et al. (2016b), who prospectively analyzed defining characteristics of *ineffective breathing pattern* (00032) among children hospitalized with acute respiratory infection, to identify markers of clinical deterioration associated with the nursing diagnosis. The authors followed 136 children for a period of ten consecutive days and, after an analysis based on the Cox model extended to time dependent covariables, identified four defining characteristics that can be interpreted as indicative of a poor prognosis for IBP.

Level 2.3.7. Generalizable validity of defining characteristics. This level includes systematic reviews of defining characteristics, and aims to identify clinical signs and symptoms that allow for a generalized interpretation of the nursing diagnosis across populations. This level of evidence criterion is based on the identification of clinical construct validation studies of the same diagnosis in different populations, using similar methods and describing measures of diagnostic accuracy of the defining characteristics. Thus, the samples are composed of well-designed studies that meet the 2.3.3. clinical construct validity criteria. To confirm generalizable validity, the study should apply meta-analysis techniques to establish summary measures of sensitivity and specificity.

An example of this type of evidence is the article by Sousa, Lopes, & Silva (2015), who completed a systematic review with meta-analysis to identify defining characteristics of *ineffective airway clearance* (00031) that presented better diagnostic accuracy in different clinical conditions. The study included a final sample of seven studies, five conducted with children and two with adults. The analysis was initially conducted for all seven studies, and later only for studies developed for children. The authors concluded that eight characteristics were valid for a generalizable interpretation for IAC.

Level 2.3.8. Diagnosis-specific causal validity. Specific causal validity refers to the degree to which clinical evidence establishes interpretations of the causal relationships between multiple factors in one diagnosis. This level of evidence criterion is based on the identification of these factors in case-control studies or using other methods that attest to their relationship with the diagnosis. This level of clinical validity refers to studies that are developed to identify multiple risk/related factors for one diagnosis. The methods commonly used include well-designed case-control studies with sufficient samples sizes to determine the magnitude of the effect of potential causal factors, as well as identification of hierarchical structures and sufficient cause for multiple related / risk factors / associated conditions / at risk populations.

The diagnostic inference for establishing subjects who will compose the case (with the nursing diagnosis) and control (without the nursing diagnosis) groups must be based on diagnostic accuracy measures established by clinical construct validity studies: level 2.3.3. criteria must be met.

This type of validity was used in the study by Medeiros et al. (2018), who completed a case-control study to identify pressure ulcer risk factors in adults in intensive care. The study was conducted with 180 patients (90 in each group). By using logistic regression analysis, the authors identified six risk factors for pressure ulcer (00249, revised to *risk for pressure injury* in this edition).

Level 2.3.9. Causal validity of exposure variable. The *causal validity of exposure variable* refers to the interpretation of a causal relationship between an etiological factor and a group of diagnoses. The level of evidence criterion is based on results obtained from cohort studies, or other methods that allow for demonstration of how such a factor can modify the interpretations (inferences) about a set of diagnoses. This type of validation allows for establishment of the importance of a related/risk factor for multiple diagnoses, using an exposure cohort design, which is based on two groups: one exposed and one not exposed to the risk/related factor. Such studies can also be useful for the establishment of causal chains, in which multiple diagnoses are clinically associated and have feedback loops, characterizing a syndrome diagnosis.

Samples should be sufficient to determine the magnitude of the risk associated with exposure to the factor, and to identify hierarchical structures that have multifactorial etiologies and/or causal chains. Finally, diagnoses believed to be caused by the same risk/related factor must be evaluated based on evidence of validity of the clinical construct; each diagnosis to be analyzed must have met the level 2.3.3. criteria for validity. The study by Reis & Jesus (2015) is an example of an exposure cohort to assess *risk for falls* (00155) among 271 institutionalized elderly.

Level 2.3.10. Generalized validity of related/risk factors. This type of validity refers to the degree to which the same set of etiological factors allows for the generation of a causal interpretation for different populations across multiple contexts. This level of evidence criterion is based on the identification of studies validating the etiological factors of the diagnosis in different populations, using similar methods, and describing measures of the effect size of these factors on the diagnosis. Thus, this level is similar to the generalizable validity of defining characteristics, but includes systematic reviews of related/risk factors. These samples will include well-designed studies that meet the level 2.3.8. criteria, and meta-analysis techniques are used to establish summary measures of the effect size of related/risk factors on the nursing diagnosis. No examples for this type of validity were found, possibly because the number of studies on related/risk factors is still very small. However, it is important to emphasize that the definition of interventions will depend on the causal factor of the diagnosis. Studies on evidence of validity are encouraged.

4.3.3 Final Considerations

These levels of evidence represent a hierarchy which depicts the degree to which observations identified as describing a diagnosis actually do describe it. The revision of the levels of evidence for the NANDA-I diagnoses should support clinicians in knowing the stage of development of the diagnoses, and their potential to represent the phenomena of the profession. In addition, this revision can help scholars to define their research, expanding the possibilities of practical application of their findings. Validation processes may accelerate the gradual development of accepted and proposed diagnoses, offering greater consistency to the terminology, in addition to improving the clinical decision making process.

In the next cycle of the terminology, work will be undertaken by the Directors of Research to reassign LOE for our diagnoses, using these new criteria.

4.4 References

American Educational Research Association. American Psychological Association. National Council on Measurement in Education. Standards for educational and psychological testing. Washington: American Psychological Association, 2014.

Cabaço SR, Caldeira S, Vieira M, et al. Spiritual coping: a focus of new nursing diagnoses. Int J Nurs Knowl 2018; 29(3): 156–164.

Chaves DBR, Pascoal LM, Beltrão BA, et al. Classification tree to screen for the nursing diagnosis Ineffective airway clearance. Rev Bras Enferm 2018; 71(5): 2353–2358.

Deeks JJ, Bossuyt PM, Gatsonis C. Cochrane Handbook for Systematic Reviews of Diagnostic Test Accuracy Version 1.0.0. The Cochrane Collaboration. 2013. Retrieved from http://srdta.cochrane.org/ on 24 June 2019.

Ferreira AM, Rocha EN, Lopes CT, et al. Nursing diagnoses in intensive care: cross-mapping and NANDA-I taxonomy. Rev Bras Enferm 2016; 69(2): 285–293

Grant JS, Kinney MR. Using the Delphi technique to examine the content validity of nursing diagnoses. Nurs Diagn 1992; 3(1): 12–22.

Gregory RJ. The history of psychological testing. In: Gregory RJ. Psychological testing: history, principles, and applications. 6th ed. London: Pearson Education, 2010.

Herdman TH, Kamitsuru S. NANDA International nursing diagnoses: definitions and classification, 2018-2020. New York: Thieme, 2018.

Lopes MVO, Silva VM, Herdman TH. Causation and validation of nursing diagnoses: a middle range theory. Int J Nurs Knowl 2017; 28(1): 53–59.

Mangueira SO, Lopes MVO. Clinical validation of the nursing diagnosis of dysfunctional family processes related to alcoholism. J Adv Nurs 2016; 72(10): 2401–2412.

Medeiros ABA, Fernandes MICD, Tinôco JDS, et al. Predictors of pressure ulcer risk in adult intensive care patients: a retrospective case-control study. Intensive Crit Care Nurs 2018; 45: 6–10.

Melo RP, Lopes MVO, Araujo TL, et al. Risk for decreased cardiac output: validation of a proposal for nursing diagnosis. Nurs Crit Care 2011; 16(6): 287–294.

Merlin T, Weston A, Tooher R. Extending an evidence hierarchy to include topics other than treatment: revising the Australian 'levels of evidence'. BMC medical research methodology 2009; 9(1): 34.

Miller S, Fredericks M. The nature of "evidence" in qualitative research methods. Int J Qual Methods 2003; 2(1): 1–27.

Oliveira MR, Silva VM, Guedes NG, et al. Clinical validation of the "Sedentary lifestyle" nursing diagnosis in secondary school students. J Sch Nurs 2016; 32(3): 186–194.

Pascoal LM, Lopes MVO, Silva VM, et al. Clinical differentiation of respiratory nursing diagnoses among children with acute respiratory infection. J Pediatr Nurs 2016a, 31 (1): 85–91.

Pascoal LM, Lopes MVO, Silva VM, et al. Prognostic clinical indicators of short-term survival for ineffective breathing pattern in children with acute respiratory infection. J Clinl Nurs 2016b, 25(5–6): 752–759.

Pearson A, Wiechula R, Court A, et al. A re-consideration of what constitutes "evidence" in the healthcare professions. Nurs Sci Q 2007; 20(1): 85–88.

Pearson A, Wiechula R, Court A, et al. The JBI model of evidence-based healthcare. Int J Evid Based Healthc 2005; 3(8): 207–215.

Pinto SP, Caldeira S, Martins JC. A qualitative study about palliative care patients' experiences of comfort: Implications for nursing diagnosis and interventions. J Nurs Educ Practice 2017; 7(8): 37–45.

Reis KMC, Jesus CAC. Cohort study of institutionalized elderly people: fall risk factors from the nursing diagnosis. Rev Lat Am Enfermagem 2015; 23(6): 1130–1138.

Sousa VEC, Lopes MVO, Silva VM. Systematic review and meta-analysis of the accuracy of clinical indicators for ineffective airway clearance. J Adv Nurs 2015; 71 (3):498–513.

Waltz CF, Strickland OL, Lenz ER. Measurement in nursing and health research. 5th ed. New York: Springer, 2017.

Zeleníková R, Žiaková K, Čáp J, Jarošová D. Content Validation of Nursing Diagnosis Acute Pain in the Czech Republic and Slovakia. Int J Nurs Terminol Knowledge 2014; 25:139-146.

Part 3
The Use of NANDA International Nursing Diagnoses

NANDA International, Inc. Nursing Diagnoses: Definitions and Classification 2021–2023, 12th Edition.
Edited by T. Heather Herdman, Shigemi Kamitsuru and Camila Takáo Lopes
© 2021 NANDA International, Inc. Published 2021 by Thieme Medical Publishers, Inc., New York.
Companion website: www.thieme.com/nanda-i.

5   Nursing Diagnosis Basics

Susan Gallagher-Lepak, Camila Takáo Lopes

5.1 Principles of Nursing Diagnosis: Introduction

Health care is delivered by various types of health care professionals, including nurses, physicians, and physical therapists, to name just a few. This is true in hospitals as well as other settings across the continuum of care (e.g., clinics, homecare, long-term care, community centers, prisons, schools). Each health care discipline brings its unique body of knowledge to the care of the client. In fact, a unique body of knowledge is a critical characteristic of a profession.

Collaboration, and at times overlap, occurs between professionals in providing care (▶ Fig. 5.1). For example, a physician in a hospital setting may write an order for the client to walk twice per day. Physical therapists focus on core muscles and movements necessary for walking. Respiratory therapists may be involved if oxygen therapy is needed to enable the patient's activity tolerance, due to an underlying respiratory condition. Social workers may be involved with insurance coverage for necessary equipment. Nurses have a holistic view of the patient, including working with the patient on balance and muscle strength related to walking, breathing pattern and oxygenation to conserve energy during activity, teaching the patient how to use accessory devices to support walking, as well as supporting the patient's confidence and motivation.

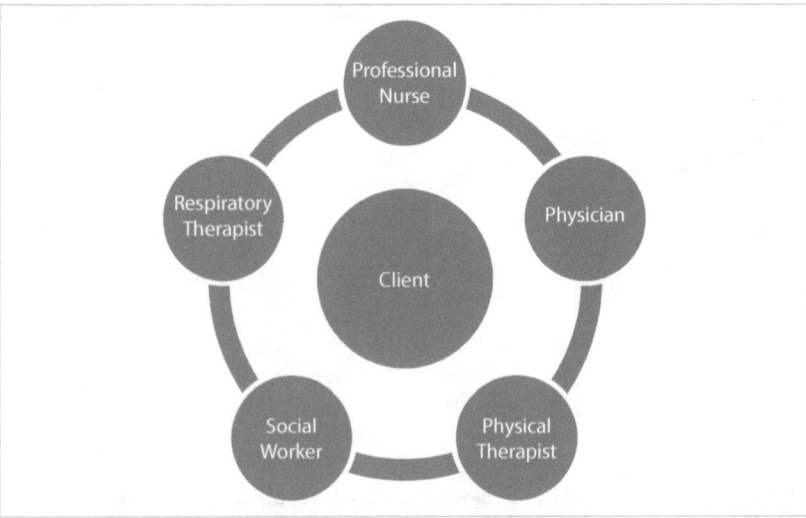

Fig. 5.1 Example of a collaborative health care team

Each health profession has a way to describe "**what**" the professional knows and "**how**" it acts on what it knows. This chapter is primarily focused on the "what". A profession may have a common language that is used to describe and code its knowledge. Physicians treat diseases and use the International Classification of Disease (ICD) taxonomy to represent and code the medical problems they treat. Psychologists, psychiatrists, and other mental health professionals treat mental health disorders, and use the Diagnostic and Statistical Manual of Mental Disorders (DSM) (American Psychiatric Association, 2013). Although nurses learn a lot about diagnoses contained in both the ICD and the DSM, it is important to remember that nurses independently diagnose and treat human responses to health problems and/or life processes, and use the NANDA International, Inc. (NANDA-I) nursing diagnosis classification. The nursing diagnosis taxonomy, the process of diagnosing, and the use of the NANDA-I terminology, will be described further.

The NANDA-I taxonomy provides a way to classify and categorize areas of concern to the nursing professional (i.e., diagnostic foci). It contains 267 nursing diagnoses grouped into 13 domains and 47 classes. A domain is a "sphere of knowledge" and the NANDA-I domains identify the unique knowledge of the nursing discipline (▶ Table 5.1). The 13 NANDA-I domains are further divided into classes (groupings that share common attributes). *Urinary function*, for example, is a class in the *Elimination and exchange* domain. Each of the classes contain relevant nursing diagnoses. *Urinary retention* (00023) is a nursing diagnosis in the class, Urinary function, within the domain of Elimination and exchange.

Table 5.1 NANDA-I domains

Domain	Name
1	Health promotion
2	Nutrition
3	Elimination and exchange
4	Activity/rest
5	Perception/cognition
6	Self-perception
7	Role relationships
8	Sexuality
9	Coping/stress tolerance
10	Life principles
11	Safety/protection
12	Comfort
13	Growth/development

Understanding the NANDA-I taxonomy helps the nurse identify and review diagnoses within the same class. For example, in the *Comfort* domain, in the *Physical comfort* class, a nurse will find nursing diagnoses related to pain, comfort, and nausea. A nursing diagnosis is a *clinical judgment concerning a human response to health conditions /life processes, or susceptibility to that response, by an individual, family, group or community*. Each nursing diagnosis has a label, definition, and diagnostic indicators. Examples of nursing diagnosis labels include *chronic pain* (00133) and *ineffective health self-management* (00276).

Nurses deal with responses to health conditions/life processes among individuals, families, groups, and communities. Such responses are the central concern of nursing care and fill the circle ascribed to nursing in ▶ Fig. 5.1. A nursing diagnosis can be focused on a problem, a potential risk, or a strength.

- **Problem-focused diagnosis** – a clinical judgment concerning an *undesirable human response* to a health condition/life process that exists in an individual, caregiver, family, group, or community
- **Risk diagnosis** – a clinical judgment concerning the *susceptibility* of an individual, caregiver, family, group, or community for developing an undesirable human response to health conditions/life processes
- **Health promotion diagnosis** – a clinical judgment concerning *motivation and desire* to increase well-being and to actualize health potential. These responses are expressed by a readiness to enhance specific health behaviors, and can be used in any health state. In cases where individuals are unable to express their own readiness to enhance health behaviors, the nurse may determine that a condition for health promotion exists and then act on the client's behalf. Health promotion responses may exist in an individual, caregiver, family, group, or community.

Although limited in number in the NANDA-I taxonomy, a **syndrome** can also be diagnosed by a nurse. A syndrome is a clinical judgment concerning a specific *cluster of nursing diagnoses* that occur together, and is therefore best addressed through similar interventions. An example of a syndrome diagnosis is *chronic pain syndrome* (00255). The nursing diagnosis, *chronic pain* (00133) is recurrent or persistent pain that has lasted at least 3 months and that significantly affects daily functioning or well-being. *Chronic pain syndrome* is differentiated from *chronic pain* in that, in addition to the chronic pain, it significantly impacts other human responses, and thus a syndrome includes other nursing diagnoses, such as *disturbed sleep pattern* (00198), *fatigue* (00093), *impaired physical mobility* (00085), or *social isolation* (00053).

5.2 Principles of Nursing Diagnosis: Diagnosing

The nursing process requires nursing knowledge (theory/nursing science/ underlying nursing concepts) (Herdman, 2013), and includes assessing, diagnosing, planning outcome(s) and interventions, implementing, and evaluating (► Fig. 5.2). Nurses use assessment and clinical judgment to formulate hypotheses or explanations about presenting problems, risks, and/or health promotion opportunities. Application of the knowledge of underlying concepts of nursing science and nursing theory are required before patterns can be identified in clinical data or accurate diagnoses can be made.

The components of the nursing process occur more or less simultaneously in the nurse's thought processes. Note that the rectangles have the closest start line on the left and the most distant end line on the right. This asymmetry represents the time period after the beginning of data collection, when the nurse uses reasoning and clinical judgment to begin to identify diagnoses, set patient-specific outcomes, and decide on interventions. While completing these operations, the nurse can start implementing these decisions and evaluating their outcomes (Bachion, 2009).

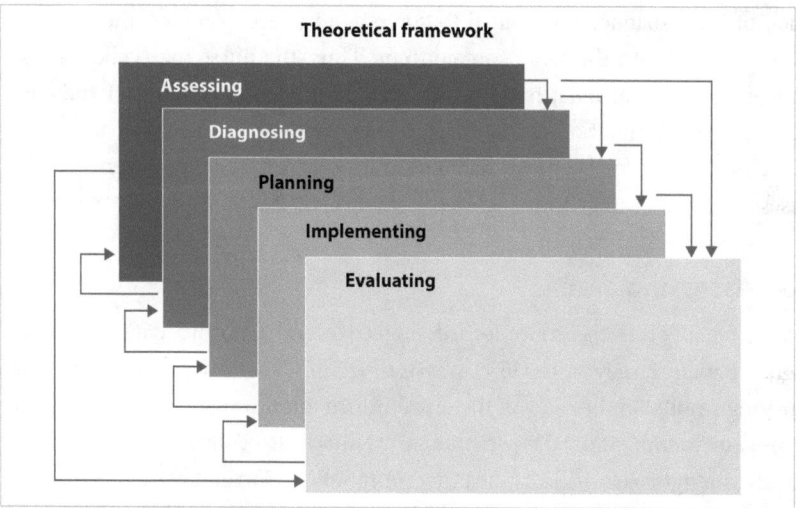

Fig. 5.2 The nursing process.
From Bachion, M.M. (2009). Intrumentos básicos do cuidar: observação, interação e mensuração. [Basic instruments for delivering care: observation, interaction and measurement]. I Simpósio Brasiliense de Sistematização da Assistência de Enfermagem, 2009. Brasília, Brazil. (Portuguese). Reproduced with the author's permission.

5.3 Principles of Nursing Diagnosis: Knowledge of Nursing Concepts

Knowledge of key concepts, or nursing diagnostic foci, is necessary before beginning an assessment. Examples of critical concepts important to nursing practice include breathing, elimination, thermoregulation, physical comfort, self-care, and skin integrity. Understanding such concepts allows the nurse to see patterns in the data and accurately diagnose. Key areas to understand within the concept of pain, for example, include manifestations of pain, theories of pain, at risk populations, related pathophysiological concepts (fatigue, depression), and management of pain. Full understanding of key concepts is needed, as well, to differentiate diagnoses.

For example, to understand issues related to coping and stress tolerance that might be specific to an immigrant population, a nurse must first understand the core concepts related to potential problems, risks, or health promotion opportunities. *In looking simply at problems that can occur with coping and stress tolerance*, the nurse may need to consider the diagnoses of *risk for complicated immigration transition* (00260), and *maladaptive grieving* (00135); concerns with resilience may lead the nurse to the diagnosis, *impaired resilience* (00210); while issues related to activity planning might lead to a diagnosis of *ineffective activity planning* (00199). As you can see, although each of these diagnoses is related to coping and stress tolerance, they are not all concerned with the same core concept. Thus, the nurse may collect a significant amount of data, but without a sufficient understanding of the core concepts of immigration transition, grieving, resilience and activity planning, the data needed for accurate diagnosis may be omitted, and patterns in the assessment data can go unrecognized.

5.4 Assessing

Assessing involves the collection of subjective and objective data (e.g., vital signs, patient/family interview, physical exam, laboratory and diagnostic imaging results) and review of historical information provided by the patient/family, or found within the patient chart. Nurses also collect data on patient/family strengths (to identify health promotion opportunities) and risks (to prevent or postpone potential problems). Assessments should be based on theoretical frameworks, including, but not limited to, nursing theories, such as Careful Nursing, Culture Care Theory, and Theory of Transpersonal Caring. The elements in the theoretical frameworks can be operationalized through assessment frameworks, such as Marjory Gordon's Functional Health Patterns

(FHPs). More information will be provided about Gordon's FHPs in the chapter on assessment (Chapter 7.3). Nursing-centric frameworks provide a way of categorizing large amounts of data into a manageable number of related patterns or categories of data. In the upcoming chapter on assessment, we will discuss this in more detail. However, it is important to consider that there are different approaches to assessment, which can range from very broad to very narrow in focus, and include risk assessment tools, patient reported assessment tools, and in-depth nursing assessment tools, to name just a few.

The foundation of nursing diagnosis is clinical reasoning. Clinical reasoning involves the use of clinical judgment to decide what is wrong with a patient, and clinical decision-making to decide what needs to be done (Levett-Jones et al 2010). Clinical judgment is "an interpretation or conclusion about a patient's needs, concerns, or health problems, and/or the decision to take action (or not)" (Tanner 2006, p. 204). Key issues, or diagnostic foci, may be evident early in the assessment (e.g., altered skin integrity, loneliness) and allow the nurse to begin the diagnostic process. For example, a patient may report insomnia, irritability, anguish, and/or show facial tension, hand tremors, and increased perspiration. The experienced nurse will recognize the client's *anxiety (00146)* based on client report and/or anxiety behaviors. Expert nurses can quickly identify clusters of clinical cues from assessment data and seamlessly progress to nursing diagnoses. Novice nurses take a more sequential process in determining appropriate nursing diagnoses.

As another example, after initial assessment of a patient experiencing breathing difficulties with activity, several potential diagnoses may be considered. Nurses might use valid and reliable instruments that measure actual responses, to further assess for these diagnoses, and confirm or refute their diagnostic hypothesis. Some examples might include use of the Multidimensional Dyspnea Scale (Kalluri et al., 2019), the International Sedentary Assessment Tool (Prince et al., 2019), or the Sedentary Behaviour Questionnaire (Rosenberg et al., 2010).

As another example, if upon initial assessment, a potential diagnosis related to coping with pain is identified, nurses might work with patients to use valid and reliable instrument or scale that measures risk or signs/symptoms of an actual response, to further assess this possibility and confirm or refute their diagnostic hypothesis. Some examples might include use of the Morse Fall Scale (Morse, 1997), Multidimensional Dyspnea Scale (Kalluri et al, 2019), or the Braden Scale (Bergstrom et al, 1987).

Table 5.2 Parts of a nursing diagnosis label

Modifier	Focus of the diagnosis
Ineffective	activity planning
Risk for	infection
Chronic	confusion
Impaired	physical mobility
Readiness for enhanced	health self-management

5.5 Diagnosing

A nursing diagnosis is a clinical judgment concerning a human response to health conditions/life processes, or susceptibility to that response, by an individual, caregiver, family, group, or community (NANDA-I DDC communication, 2019). It is the outcome of diagnostic reasoning (Gordon, 1994) and it is typically stated in two parts: (1) descriptor or modifier and (2) focus of the diagnosis or its key concept, such as with the diagnosis, *ineffective activity planning* (00199) (▶ Table 5.2). There are some exceptions in which a nursing diagnosis is only one word, such as *anxiety* (00146), *constipation* (00011), *fatigue* (00093), and *nausea* (00134). In these diagnoses, the modifier and focus are inherent in the one term.

Nurses diagnose health problems, risk states, and readiness for health promotion. Problem-focused diagnoses should not be viewed as being more important than risk diagnoses. Sometimes a risk diagnosis can be the diagnosis with the highest priority for a patient. An example may be a patient who has the nursing diagnoses of *impaired oral mucous membrane integrity* (00045), *impaired memory* (00131), *readiness for enhanced health self-management* (00293), and *risk for adult pressure injury* (00304), and has been newly admitted to a skilled nursing facility. Although *impaired oral mucous membrane integrity* and *impaired memory* are the problem-focused diagnoses, the patient's *risk for adult pressure injury* may be the number one priority diagnosis. This may be especially true when related risk factors are identified during the assessment (e.g., decreased physical mobility, protein-energy malnutrition, dehydration, inadequate caregiver knowledge of pressure injury prevention strategies) in an individual known to be part of an at risk population (elderly; Individuals in community, aged care, and rehabilitation settings; wheelchair bound).

Each nursing diagnosis has a label and a clear definition. It is important to state that merely having a label or picking from a list of labels is insufficient. It is critical that nurses know the definitions of the diagnoses they most commonly use. In addition, they need to know the "diagnostic indicators" – the

Table 5.3 Key terms at a glance

Term	Brief description
Nursing diagnosis	A clinical judgment concerning a human response to health conditions/life processes, or a susceptibility to that response, by an individual, caregiver, family, group, or community. A nursing diagnosis provides the basis for selection of nursing interventions to achieve outcomes for which the nurse has accountability
Defining characteristic	Observable cues/inferences that cluster as manifestations of a problem-focused, health promotion diagnosis or syndrome. This implies not only those things that the nurse can see, but also things that are seen, heard (e.g., the patient/family tells us), touched, or smelled.
Related factor	Antecedent factor that appears to show some type of patterned relationship with the human response (etiological factors). These factors must be modifiable by independent nursing interventions, and whenever possible, interventions should be aimed at these etiological factors.
Risk factor	Antecedent factor that increases the susceptibility of an individual, caregiver, family, group, or community to an undesirable human response. These factors must be modifiable by independent nursing interventions, and whenever possible, interventions should be aimed at these factors.
At risk populations	Groups of people who share sociodemographic characteristics, health/family history, stages of growth/development, exposure to certain events/experiences that cause each member to be susceptible to a particular human response. These are characteristics that are not modifiable by the professional nurse.
Associated conditions	Medical diagnoses, diagnostic/surgical procedures, medical/surgical devices, or pharmaceutical preparations. These conditions are not independently modifiable by the professional nurse.

information that is used to diagnose and differentiate one diagnosis from another. These diagnostic indicators include defining characteristics and related factors or risk factors (▶ Table 5.3). **Defining characteristics** are observable cues/inferences that cluster as manifestations of a diagnosis (e.g., signs or symptoms). An assessment that identifies the presence of a number of defining characteristics lends support to the accuracy of the nursing diagnosis. **Related factors** are an integral component of all problem-focused nursing diagnoses. Related factors, also called etiological factors, are antecedent factors shown to have a patterned relationship with the human response (e.g., cause, contributing factor). These factors must be modifiable by independent nursing interventions, and whenever possible, interventions should be aimed at these etiological factors. A review of client history often helps to identify related factors. Whenever possible, nursing interventions should be aimed at these etiological factors in order to remove the underlying cause of the nursing diagnosis. **Risk factors** are antecedent factors that increase the susceptibility of an individual, caregiver, family, group, or community to an undesirable human response (e.g., environmental, psychological).

Observable cues/inferences cluster as manifestations of a problem-focused or health promotion diagnosis. This implies not only those things that the nurse can see, but also things that are heard (e.g., the patient/family tells us), touched, or smelled.

A nursing diagnosis does not need to contain all types of diagnostic indicators (i.e., defining characteristics, related factors, and/or risk factors). Problem-focused nursing diagnoses contain defining characteristics and related factors. Health promotion diagnoses usually have defining characteristics only; related factors could be used if they would improve the clarity of the diagnosis. Only risk diagnoses have risk factors.

A nursing plan of care does not need to contain each type of nursing diagnosis. The example below illustrates the use of problem and risk diagnoses, as well as the dynamic process of determining nursing diagnoses.

The plan of care for an 82-year-old female in the hospital includes the diagnoses, *risk for adult falls* (00303), *acute pain* (00132), and *deficient fluid volume* (00027). The nurse indicates to her colleague during an end of shift hand-off that her interview with the woman's husband suggests that he is overwhelmed by her increased care needs over the past year, and he is providing all her care by himself. The nurse states she will be adding *risk for caregiver role strain* (00062) to the plan of care.

A common format used by students when learning to document nursing diagnoses includes: _____ [nursing diagnosis] related to _____ [cause/related factors] as evidenced by _____ [symptoms/defining characteristics]. For example, *ineffective breastfeeding (00104)* related to *maternal anxiety, inadequate family support,* and *pacifier use* as evidenced by *infant crying at breast / inability to latch on to maternal breast correctly / sustained weight loss.* Many nurse educators support this method as a helpful method for students to learn to think critically, while it a also provides faculty members with a way to evaluate clinical reasoning. Further, some argue that all nursing diagnoses should be documented in the patient chart using this three-part format. However, it has always been the position of NANDA-I that it is appropriate to document the label only, provided that the related/risk factors and defining characteristics can be recognized in the assessment data, nursing notes, or plan of care sections within the patient record, in order to provide support for the nursing diagnosis.

Additionally, most electronic health records (EHRs) in use today will not include the "related to" and "as evidenced by" components. Therefore, it is important that the nursing assessment tool within the EHR system contains the diagnostic indicators necessary for diagnosis, to allow for documentation of the nursing diagnosis label only within the patient problem list. After all, simply documenting a diagnosis does not prove its accuracy. As with our colleagues in medicine, we must have our diagnostic indicators appear within the patient record to support our diagnoses. Without this information, it is impossible to verify diagnostic accuracy, which puts the quality of nursing care in question.

5.6 Planning/Implementing

Once diagnoses are identified, prioritizing of selected nursing diagnoses must occur to determine care priorities. High-priority nursing diagnoses need to be identified (i.e., urgent need, diagnoses with high level of congruence with defining characteristics, related factors, or risk factors) so that care can be directed to resolve these problems or lessen the severity or risk of occurrence (in the case of risk diagnoses).

Nursing diagnoses are used to identify intended outcomes of care and plan nursing-specific interventions sequentially. A nursing outcome, according to the authors of the Nursing Outcome Classification (NOC), refers to "a measurable individual, family, or community state, behavior or perception that is measured along a continuum in response to nursing interventions". The NOC is one example of a standardized nursing language that can be used when planning care, to represent outcome measures related to a nursing diagnosis (Moorhead, Swanson, Johnson, & Maas, 2018, p. 3). Nurses often, and incorrectly, move directly from nursing diagnosis to nursing intervention without consideration of desired outcomes. Instead, outcomes need to be identified before interventions are determined. The order of this process is similar to planning a road trip. Simply getting in a car and driving will get a person somewhere, but that may not be the place the person really wanted to go. It is better to first have a clear location (outcome) in mind, and then choose a route (intervention), to get to a desired location.

An intervention, according to the authors of the Nursing Interventions Classification (NIC), is defined as "any treatment, based upon clinical judgment and knowledge that a nurse performs to enhance patient/client outcomes" (Butcher, Bulechek, Docterman, & Wagner, 2018, p.xii). The NIC is an example of a standardized nursing intervention language that nurses may use across various care settings. Using nursing knowledge, nurses perform both independent and interdisciplinary interventions. These interdisciplinary interventions overlap with care provided by other health care professionals (e.g., physicians, respiratory and physical therapists).

Hypertension is a medical diagnosis, yet nurses perform both independent and interdisciplinary interventions for these clients who have various types of problems or risk states. Often nurses initiate standing protocols to manage medical diagnoses for patients, and may believe that they are providing independent nursing interventions because they do not require a direct order from a physician to begin the protocol. However, these standing protocols are, in fact, dependent medical orders that are performed and monitored by nurses; they are not independent nursing interventions. However, nurses do perform independent interventions for those clients diagnosed with nursing diagnoses, such as *risk for unstable blood pressure* (00267), which is a common nursing diagnosis in many settings. In reviewing the related (etiological factors) for this diagnosis, the nurse would determine an appropriate outcome for this patient, and then determine what nursing intervention(s) might be initiated to achieve this outcome, aimed at the related factors of the diagnosis.

5.7 Kamitsuru's Tripartite Model of Nursing Practice

Kamitsuru's Tripartite Model of Nursing Practice provides nurses with a clear understanding of the types of interventions nurses perform, and the basis of knowledge that underlies those different types.

Nurses often work with a patient who has medical problems. However, from a legal point of view, physicians are responsible for the diagnosis and treatment of these medical problems. In the same way, nurses are responsible for the diagnosis and treatment of nursing problems. The important point is that nursing problems are different from medical problems. Moreover, we do not rename medical diagnoses or terms to create nursing diagnoses, nor do we need a nursing diagnosis for every nursing intervention or action.

To make these points clear, let's examine how nursing practice exists within health care, from a broader perspective, based on the *Three Pillar Model of Nursing Practice* (Kamitsuru, 2008), ▶ Fig. 5.3. This model depicts three major components of nursing practice, which are distinct but interrelated. In clinical practice, nurses are expected to perform various actions.

First, we have practices/interventions that are driven by medical diagnoses. Nursing actions may be related to related to medical treatments, patient surveillance and monitoring, as well as interdisciplinary collaboration. For

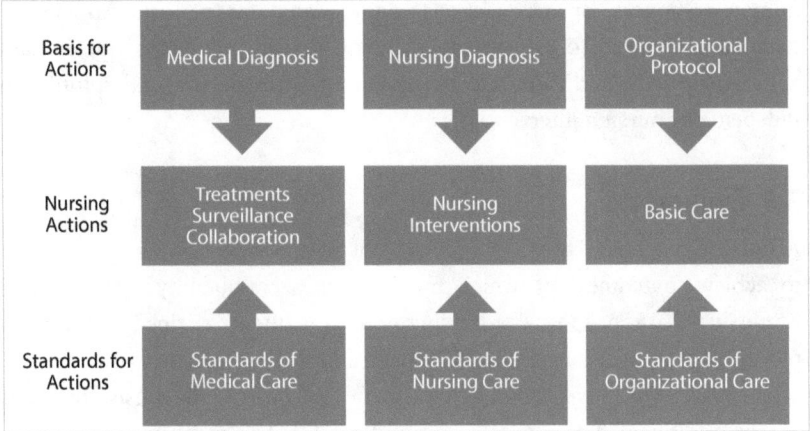

Fig. 5.3 Kamitsuru's Tripartite Model of Nursing Practice

instance, when a physician diagnoses an unconscious patient as having a cerebral infarction and orders intravenous (IV) medications, the nurse implements the IV order as directed and carefully monitors the patient's response to the medications. Nurses take these actions in response to medical diagnoses, and use medical standards of care as the basis for these nursing actions.

Secondly, practice may be driven by nursing diagnoses. Independent nursing interventions do not require physician approval or permission. For instance, for the above patient with a cerebral infarction, the nurse positions the patient in a careful manner to prevent aspiration, as well as pressure injury. Supportive care may also be provided to the patient's spouse, who is also taking care of an elderly person with dementia at home. Nurses take these actions based on nursing diagnoses, and use nursing standards of care as the basis for these nursing actions.

Finally, practice may be driven by organizational protocols. These can be actions related to basic care, such as changing linen, providing hygiene and daily care. These actions are not specifically related to either medical diagnoses or nursing diagnoses, but they are based on organizational standards of care.

All three actions combine to form the practice of nursing. Each has a different knowledge base, and different responsibilities. The three parts are equally important for nurses to understand, but only one of them relates to the unique disciplinary knowledge of nursing – and that is the area we know as nursing diagnosis. This model also shows why we do not need to rename medical diagnoses as nursing diagnoses. Medical diagnoses already exist in the medical domain. However, medical diagnoses do not always explain everything that nurses understand about patients, judgments made about their human responses, or interventions implemented for patients. So, nursing diagnoses are used to explain independent clinical judgments nurses make about their patients. Thus, nursing diagnoses provide the underpinning of independent nursing interventions.

5.8 Evaluating

A nursing diagnosis "provides the basis for selection of nursing interventions to achieve outcomes for which nursing has accountability" (Herdman & Kamitsuru 2018, p. 133). The nursing process is often described as a stepwise process, but in reality a nurse will go back and forth between steps in the process. Nurses will move between assessment and nursing diagnosis, for example, as additional data are collected and clustered into meaningful patterns and the accuracy of nursing diagnoses is evaluated. Similarly, the effectiveness of interventions and achievement of identified outcomes is continuously evaluated as the client status is assessed. Evaluation should ultimately occur at each step in the nursing process, as well as once the plan of care has been implemented. Several questions to consider include the following: "What data might I have missed? Am I making an inappropriate judgment? How confident am I in this diagnosis? Do I need to consult with someone with more experience? Have I confirmed the diagnosis with the patient/family/caregiver/group/community? Are the expected outcomes appropriate for this client in this setting, given the regulations governing nursing practice in the country/state/region, the reality of the patient's condition, the patient's values/beliefs, professional expertise, and resources available? Are the interventions based on research evidence or tradition (e.g., "what we always do")?

5.9 Principles of Nursing Diagnosis: Clinical Application

This description of nursing diagnosis basics, although aimed primarily at novices, can benefit many nurses in that it highlights critical steps in using nursing diagnosis and provides examples of areas in which inaccurate diagnosing can occur. An area that needs continued emphasis, for example, includes the process of linking knowledge of underlying nursing concepts to assessment, and ultimately nursing diagnosis. The nurse's understanding of key concepts (or diagnostic foci) directs the assessment process and interpretation of assessment data. Relatedly, nurses diagnose problem, risk and strength responses. Any of these types of diagnoses can be the priority diagnosis (or diagnoses), and the nurse makes this clinical judgment.

In representing the knowledge of nursing science, the NANDA-I taxonomy provides the structure for a standardized language in which to communicate nursing diagnoses. Using the NANDA-I terminology (the diagnoses themselves), nurses can communicate with each other, as well as professionals from other health care disciplines, about "what" nurses uniquely know. The use of nursing diagnosis in our interactions with patients/family members can help them to understand the issues on which nurses will be focusing, and can engage them in their own care. The terminology provides a shared language for nurses to address health problems, risk states, and health promotion opportunities. NANDA-I's nursing diagnoses are used internationally, with translation into more than 20 languages. In an increasingly global and electronic world, NANDA-I also allows nurses involved in scholarship to communicate about phenomena of concern to nursing in manuscripts and at conferences, in a standardized way, thus advancing the science of nursing.

Nursing diagnoses are peer reviewed, and submitted for acceptance/revision to NANDA-I by nurses in practice, nurse educators, and nurse researchers around the world. Submissions of new diagnoses and/or revisions to existing diagnoses have continued to grow in number over the nearly 50 years of the NANDA-I nursing diagnosis terminology. Continued submissions (and revisions) to NANDA-I will further strengthen the scope, extent, and supporting evidence of the terminology.

5.10 Brief Chapter Summary

This chapter describes types of nursing diagnoses (i.e., problem-focused, risk, health promotion) and steps in the nursing process. The nursing process begins with an *understanding* of underlying concepts of nursing science, and nursing theories. *Assessing* follows and involves collection and clustering of data into meaningful patterns. *Diagnosing* involves clinical judgment about a human response to a health condition or life process, or susceptibility to that response, by an individual, caregiver, family, group, or a community. The nursing diagnosis components were reviewed in this chapter, including the label, definition, and diagnostic indicators (i.e., related factors, risk factors, at risk populations, and associated conditions). Given that a patient assessment will typically generate a number of nursing diagnoses, prioritizing of nursing diagnoses is needed to direct care delivery. Critical next steps in *planning/ implementing* include identification of nursing outcomes and nursing interventions to eliminate the causative or risk factors of a diagnosis, or to minimize their impact on the individual's, caregiver's, family's, group's, or community's well-being. *Evaluating* occurs throughout the nursing process, and at the conclusion of patient care.

5.11 References

American Psychiatric Association. Diagnostic and Statistical Manual of Mental Disorders. 5th ed. Arlington, VA: American Psychiatric Association; 2013. Available at: dsm.psychiatryonline.org

Bachion MM. [Basic instruments for delivering care: observation, interaction and measurement]. I Simpósio Brasiliense de Sistematização da Assistência de Enfermagem. Brasília, Brazil, 2009 (Portuguese).

Butcher HK, Bulechek GM, Dochterman JM, Wagner CM (eds.). Nursing Interventions Classification (NIC). 7th ed. St. Louis, MO: Elsevier, 2018.

Butryn ML, Arigo D, Raggio GA, Kaufman AI, Kerrigan SG, Forman EM. Measuring the Ability to Tolerate Activity-Related Discomfort: Initial Validation of the Physical Activity Acceptance Questionnaire (PAAQ). Journal of physical activity & health 2015; 12(5): 717–726.

Herdman TH. Manejo de casos empleando diagnósticos de enfermería de la NANDA Internacional [Case management using NANDA International nursing diagnoses]. XXX Congreso FEMAFEE 2013. Monterrey, Mexico.

Kalluri M, Bakal J, Ting W, Younus S. (2019). Comparison of MRC breathlessness scale to a novel multidimensional dyspnea scale (MDDS) for clinical use. In: B46. Idiopathic interstitial pneumonia: natural history (pp. A3371-A3371). American Thoracic Society International Conference, 2019.

Kamitsuru, S. Kango shindan seminar shiryou [Nursing diagnosis seminar handout]. Kango Laboratory, 2008 (Japanese).

Leininger M. Culture care theory: a major contribution to advance transcultural nursing knowledge and practices. J Transcult Nurs 2002; 13(3): 189–201.

Levett-Jones T, Hoffman K, Dempsey J. The "five rights" of clinical reasoning: an educational model to enhance nursing students' ability to identify and manage clinically "at risk" patients. Nurse Educ Today 2010; 30 (6): 515–520. https://pubmed.ncbi.nlm.nih.gov/19948370/.

Meehan TC, Timmons F, Burke J. Fundamental care guided by the Careful Nursing Philosophy and Professional Practice Model. Journal of Clinical Nursing 2018; 27: 2260–2273.

Moorhead S, Swanson E, Johnson M, Maas ML (eds.). Nursing Outcomes Classification (NOC): Measurement of health outcomes. 6th ed. St. Louis, MO: Elsevier, 2018.

Prince SA, Butler GP, Roberts KC, Lapointe P, MacKenzie AM, Colley RC, et al. Developing content for national population health surveys: an example using a newly developed sedentary behaviour module. Archives of Public Health 2019; 77(1): 53.

Rosenberg DE, Norman GJ, Wagner N, Patrick K, Calfas KJ, Sallis JF. Reliability and validity of the Sedentary Behavior Questionnaire (SBQ) for adults. Journal of Physical Activity & Health 2010; 7(6): 697–705.

Tanner CA. Thinking like a nurse: a research-based model of clinical judgment in nursing. J Nurs Educ 2006; 45 (6): 204–211. https://pubmed.ncbi.nlm.nih.gov/16780008/.

Watson, J. Caring science as a sacred science. In: McEwen M, Wills E (eds.). Theoretical basis for nursing. Lippincott Williams & Wilkins, 2005.

6 Nursing Diagnosis: An International Terminology

Susan Gallagher-Lepak, T. Heather Herdman

6.1 Nursing Commonalities Around the Globe

There are approximately 19 million nurses and midwives in the world, according to the World Health Organization (WHO, 2013). Visualize this large number of nurses providing nursing care across the world in various types of healthcare settings, speaking different languages, using a range of equipment and technologies, and following countless and varied institutional protocols. Although differences are evident, commonalities are numerous among this professional group and its members' collective provision of nursing care.

Nurses have similar professional values (e.g., caring, dignity of the patient, collaboration) and share foundational nursing knowledge. The individual (or recipient of care) is the central focus of nursing. Nurses deal with individuals' responses to health problems and life processes among individuals, caregivers, families, groups, and, communities.

Nurses use NANDA-I nursing diagnoses to communicate their clinical judgments about human responses/life processes, or susceptibilities for these responses, that their patients are experiencing. The nurse's clinical judgment "provides the basis for selection of nursing interventions to achieve outcomes for which nursing has accountability" (Herdman & Kamitsuru, 2018, p. 133).

6.2 Nursing Education and Practice

Many schools of nursing have curricula that integrate nursing diagnosis, and linkages to outcomes and interventions. Critical in the curricula is the importance of assessment to guide identification and validation of nursing diagnoses. Also important is that members of the faculty and administrative staff value and have knowledge of nursing diagnosis terminology.

The *NANDA-I Nursing Diagnoses: Definitions and Classification* publication is a core textbook for many nursing education programs, and is published in over 20 languages (► Table 6.1). Newer language translations and distribution in the last book cycle reflect broader interest in our work within, countries in Africa, Asia, Eastern Europe, and the Indian subcontinent. A number of countries have shown recent interest in adopting NANDA-I via activities such as international workshops, developing a NANDA-I Network Group, attending NANDA-I conferences, requesting online seminars, or other

Table 6.1 NANDA International nursing diagnoses: definitions and classification. Translations

Complex Chinese	Croatian	Czech	Dutch
English	Estonian	European Spanish	French
German	Hispanoamerican Spanish	Indonesian	Italian
Japanese	Korean	Latvian	Polish
Portuguese	Romanian	Simplified Chinese	Slovenian
Swedish	Turkish		

learning activities to build knowledge of the NANDA-I taxonomy and terminology.

Exposure to and application of the nursing process, and in-depth understanding of nursing diagnosis, in nursing education equips each aspiring nurse with knowledge and skills necessary for professional nursing practice. Integrating NANDA-I nursing diagnoses throughout the curriculum involves content threaded into lecture courses, skills courses, and simulation and clinical experiences. There are numerous ways to integrate standardized nursing languages (SNL), including NANDA-I nursing diagnoses, into the curriculum. Developing plans of care as clinical assignments are very common, and can be an effective learning opportunity after students have been exposed to diagnosing. Problematic approaches include teaching nursing diagnoses in a way that links them directly to medical diagnoses, using standardized care plans for specific nursing diagnoses without linking assessment data to diagnosis, and/or without customization of interventions and outcomes for the patient. A medical diagnosis should be considered by the nurse as part of the assessment, but should never be used exclusively as the rationale for a nursing diagnosis. Similarly, a standardized care plan can be a starting template, but must be customized to the patient and the specific concerns or needs of each patient, as identified through nursing assessment.

Healthcare settings use nursing diagnoses or "patient problems" to identify and prioritize the areas of concern to nursing. Many healthcare organizations have moved from paper medical records to electronic health records (EHR) to document nursing care. NANDA-I contracts with major EHR vendors to license the NANDA-I terminology, and EHR vendors then customize the terminology for each unique healthcare institution's HER, and customized builds can link assessment data to diagnoses. NANDA-I also contracts directly with organizations (e.g., hospitals, home health, long-term care) for the use of the terminology, through its publishing partners. With the popularity of EHRs, it is important to note that it is a violation of copyright law to use NANDA-I terminology in an EHR without permission from NANDA-I, in the form of a written contract from the publishing partner that manages digital rights in the language of the user.

The presence of SNLs in EHRs offers new ways to study diagnostic accuracy (correspondence between assessment data and the patient's current condition) and nursing documentation. Studies have shown a need to improve diagnostic reasoning and accuracy among students and nurses in practice (Johnson, Edwards, & Giandinoto, 2017; Larijani & Saatchi, 2019; Freire, Lopes, Keenan, & Lopez, 2018). A wealth of clinical information can be mined when SNLs are contained within the EHR, and when diagnoses can be validated through the use of data within standardized nursing assessments.

6.3 Professional Associations and Nursing Classifications

The NANDA-I professional association connects nurses (and others with interest in nursing diagnosis) with interest in the pursuit of diagnostic terminology development and refinement, as well as best practices for education, research, and use of the NANDA-I terminology. Members of the association include students, nurses in practice, administrators, educators, informaticists, and researchers. Members are connected through its website and social media channels, as well as having the opportunity to present their research and share experiences at NANDA-I conferences. The NANDA-I journal, *International Journal of Nursing Knowledge*, publishes research on worldwide efforts to identify nursing knowledge, develop and apply SNLs in practice, education, informatics and research.

NANDA-I has been linked to several nursing classifications, and, with permission, several have incorporated NANDA-I diagnoses within their development (assigned *) over the years, for the purposes of practice, education, or research. These include:

- Belgium's **Nursing Minimum Data Set** (NMDS)
- **Clinical Care Classification** (CCC) System*
- **European Nursing care Pathways** (ENP)
- **International Classification of Function** (ICF)
- **International Classification of Nursing Practice** (ICNP)*
- **Leistung Erfassung des Pflegeaufwandes** (LEP)
- **Nursing Intervention Classification** (NIC), University of Iowa
- **Nursing Outcome Classification** (NOC), University of Iowa
- **Omaha System** (Omaha)*

- **Perioperative Nursing Data Set** (PNDS)*
- **Sundheds-væsenets Klassifikations System** (SKS), Danish Nursing Intervention Classification.

Most research in the area of SNLs has been conducted on NANDA-I diagnoses, followed by "NNN", which is the combined use of NANDA-I, the Nursing Outcomes and Nursing Interventions Classifications (NOC and NIC, respectively), and their linkages (Tasten et al, 2014; Herdman & Kamitsuru, 2018; Moorhead, Swanson, Johnson, & Maas, 2018; Butcher, Bulechek, Dochterman, & Wagner, 2018).

Many of the NANDA-I terms are contained within SNOMED CT (Systematized Nomenclature of Medicine-Clinical Terms), an international clinical reference terminology. At the time of this writing, NANDA-I is collaborating with members of SNOMED to consider the possibilities of developing a reference set within SNOMED CT so that its users could access NANDA-I terms within their EHRs.

6.4 International Implementation

There are many ways that colleges and universities, healthcare organizations, professional associations, and even government entities have worked together to educate and implement nursing diagnosis terminology. Widespread implementation of nursing diagnosis terminology has been advanced in some countries by mandates for use. Several countries in Latin America (e.g., Peru, Mexico, Brazil) have included the use of nursing process and nursing diagnosis in professional nursing regulations or governmental laws. The following exemplars, in alphabetical order of country, provide a global perspective on the status of implementation in some parts of the world of the NANDA-I terminology.

6.4.1 Brazil

The Federal Nursing Council (COFEN) has regulated nursing since 1986, and requires that nursing care be performed according to the nursing process elements in every healthcare institution, and states that nurses have the right to do so (Brasil, 1986, 1987; COFEN, 2002, 2009, 2017). Prior to these regulations, nurses in Brazil promoted the scientific advancement of nursing. In the 1960s and 1970s, Dr. Wanda de Aguiar Horta, from the University of São Paulo (EEUSP), promoted scientific methods and the use of nursing diagnosis and the nursing process (Paula, Nara, & Horta, 1967; Horta, Hara, & Paula, 1971; Horta, 1972; Horta, 1977). In the late 1980s, two groups adopted

NANDA diagnoses, the EEUSP (led by Dr. Edna Arcuri) and Federal University of Paraíba (UFPB) (led by Dr. Marga Coler) (Coler, Nóbrega, Garcia, & Coler-Thayer, 2009; Cruz, 1991).

Knowledge of the NANDA taxonomy and terminology was further disseminated through publications and conferences. In 1990, publication of the manual, *Nursing diagnosis: a conceptual and practical approach,* contained a translation of the revised NANDA-I Taxonomy 1 (Farias, Nóbrega, Perez, & Coler, 1990). The first National Symposium on Nursing Diagnoses was promoted in 1991 by Dante Pazzanese Cardiology Institute (IDPC) and the current Paulista Nursing School (EPE-Unifesp); the first International Symposium on Nursing Diagnoses followed, in 1995, promoted by EEUSP. The first official translation of the NANDA classification was completed in 1999. In 2002, EPE-Unifesp held the 6th National Symposium on Nursing Diagnoses occurred along with the first International Symposium on Nursing Classifications. The events helped nurses to understand the linkages between NANDA, NOC and NIC.

The nursing process is taught across all nursing programs. This stems in part from the National Curricular Guidelines of Undergraduate Nursing Courses, established in 2001, which affirmed that nurses can diagnose (Conselho Nacional de Educação, 2001). The Commission on the Organization of Nursing Practice (COMSISTE ABEn Nacional), established in 2006 by the Brazilian Nursing Association (ABEn), educates nurses on the nursing process, and promotes effective implementation of the nursing process and SNL in practice (ABEn, 2017a; ABEn 2017b). Graduate programs have contributed widely to the use of nursing diagnosis in Brazil, and during the period of 2006–2016, 85% of 216 accessible theses and dissertations focused on nursing diagnoses and NANDA-I nursing diagnoses (Hirano, Lopes, & Barros, 2019). Other educational initiatives include the distance learning Update Program on Nursing Diagnoses (PRONANDA) produced in Brazil since 2013 (NANDA International, Herdman, & Carvalho, 2013). Implementation of SNL in EHRs has contributed to the expanded use of NNN. Since 2013, nearly 400 licensed sales have been made by Grupo A to a total of 32 health care settings.

Despite this favorable scenario, implementation and use of the nursing process and SNL remain inconsistent in the country. For example, in 416 sectors with 40 institutions in São Paulo State, 78.8% documented assessment, 78.8% documented diagnoses, but only 56.0% documented assessment, diagnosis, interventions and outcomes, whereas 5.8% documented no phase of the nursing process or nursing notes (Azevedo, Guedes, Araújo, Maia, & Cruz,

2019). In 2020, the Nursing Process Research Network (REPPE) was created by researchers from several regions in the country, aimed at generating, synthesizing, and sharing knowledge on the nursing process and SNL (REPPE, n.d.). The continuous promotion of events by ABEn, COMSISTE's actions and bedside discussions using SNL, such as those promoted by IDPC, Hospital de Clínicas de Porto Alegre (HCPA), and Hospital Universitário da USP, are valuable initiatives for the advancement of the nursing process and SNL implementation in practice in Brazil.

6.4.2 Japan

In the 1990s, nursing diagnosis fascinated many Japanese nurses who sought independent practice based upon professional knowledge. Although there is no regulation mandating nursing diagnosis use, it is used or taught by nearly 60% of hospitals and 50% of nursing schools. Nursing diagnosis is not included in the standard nursing curriculum. Whether nursing diagnosis is taught in undergraduate programs depends on the expertise and perspective of the instructors at each nursing school. Since there are no guidelines for nursing diagnosis education, instructors are often confused about what or how to teach.

In the last 20 years, the introduction of EHR systems has spread throughout the country, and nursing diagnosis is viewed as an essential standardized language. Hospitals that use nursing diagnosis terminology incorporate its training into in-service education. Some hospitals invite outside instructors to provide such training periodically, while others utilize internal and external instructors to enhance staff members' diagnostic skills and knowledge. It is a challenge for many hospitals to develop and retain their own instructors.

Although present in EHRs, nursing leadership has not taken full advantage of nursing diagnosis data for healthcare improvement (e.g., staffing, patient outcomes). Continued efforts are needed in Japan to strengthen the knowledge and confidence of nurses in their diagnostic judgments. Nursing diagnosis is used most effectively in hospitals where nurse administrators value its use in the EHR, and are committed to staff development with a long-term perspective.

6.4.3 Mexico

Since the early 1970's, educational activities focused on the nursing process were promoted by educational and service organizations and institutions, especially the National Association of Nursing Schools, the National Association of Universities and Higher Education Institute, and National Nurses Association. Collaborations resulted in guidance and unified criteria for standardized care plans, and criteria for teaching and application of the nursing process to improve nursing performance (Moran, nd).

In 2007 the creation of the Permanent Nursing Commission (PNC) was reported in the official newspaper of the Federation (government), Diario Oficial de la Federación. The PNC is the nursing advisory body of the Federal Government, with the purpose of establishing policies for the practice and training of nurses. The PNC developed nine recommendations to strengthen the culture of quality in the nursing services of health facilities and standardization of nursing care. The most significant were related to the nursing process (NP) and implementation of the NP in medical units (Recommendation 1); standardization of nursing care through nursing care plans for main health problems using diagnostic labels (Recommendation 2); and proposed development of a catalog of nursing care plans (Recommendation 9) (Hernández, 2011).

The nursing process has been incorporated into nursing curricula. There remains, however, a gap between theory and practice, as well as a minimal implementation in healthcare settings. Professionals apply knowledge mediated by a series of values inherent to the profession, however there is a difference between how the academic area applies the nursing process, and how it is implemented in the clinical area. In hospital practice, there are few nursing professionals who apply NNN as a helpful tool for the development of professional practice. Nurses typically put more emphasis on the development of technical skills than on the methodological knowledge of necessary for planning care. The collection of data, or assessment, is conducted quickly, and often incompletely, which limits decision-making regarding human responses, with greater weight attributed to pathophysiological responses of patients, with the predominant biomedical model prevailing in the hospital setting.

Nursing in Mexico has made progress in terms of the nursing care modalities and the use of standardized language. More research is needed in Mexico to contribute to the development of nursing diagnosis terminology.

6.4.4 Peru

Nursing in Peru has gone through a process of development and transition in both education and clinical practice. Since the adoption of the *Peruvian University Law* in 1983, only universities can offer a professional degree, and the curriculum for nursing schools has been strengthened. The nursing process was incorporated into nursing courses, which includes identification of problems and/or needs of the patient. In this context, three stages were taught: assessing, implementing and evaluating, which allowed the nurse to identify patient needs, to develop individual, caregiver, group, family, or community care plans.

In the 1980s, further development of the nursing process led to use of five stages: assessing, diagnosing, planning, implementing, and evaluating. The role of universities was essential for education and outreach of this process. The NANDA-I diagnosis classification began to spread, and Universidad Peruana Cayetano Heredia, started the first collaborative work between a university and a hospital (State Hospital Arzobispo Loayza). Professors from the university began educating nurses at this hospital on the NANDA-I diagnosis classification. This was replicated at three additional state hospitals.

The support of the College of Nursing Professionals and approval of the *Peruvian Nurse Law* in 2002 further increased the use of nursing diagnosis terminology, as the Law required inclusion of the nursing process in the nursing documentation system. Teaching methodologies have varied among universities, hospitals, and regions. In some settings the NANDA-I classification has been implemented, and in others, this is still in process. Professional Certification by the College of Nursing Professionals began in 2010, and was implemented by the Professional Competencies Assessments, Evaluation Centers, which are accredited by the National System for the Evaluation, Accreditation, and Certification of University Quality. In addition, the use of NANDA-I nursing diagnosis was formalized by the *Professional Competences' regulations* in 2015. This included the use of the NANDA-I classification in the evaluation instruments used in the process, such as the nursing progress notes, which shows the importance of the use of the SNL in the safe care of the patient. Moreover, policy entities, such as the Ministry of Health, approved Nursing Intervention Guides that strengthened the use of the NANDA-I classification in the clinical area of the State Hospitals nationwide, as well as "Nursing Progress Notes", which have been approved and published at the entities' web pages.

Significant integration of NANDA-I diagnoses has occurred at multiple state hospitals. Electronic health records are currently being implemented, based on the National Registry of Electronic Clinical Records implementation plan.

The acquisition of NANDA-I diagnosis knowledge by university professors, and their interest in promoting this knowledge in the education of nurses, is the primary force driving the implementation of NANDA-I diagnosis forward. The NANDA-I Network: Peru continues to strengthen the understanding and implementation of SNLs. This network meets with stakeholders to make nursing visible for the benefit of society and nursing professionals.

6.4.5 Republic of Ireland

The Republic of Ireland serves as an interesting exemplar of how NNN is being integrated into educational and healthcare settings (Murphy, McMullin, Brennan, & Meehan, 2017). Implementation of the Careful Nursing Philosophy and Professional Practice Model (Careful Nursing) has been underway since 2009. Central to nursing practice is the Practice Competence and Excellence dimension, which includes the concept, diagnoses–outcomes–interventions, as well as a care planning structure using NANDA-I. An essential first step in this care planning structure is the identification of the patient's NANDA-I nursing diagnoses. At this time, Careful Nursing is being implemented in ten hospitals and four nursing schools, primarily in the southwest and southern areas of the Republic of Ireland.

NANDA-I is implemented in the Republic of Ireland because nurses in hospital practice want to or are required to use it (initially because of Careful Nursing), but also because hospital Directors of Nursing have found that NANDA-I is usable "at the bedside". Nurses in practice recognize that NANDA-I nursing diagnoses give them the ability to name what they know, and diagnose nursing needs of people for whom they provide care. This encourages nurse educators to prioritize and thread knowledge of NANDA-I through all levels of the undergraduate curriculum. The shared perspectives of practicing nurses and nurse educators is truly helping to narrow the theory-practice gap.

6.4.6 Spain

Implementation of SNL in Spain occurred more than 20 years ago. Nurses began to use SNL in practice, mainly with the incorporation of the EHR and, as a consequence, the Health Ministry created legislation on the necessity to use SNL, specifically NNN, for nursing documentation. There was collaboration between clinical nurses and university nursing faculty to decide how SNL would be included in the electronic systems. From the beginning of electronic system implementation in the Spanish Territory, the efforts have multiplied. The use of NANDA-I nursing diagnoses in nursing practice is not questioned. The Spanish Health Ministry includes NNN languages in updates made to any nursing protocol.

Nursing colleges, and many clinical nurses working in hospitals or primary healthcare, have been part of the change forces regarding SNL. The development of primary healthcare services was a major impetus for SNL to be taught at all levels, through continuing education for nursing professionals and at the colleges of nursing. The creation of the Spanish Association for Nomenclature,

Taxonomy and Nursing Diagnoses (AENTDE) in 1996 was crucial for thousands of Spanish nurses to learn and discuss with colleagues from NANDA-I, and other international associations, the significance of using SNL in general, and nursing diagnoses in particular.

The Spanish Health Ministry has been very involved in the implementation and use of SNL. One of the first projects, together with the *Consejo General de Enfermería* (National Organization of Spanish Nurses) and AENTDE, was the calculation of the cost of nursing care using standardized nursing care plans that included NNN for different clinical processes, both at hospitals and in Primary Health Care (Ministerio de Sanidad y Consumo, n.d.). By 2010, there were more than 100 Spanish hospitals using the same electronic system, called "GACELA", that incorporated NANDA-I nursing diagnoses. Some parts of the Spanish territory were using the system at all levels of clinical care.

Electronic systems have clearly facilitated the implementation of NANDA-I nursing diagnoses. In the EHR, nursing has the most complete SNL and it is also the most complex, including assessments, diagnoses, outcomes, outcome indicators, interventions, activities, etc., and all of these are interrelated. The electronic record is a tool that **must** facilitate the work of professionals who use it and, indeed it does this. The EHR facilitates planning and recording of care, while producing data to foster management.

The future is positive for continued use of SNL in general and NANDA-I nursing diagnosis terminology, specifically. Another important area to consider is the incorporation of the Systemized Nomenclature of Medicine Clinical Terms (SNOMED CT) in the electronic systems of many of the European Countries, which will occur in Spain in the not too distant future. Information technology innovations will continue to improve nursing software and information management, along with the use of innovations such as business intelligence or data warehouses, which allow analysis of huge amounts of data and can enhance areas of nursing, such as management and leadership, research, evidence-based nursing interventions, and practice improvement.

6.4.7 United States

The American Nurses Association (ANA) recommends that nurses document using the nursing process within the patient record, and recognizes 13 SNLs. NANDA-I is the most recognized and researched of the languages on the ANA's list (Tastan, Linch, Keenan, Stifter, McKinney, Fahey, Lopez, Yao & Wilkie, 2014). The unwillingness of the ANA to take a stand in terms of which SNLs should be used in clinical practice has led to a lack of consensus nationally, which has undermined the importance of diagnostic reasoning, and overall clinical reasoning related to the nursing process, within education and practice. Unfortunately, because there are no professional regulations or requirements guiding use of nursing diagnosis, or SNLs related to outcomes or interventions, it remains the decision of each individual nursing school as to the degree to which it includes NANDA-I nursing diagnosis terminology – and that of other SNLs – in the curriculum. This leaves the USA at a distinct disadvantage due to its inability to harvest data from EHRs to better understand nurses' impact on patient care, what the actual cost of nursing care is, and which nursing diagnoses may prolong hospital stays, lead to increased readmissions, or result in preventable sequelae.

It is not known how many healthcare institutions have implemented the use of SNLs for electronic nursing documentation in the United States. In a rare study, usage of EHRs in the state of Minnesota (USA) was examined, with 92% of healthcare systems (e.g., hospitals, clinics, public health) in the state using EHRs. Of these organizations, only 30% used a SNL (Huard & Monsen, 2017). However, it is well known that many organizations do indeed incorporate NANDA-I nursing diagnoses labels into documentation systems, without procuring a license. In many of these cases, nurses are unaware that they are documenting with NANDA-I labels, because they are not properly referenced, and many nurses, especially those with associate degree education, have not learned nursing diagnosis content in their curricula. This problem is certainly not unique to the USA, and is probably a reflection of the continued lack of economic support for nursing as a professional, independent discipline.

The EHR is part of the healthcare landscape in the USA. Incentives in the federal Health Information Technology for Economic and Clinical Health (HITECH) Act of 2009 put adoption of EHRs on the fast track for healthcare organizations. Standards issued by the government (Department of Health and Human Services) require that EHRs contain an up-to-date problem list of current diagnoses that users can electronically enter and modify. However, there are no standards for languages that must be used in problems lists, and thus problem lists vary widely among healthcare institutions, and often the problem lists include only medical diagnoses. Again, this lack of consistency significantly limits the availability of well defined, high quality big data sets for nursing research.

The apparent lack of use of SNLs creates a gap between what knowledge nursing schools use to prepare nurses for practice, and what nurses actually see and use in healthcare settings. That said, many undergraduate schools of nursing do teach NANDA-I nursing diagnosis in the curriculum, but it is often taught in an early course and not well integrated into advanced content as students move through their programs. Furthermore, it is often incorrectly linked to medical diagnosis, with little to no education provided on diagnostic reasoning, or how assessment should drive nursing diagnosis. Nursing faculty members often received little or confusing education themselves on diagnosing, and therefore are often unsure about how to teach nursing diagnosis. One very positive aspect is the new relationship between Boston College and NANDA-I, which cofounded the Marjory Gordon Program for Knowledge Development and Clinical Reasoning. This partnership will advance development of educational materials, tools, and learning strategies to support nursing educators as they teach diagnostic reasoning and nursing diagnosis terminology, as well as foster the development of nursing knowledge.

6.5 Summary

It takes a global community to inform, teach, and implement NANDA-I nursing diagnosis terminology. Indeed, it is a global phenomenon! The NANDA-I taxonomy provides a way to classify areas of concern (diagnostic foci) to nurses and the patients for whom we provide care. The NANDA-I nursing diagnoses describe human responses to health problem/life processes and inform the identification of outcomes and interventions. What is clear is that NANDA-I nursing diagnoses support the clinical reasoning process and provide a discipline-specific language to describe the unique knowledge of the nursing discipline.

Innovative practices for implementation of nursing diagnosis are occurring in many places across the globe (e.g., Estonia, Slovenia, Italy, Spain, Brazil) – too many to name! There are many professionals dedicated to these efforts, including clinical nurses, nurse educators, administrators, informaticists, and researchers.

The NANDA-I nursing terminology is the only SNL that is continually updated with current evidence, and assigned level of evidence criteria, to best reflect the full scope of nursing practice. Nursing diagnoses are submitted for acceptance (new diagnoses) or revision (existing diagnoses) to NANDA-I by practicing nurses, nurse educators, graduate students, and nurse researchers. It is clear that NANDA-I has a global reach to support the millions of nurses making clinical judgments (nursing diagnoses) related to patient health problems, risks, and strengths, and to drive relevant interventions and outcomes.

6.6 Acknowledgment of Contributors to This Chapter

Thank you to the following experts who provided content about nursing diagnosis in their area of the world.

Brazil

- Camila Takáo Lopes, PhD, RN, FNI, Director of the Diagnosis Development Committee of NANDA International, and Adjunct Professor at *Escola Paulista de Enfermagem, Universidade Federal de São Paulo* (EPE-Unifesp)
- Alba Lucia Bottura Leite de Barros, PhD, RN, FNI, Full Professor at EPE-Unifesp, Coordinator of the Research Network on the Nursing Process (REPPE) and Researcher of the National Council for Scientific and Technological Development (CNPq)
- Diná de Almeida Lopes Monteiro da Cruz, BSN, PhD, FNI, Full Senior Professor at Escola de Enfermagem da Universidade de São Paulo (EEUSP), CNPq Researcher
- Emilia Campos de Carvalho, PhD, RN, FNI, Director at Large of NANDA International (2012–2016), Full Senior Professor at *Escola de Enfermagem de Ribeirão Preto, Universidade de São Paulo* (EERP-USP), CNPq Researcher (1987–2019)
- Marcos Venícios de Oliveira Lopes, PhD, RN, FNI, member of the Education and Research Committee of NANDA International since 2014, Associate Professor at *Faculdade de Farmácia, Odontologia e Enfermagem, Universidade Federal do Ceará* (UFC), member of the Nursing Assessor Committee of CNPq
- Miriam de Abreu Almeida, PhD, RN, FNI, member of the Diagnosis Development Committee of NANDA International (2010–2018), Full Professor at *Escola de Enfermagem, Universidade Federal do Rio Grande do Sul* (UFRGS), CNPq Researcher
- Viviane Martins da Silva, PhD, RN, FNI, member of the Education and Research Committee of NANDA International since 2018, Associate Professor at *Faculdade de Farmácia, Odontologia e Enfermagem, Universidade Federal do Ceará* (UFC), CNPq Researcher.

Japan

- Shigemi Kamitsuru, PhD, RN, FNI, Nurse Consultant, President of NANDA International

Mexico

- Prof. Dr. Hortensia Castañeda-Hidalgo

- Prof. Ángeles Fang Huerta
- Prof. Dr. Florabel Flores Barrios
- Prof. Dr. Rosalinda Garza Hernández
- Prof. Dr. Nora Hilda González Quirarte
- Prof. Dr. Dolores Eunice Hernández
- Prof. Dr. Concepción Meléndez Méndez

Peru
- Dr. Ruth Aliaga Sánchez
- Dr. Roxana Obando Zegarra
- Mg. Rossana Gonzáles de la Cruz
- Lic. Elver Luyo Valera

Republic of Ireland
- Therese Meehan, PhD, RGN, Adjunct Associate Professor of Nursing, University College Dublin
- Mary Kemple, MSc., RGN, Assistant Professor of Nursing, University College Dublin
- Catherine (Kay) O'Mahony, MBA, RGN, Assistant Director of Nursing, South/South West Hospital Group

Spain
- Carme Espinosa i Fresnedo, MSN, FNI, President Elect NANDA International
- Rosa González Gutiérrez-Solano, European Master in Quality, FNI, Former President of AENTDE (Spanish Association of Nomenclature, Taxonomy and Nursing Diagnoses)
- Rosa Rifà Ros, PhD, Professor of Fundamental Concepts in Nursing. Ramon Llull University, Barcelona

6.7 References

Associação Brasileira de Enfermagem. Regimento Interno. 2017a. Available from: http://www.abennacional.org.br/site/wp-content/uploads/2019/01/regimento_COMSISTE.pdf.

Associação Brasileira de Enfermagem. Comissão Permanente de Sistematização da Prática de Enfermagem Relatório 2017. 2017b. Available from: http://www.abennacional.org.br/site/wp-content/uploads/2019/01/relatorio_COMSISTE_ABEn-Nacional2017-1.pdf.

Azevedo OA, Guedes ES, Araújo SAN, Maia MM, Cruz DALM. Documentation of the nursing process in public health institutions. Revista da Escola de Enfermagem da USP. 2019; 53: e03471. https://doi.org/10.1590/s1980-220x2018003703471.

Brasil. Presidência da República. 1986. Lei n. 7498, de 25 de Junho de 1986. http://www.cofen.gov.br/lei-n-749886-de-25-de-junho-de-1986_4161.html.

Brasil. Presidência da República. 1987. Decreto n. 94.406/87 de 08 de Junho de 1987. http://www.cofen.gov.br/decreto-n-9440687_4173.html.

Butcher HK, Bulechek GM, Dochterman JM, Wagner CM (eds.). Nursing Interventions Classification (NIC). 7th ed. St. Louis, MO: Elsevier, 2018.

Coler MS, Nóbrega MML, Garcia TR, Coler-Thayer M. Linking the nature of the person with the nature of nursing through nursing theory and practice and nursing language in Brazil. In: Roy C, Jones DAA. Nursing Knowledge Development and Clinical Practice. New York: Springer, 2007, p.79–91.

Conselho Federal de Enfermagem [COFEN]. 2002. Resolução COFEN-272/2002. http://www.cofen.gov.br/resoluo-cofen-2722002-revogada-pela-resoluao-cofen-n-3582009_4309.html.

Conselho Federal de Enfermagem [COFEN]. 2009. Resolução COFEN-358/2009. http://www.cofen.gov.br/resoluo-cofen-3582009_4384.html.

Conselho Federal de Enfermagem [COFEN]. 2017. Resolução COFEN-564/2017. http://www.cofen.gov.br/resolucao-cofen-no-5642017_59145.html.

Conselho Nacional de Educação. 2001. Resolução CNE/CES Nº 3, de 7 de Novembro de 2001. Institui Diretrizes Curriculares Nacionais do Curso de Graduação em Enfermagem. Available from: http://portal.mec.gov.br/cne/arquivos/pdf/CES03.pdf

Cruz DALM. Classificações em enfermagem: tensões e contribuições. Revista Saúde 1991; 1(1): 20–31. http://revistas.ung.br/index.php/saude/article/view/65/104.

Farias JN, Nóbrega MML, Perez VLAB, Coler MS. Diagnóstico de enfermagem: uma abordagem conceitual e prática. João Pessoa: Ccs/UFPB, 1990.

Freire VECS, Lopez MVO, Keenan GM, Lopez KD. Nursing students' diagnostic accuracy using computer-based clinical scenario simulation. Nurse Education Today 2018; 71: 240–246. https://pubmed.ncbi.nlm.nih.gov/30340106/.

Herdman TH, Kamitsuru S (eds). NANDA International nursing diagnoses: Definitions and Classification, 2018–2020. New York: Thieme, 2018.

Hernández E. 2011. Proceso enfermero en México y generalidades del proyecto places. Available in: http://www.enlinea.cij.gob.mx/Cursos/Hospitalizacion/pdf/proceso.PDF.

Hirano GSB, Lopes CT, Barros ALBL. Development of research on nursing diagnoses in Brazilian graduate programs. Revista Brasileira de Enfermagem 2019; 72(4): 926–932. https://doi.org/10.1590/0034-7167-2018-0259.

Horta WA. Diagnósticos de enfermagem: estudo básico da determinação da dependência de enfermagem. Revista Brasileira de Enfermagem 1972; 25(4): 267–273. https://www.scielo.br/pdf/reben/v25n4/0034-7176-reben-25-04-0267.pdf.

Horta WA. Diagnóstico de enfermagem-representação gráfica. Revista enfermagem em novas dimensões 1977; 3(2): 75–77.

Horta WA, Hara Y, Paula NS. O ensino dos instrumentos básicos de enfermagem. Revista Brasileira de Enfermagem 1971; 24(3): 159–169.

Huard RJC, Monsen KA. Standardized Nursing Terminology Use in Electronic Health Records in Minnesota. Modern Clinical Medicine Research 2017; 1(1). https://dx.

doi.org/10.22606/mcmr.2017.11003. Retrieved from http://www.isaacpub.org/images/PaperPDF/MCMR_100004_2017052511033162338.pdf.

Johnson L, Edwards KL, Giandinoto J. (2017). A systematic literature review of accuracy in nursing care plans and using standardised nursing language. 2017. Retrieved from https://doi.org/10.1016/j.colegn.2017.09.006.

Larijani TT, Saatchi B. Training of NANDA-I nursing diagnoses (NDs), Nursing Interventions Classification (NIC) and Nursing Outcome Classification (NOC), in Psychiatric Wards: A randomized controlled trial. Nurs Open 2019; 6(2): 612–619. DOI: 10.1002/nop2.244

Ministerio de Sanidad y Consumo, Consejo General de Enfermería. NIPE Project; Normalización de las Intervenciones para la Práctica de la Enfermería. 2002. Retrieved from https://www.mscbs.gob.es/estadEstudios/estadisticas/normalizacion/proyec-NIPE.htm.

Moorhead S, Swanson E, Johnson M, Maas ML (eds.). Nursing Outcomes Classification (NOC): Measurement of health outcomes. 6th ed. St. Louis, MO: Elsevier, 2018.

Moran Aguilar Victoria (n.d.). El proceso de atención de enfermería Asociación Nacional de Escuelas de Enfermería, A. C. Undated. Available from: http://publicaciones.anuies.mx/pdfs/revista/Revista19_S2A1ES.pdf.

Murphy S, McMullin R, Brennan S, Meehan TC. Exploring implementation of the Careful Nursing Philosophy and Professional Practice Model in hospital-based practice. J Nurs Manag 2018; 26:263–273. https://doi.org/10.1111/jonm.12542.

NANDA International, Inc.; Herdman TH, Carvalho EC, organizadoras. PRONANDA Programa de Atualização em Diagnósticos de Enfermagem: Ciclo 1. (Sistema de Educação Continuada a Distância, v. 1). Porto Alegre: Artmed Panamericana, 2013, p.11–145.

North American Nursing Diagnoses Association. Diagnósticos de Enfermagem da NANDA: Definições e Classificação 1999–2000. Porto Alegre: Editora Artes Médicas Sul, 2000.

Paula NS, Nara Y, Horta WA. Ensino do plano de cuidados em fundamentos de enfermagem. Revista Brasileira de Enfermagem 1967; 20(4): 249–263. http://www.teses.usp.br/teses/disponiveis/5/5131/tde-09032010-181608/en.php.

Rede de Pesquisa em Processo de Enfermagem [REPPE]. Undated. Available from: https://repperede.org/.

Tastan S, Linch GCF, Keenan GM, Stifter J, McKinney D, Fahey L, Lopez KD, Yao Y, Wilkie DJ. Evidence for the existing American Nurses Association-recognized standardized nursing terminologies: A systematic review. International Journal of Nursing Studies 2014; 51: 1160–1170. https://doi.org/10.1590/S0080-62342010000200008.

World Health Organization [WHO]. World Health Statistics 2013. 2013. Retrieved from https://www.who.int/gho/publications/world_health_statistics/2013/en/.

7 Clinical Reasoning: From Assessment to Diagnosis

Dorothy A. Jones, T. Heather Herdman, Rita de Cássia Gengo e Silva Butcher

7.1 Clinical Reasoning: Introduction

Clinical reasoning has been defined in a variety of ways within health care disciplines. Koharchik et al (2015) indicate that it requires the application of ideas and experience to arrive at a valid conclusion; in nursing, it is used to describe the way a nurse "analyzes and understands a patient's situation and forms conclusions" (p. 58). Tanner (2006) sees it as the process by which nurses make clinical judgments by selecting from alternatives, weighing evidence, using intuition and pattern recognition. Similarly, Banning (2008) defined clinical reasoning as the application of knowledge and experience to a clinical situation, in a concept analysis of clinical reasoning, dating from 1964 to 2005. The study identified the need for tools to measure clinical reasoning in nursing practice.

It is important to note that clinical reasoning is a process, informed and reformed by new data or evidence. It is not a step-by-step, linear process, but rather an evolving one. It occurs over time, often across multiple patient/family encounters. The process is also an iterative one. The more information we obtain, the more information we are able to synthesize, uncovering the problem(s) and discovering pattern formation. For the more novice nurses early in their careers, this process may take time. Nurses with more experience may move through the process more quickly, having developed knowledge from seeing many patients over time. Nevertheless, each patient situation is unique and requires nurses to fully engage in all of the components of the reasoning process to uncover pattern formation or problem identification.

7.2 Clinical Reasoning within the Nursing Process

Many authors focus on the nursing process, without taking the time to ensure that we understand the concepts of nursing science; yet, the nursing process begins with - and requires - an understanding of these underlying concepts of nursing and the human experience. If we do not understand our disciplinary concepts (or ideas defined by our knowledge), we will struggle to identify how pattern formation of the whole is experienced by our patients, families, and communities.

A concept is as an image or an abstract idea. Central concepts of the discipline of nursing include environment, health, nursing, and person (Walker & Avant, 2019). Other concepts emerge as we describe phenomena of concern to nursing, such as well-being, stress, or activity. It is critical that we know (and teach) these concepts so that nurses can recognize normal human responses and patterns inconsistent with usual responses, identify risks or threats to health, and promote health and wellness. Engaging in the nursing process (assessing, diagnosing, planning, intervening, and evaluating) is meaningless if we do not understand underlying nursing concepts and if we cannot identify them from the individual patterns manifested within the data we collect during assessment.

Without a solid grounding in concepts, the knowledge or phenomena of concern to nursing, it is difficult to articulate hypotheses or statements of probability about patients and their experiences. Without this knowledge, we lack the ability to engage in a more in-depth assessment and obtain new data that will confirm or eliminate a tentative problem or diagnosis. Although conceptual knowledge has not generally been included within the nursing process, knowing this information enhances our ability to understand the human experience to its fullest.

Example. What do we mean by pattern formation or data synthesis? We are talking about how our minds pull together information from a variety of data points to form a picture of what we are seeing, and then recognize a name. Let us first look at a nonclinical scenario.

Assume you are out for a walk, and you go past a group of men seated at a picnic bench at a park. You notice that they are doing something with little rectangular objects, and they are speaking in very loud voices – some are even shouting – as they slam these objects on the table between them. The men seem very intense, and it appears they are arguing about these objects, but you cannot understand what these objects are or what exactly the men are doing with them. As you slow down to watch them, you notice a small crowd has gathered. Some of these individuals occasionally nod their heads or comment in what seems to be an encouraging manner, some seem concerned, and others appear to be as confused by what they are watching as you are.

Linking concepts and data. What is happening here? What is it that you are observing? It may be hard for you to articulate what you are seeing if it is something with which you have no experience. When we do not understand a concept, it is hard to move forward with our thinking process. Suppose that we told you that what you were observing was men playing Mahjong, a type of tile-based board game. The tiles are used like cards, only they are small, rectangular objects traditionally made of bone or bamboo. Although you may not know anything about Mahjong, you can understand the concept "game". With this understanding, you might begin to look at the scene unfolding before you in a different way. You might begin to see the four men as competitors, each hoping to win the game, which might explain their intensity. You might begin to consider their raised voices as a form of good-natured taunting of one another, rather than angry shouting. Once you understand the concept of "game", you can begin to paint a picture in your mind as to what is happening in this scene, and you can begin to interpret the data you are collecting (cues) in a way that makes sense within the context of a game. Without the "game" concept, though, you might continue the struggle to make sense of your observations.

Now let us look at the idea of nursing concepts (knowledge) using a clinical scenario. Lisa is on her first clinical placement as a nursing student, under the supervision of Prof. Leonard, a faculty member in an elderly independent/ assisted living facility. On one of her placement days, Lisa is assessing Mr. Smith, while assisted by her professor. Mr. Smith is 75 years old and has lived in the facility for 12 months. He tells Lisa that he feels that he is lacking energy all the time, he cannot concentrate, and most days he has not even brushed his teeth. He is very concerned that there is something wrong with his heart. Lisa begins by taking his vital signs, but as she is doing this, she asks Mr. Smith to tell her what has been happening in his life since he began living at the facility. He indicates that he had to move in after his wife died from a heart attack, because he could not take care of the house chores and run errands all by himself, and his only daughter lived abroad with her husband and 4 children. He denies any chest pain, heart palpitations, or shortness of breath. When Prof. Leonard asks him why he's worried about his heart, he says "well, this thought keeps repeating in my mind every day, that my wife wouldn't have died if I had insisted that she went to see a cardiologist earlier".

Lisa asks him how often his daughter gets to visit him. Mr. Smith indicates that she had to leave immediately after his wife's funeral, because she and her husband had a lot of work activities, and they had not been able to visit him since then, but they usually spoke on the phone once a week. He notes that he doesn't really have an interest in the living facility activities, and it was hard to leave his neighborhood because there was a couple who lived across the street and they were very good friends. They met at least three times a week for dinner, or they watched TV or played board games, and they even traveled together a couple of times. Now they only talk by phone. Although he is glad he gets to talk with them, he says it isn't the same as enjoying dinner with his wife and them. He points out that his wife was the strong link to the relationship with the neighbors, because she was always proposing and planning different activities. He even has a voice message from her on his phone that he listens to every day, proposing that they all should go to a party together that weekend.

Lisa tells Mr. Smith that his vital signs are very good. Prof. Leonard suggests to Lisa that he may be suffering from a change in his grieving process, and suggests that they try a few adjustments to see if that can impact Mr. Smith's feelings of restfulness and being at peace with himself. First, he recommends that they speak with Mr. Smith, and then with the environmental services director to get him enrolled in a bereavement support group, and begin counseling with mental health staff at the nursing home, so that he can express his grieving process. He also tells her that Mr. Smith should be assessed for the development of clinical depression. Finally, he suggests talking with Mr. Smith about reconnecting with his neighborhood friends, in person, and to the director of resident life to find out how he might be able to visit his friends, or have them come to the facility to see his new apartment to slowly get Mr. Smith involved in his new community.

Lisa is amazed that Prof. Leonard almost immediately identified a potential problem with Mr. Smith. Prof. Leonard draws Lisa's attention to the nursing diagnosis, *maladaptive grieving (00301),* and she realizes that his assessment data are defining characteristics and related factors of this diagnosis. Lisa's professor talks with her about the grieving process, and the things that can impact it, such as inadequate social support (Mr. Smith's recent move; lack of connection with his daughter and friends). He quickly considered this nursing diagnosis because he understood the normal grieving process, and identified factors that contribute to a disturbance in this normal pattern. Further, he identified probable etiological (related) factors. Lisa, as a nursing student, did not yet have the conceptual knowledge from which to draw; for her, this diagnosis did not seem obvious.

This is the reason why studying concepts underlying diagnoses is so important. We cannot understand an individual's usual human response patterns without drawing on conceptual knowledge throughout the nursing process.

7.3 The Nursing Process

Without a complete nursing assessment, there can be no patient-centered nursing diagnosis, nor can we identify evidence-based, patient-centered, independent nursing interventions. Assessment should not be conducted to fill in the blank spaces on a form or computer screen. If this form of rote assessment rings a bell for you, it is time to take a new look at the purpose of assessment!

Assessing. Nurses engage in assessment to come to know the person and his experiences, accurately identify patient concerns, and implement nursing interventions with the purpose of achieving optimal patient care outcomes. As a discipline, nursing has developed knowledge that comprises nursing science. Nursing diagnosis, which is a clinical judgment, is the outcome of a nursing assessment that describes health conditions/life processes, or a susceptibility for that response. That diagnosis then provides the basis for selection of nursing interventions to achieve outcomes *for which the nurse has accountability*: the focus here is "human response".

Assessment of *human responses* within a nursing assessment framework is a way to identify nurse-focused phenomena of concern and address problems within the scope of professional nursing practice. Human beings are complex and dynamic, and will respond uniquely to the same situation. Human responses are influenced by many factors, including genetics, physiology, health conditions, and experiences with illness/injury. These responses are also influenced by the patient's age, culture, ethnicity, religion/spiritual beliefs, economics, gender, and family experiences.

A comprehensive nursing assessment framework provides for a person's unique response to illness, health, or wellness to be shared with others. Nursing diagnoses provide standardized terms to describe human responses, with clear definitions and assessment criteria that represent nursing knowledge.

Nurses view assessing as an opportunity to engage with a patient, in a process where data is shared, transformed into information, and organized into meaningful categories of nursing content, also known as nursing diagnoses. Assessing provides an important opportunity for nurses' knowledge and contributions to patient care to be realized.

Nurse-patient relationship. The relationship between the nurse and patient is core to optimal nursing practice (Roy & Jones, 2007, Watson, Smith, 2019). Within this relationship, the nurse comes to know the individual as a whole person and to view illness as part of health (MacLeod, 2011; Smith, 2011, Jones, 2013). Dossey and Keegan (2013, p. 17) describe the relationship between the nurse/patient/family/community as one of "self-awareness, patient experiences of health and illness, and developing and maintaining a caring relationship and effective communication".

Nursing knowledge, expertise, skills, and values contribute to establishing trust and connecting with a person in a meaningful way. Within the practice setting, the environment of care enables the nurse to come to know the person through relationship. Being with patients and families requires presence, awareness, careful listening, and observing. These responses help to actualize the professional role of the nurse in delivery of cost effective, high quality, safe, knowledge-driven patient care (Jones, 2013).

The engagement of the nurse and patient is a mutual care experience (Newman, 2008). It moves nursing beyond *doing* (focusing on tasks that help to manage care) to *understanding* the patient experience holistically, *identifying* mutual areas of concern, and *providing* information to assist the person to engage in changes and take actions that can be transforming (Newman, 2008; Jones, 2013).

Intentional authentic presence. Intentional presence requires a "genuine dialogue, commitment, full engagement and openness, free flowing attentiveness and transcendent oneness" (Smith, 2011). When nurses are present with a person, they are engaged in the moment and consciously aware of their environment.

The authentic presence of the nurse in a patient caring experience promotes engagement and enhances relationship (Newman, 2008; Newman, Smith, Pharris and Jones, 2008). The experience can be transformational for both the nurse and the patient. Presence is a matter of consciousness and is reflected in the holistic beings that are both nurse and patient (Chase, 2011).

Intentional presence allows the nurse to experience verbal and non-verbal expressions and responses to a situation, in the moment. Exploring patient experiences helps to uncover what is meaningful to the individual, fosters reflection, increases awareness about choices, actions and behaviors that enhance health, and provides insights that can lead to discovery, change, and personal transformation (Jones, 2013, 2006; Newman, 2008; Jones & Flanagan, 2007; Doona, Chase & Haggerty, 1999).

When the nurse is able to create a safe space, the patient may feel free to disclose his concerns and freely express his fears (Jones, 2013). As the nurse and patient engage in the process of assessing, the patient may experience new awareness and insights (Newman, 2008) and recognize new opportunities for making personal changes in his life, and engage in health promotion actions.

According to Willis et al., "meaning is a human's arrived-at understanding of life experiences and their significance that comes from processing those experiences" (2008, p. E34).

Knowing the person. "Knowing the patient encompasses the complex processes whereby the nurse acquires understanding of a specific patient as a unique individual, which enhances clinical decision-making" (Whittemore, 2000, p. 75). Benner (1984) initially describes nurses' skill in being mindful of the person and his environment, and experiencing an "intuitive" response to assess a situation. Often this is associated with a nurse's clinical expertise. The nurse may describe an experience as, "I don't know what it is, but I just know something is wrong". Some call this *intuitive knowing*, when the nurse is able to recognize a complex set of clues that draws attention to a potential problem or situation, without necessarily being able to name the response.

As nurses gain experience and observe responses in populations over time, they expand their knowledge and process information (cues) more rapidly, as they recognize responses as being usual or problematic. As nurses care for a patient over time, they can become increasingly sensitive to changes in the patient's response pattern. As the nurse engages in assessing, there is an accumulative knowledge about the patient's pattern of responses and she is able to quickly make judgments (Gordon, 1994). It is essential that nurses engage in obtaining adequate assessment data to validate clinical judgments, or nursing diagnoses, in all situations.

Nursing assessment and the nurse-patient relationship promote patient satisfaction and enhance nursing visibility in practice. Watson & Smith (2004) discussed the importance of a caring relationship, describing it as the hallmark of the discipline. In a study conducted by Somerville (2009), patients described a feeling of being known by their nurse when they were "recognized as a unique human being, felt safe within the care environment, experienced a connection with the nurse they perceived as meaningful, and felt empowered by the nurse to actively participate in their care" (p.3). Data from this initial qualitative study informed the development of the *Patients' Perceptions of Feeling Known by Their Nurse Scale* (PPFKNS, Somerville, 2009). The PPFKNS is a valid and reliable, four component scale that can be used to evaluate patients perceptions of "being known" by the nurse.

Nursing Assessment: a holistic process. "There are multiple approaches that can be used by nurses to understand the person's response to illness and the behaviors they engage in to promote a healthy lifestyle" (Jones, 2013, p. 95). Nursing theories (Newman, 2008; Roy, 2007) offer unique approaches to understanding the human experience, and can be used alone or integrated into an assessment framework, such as the Functional Health Pattern (FHP) Assessment (Gordon, 1994). Each theory offers a framework within which data representing the patient's experiences are studied. Organizing patient responses within the FHP framework may be a way to complement knowledge generated by the theory with knowledge gained from nursing practice. The knowledge gained may help to expand nursing science.

Approaches to assessing and data collection. Process/dialogue and problem solving are two approaches that can help the nurse come to know the patient's experience. These approaches offer different ways of accessing and analyzing data, and the interventions and outcomes vary in structure and description. They are both designed to understand how life experiences affect living and impact health and well being.

Assessing as a dialogue process. Assessing, as a process, occurs within the context of a dialogue or discussion. This approach to assessing is inductive and focuses on "the nature of a relationship that is transformative for both nurse and patient" (Newman et al., 2008). Data collection is less systematic, and content evolves through purposeful discussions within the nurse-patient relationship. The nurse may begin the conversation with an open-ended question, such as: "Can you tell me what your day was like for you?"

As the nurse is present in the moment and carefully listening, the patient's story unfolds. When needed, the nurse may ask questions to seek additional information to uncover new information or seek clarification. Events and people who are part of the individual's experiences help give meaning to life events and responses. The dialogue involves a mutual interaction between the nurse and the patient. Meaningful data discussed within the dialogue helps to inform an unfolding pattern of the whole (Flanagan, 2009; Newman, 2008). Margaret Newman's theoretical framework within Health as Expanding Consciousness (HEC) is an example of a process assessment. The goal of the process/dialogue approach is to "grasp meaning" and come to know the pattern of the whole. Reflection and discussion promotes increasing awareness, reflection, and opportunities for change (Newman, 2008).

Assessing as problem solving. Problem solving is a deductive reasoning process that involves a systematic approach to data collection. Though some might consider the process linear, others argue that as new data becomes available, clinical judgments are revised and diagnoses are re-evaluated (Gordon, 1994). The problem-solving assessment perspective views humans as holistic, bio-psychosocial beings interacting (functioning) within the environment and shaped by age, developmental stage, health status and culture and ethnicity (Jones, 2007).

The problem solving approach to assessing incorporates both subjective and objective data to inform the assessment and subsequent problem identification. The naming of the problem (nursing diagnosis) and identification of the probable cause (related factors) direct interventions designed to eliminate or relieve the originating problem and reduce risk. The Functional Health Pattern Assessment is an example of a problem-solving approach to assessment.

Subjective and objective data. Nurses collect and document two types of data related to the patient experience: subjective and objective data. While physicians value objective over subjective data for medical diagnoses, nurses value both types of data for nursing diagnoses (Gordon, 2008). Nurses collect these subjective data through the assessment process or interview.

Subjective data is information obtained from patients' verbal reports about their perceptions, thoughts, and experiences related to their health, daily life, comfort, relationship, and so on. For instance, a patient may report, "I need to manage my health better", or "My partner never talks about anything important with me".

Family members/close friends can also provide this type of data, although patient data should be obtained from the person (family, community) whenever possible, because it is the patient's data. Sometimes, however, the patient is unable to provide subjective data, so we must rely on these other sources. For example, a patient with significant dementia who is no longer verbally competent may require family members to provide subjective information, based on their knowledge of the individual's behavior. An example might be an adult child of the patient telling the nurse, "She always likes to listen to soft music when she eats, it seems to calm her".

Objective data is information that nurses observe about the patient. These data are sometimes referred to as empirical or measurable evidence. Objective data is obtained through physical examinations and diagnostic test results. Here, "to observe" does not only mean the use of eyesight: it requires the use of all senses and forms of measurement. For example, nurses look at the patient's general appearance, listen to his lung sounds, they may smell foul wound drainage, and feel the skin temperature using touch. Additionally, nurses use various instruments and tools with the patient to collect numerical data (e.g., body weight, blood pressure, oxygen saturation, pain level). To collect reliable and accurate objective data, nurses must have appropriate knowledge and skills to perform physical assessment and to use standardized tools or monitoring devices.

Problem solving and nursing assessment. To date, nursing lacks a standardized approach to assessment. There are multiple assessment forms created by nurses to collect data but, unlike the review of systems in medicine, nurses use a variety of strategies to obtain patient information. In some settings nurses use a head to toe approach, others use an assessment checklist, while some nurses develop focused assessment forms (e.g., assessment for pain or fall risk).

These tools provide data, but often the information is incomplete and focuses on the illness experience by discussing the patient's chief complaint or presenting health concern(s). These approaches also lack a holistic approach to understanding the patient responses to health and illness within the nurse patient relationship. Within a problem-solving approach to assessment, Gordon's eleven Functional Health Patterns (Gordon, 1994) offer a nurse-driven, organized approach to understanding the person's response to illness and health promotion.

Functional Health Pattern Assessment Framework. Gordon (1994) notes that a structured assessment helps the nurse to focus, organize, and synthesize subjective and objective clinical data. The Functional Health Pattern (FHP) assessment provides nurses with a standardized, holistic approach to care that is useful for the collection of subjective and objective data across clinical settings, cultures, populations, ages, and health conditions. Data is collected within a nursing framework and used by the nurse within the nurse-patient care experience to develop patient problems (tentative hypotheses), test and validate clinical judgments/nursing diagnoses. The goal of assessment is to determine an individual's perception of optimal functional health, as determined by assessing the eleven FHPs (Gordon, 2008, 1994).

The FHP assessment describes client strengths and functions, lifestyle management, and overall health status for each pattern. ▶ Table 7.1 shows the FHP and some potential questions that could be explored at each pattern. Phenomena of concern identified by the nurse help to guide care and increase the visibility of nursing's contribution to patient outcomes.

During the assessment, data obtained within each pattern create a story that incorporates information about the patient's health, including her response to acute and chronic illnesses. When nurses engage the individual in a

Table 7.1 Functional Health Patterns (FHP) and sample questions

Pattern	Sample Questions
Health Perception / Health Management Pattern	– In general how would you rate your health and why? – What is the meaning of health to your life? – Are you satisfied with your current health? – What do you do regularly to maintain your health?
Nutritional – Metabolic Pattern	– Describe your usual eating pattern and food and fluid intake daily? – Do you eat 3 meals each day? – Do you have access to adequate food? – Do you snack during the day? – Do you eat when you are under stress? discuss
Elimination Pattern	– How often do you urinate during a 24-hour period? – Do you usually wake up during the night to urinate? Describe your normal (usual) bowel pattern. – Do you take laxatives regularly?
Activity – Exercise Pattern	– Describe your usual daily activities. – Do you exercise regularly each week? Describe. – How do you feel after exercising? – What is it like for you to climb a flight of stairs?
Cognitive – Perceptual Pattern	– How do you learn best? – Do you experience pain regularly? – How do you manage your pain?
Sleep – Rest Pattern	– How many hours of sleep do you get each night? – Do you wake up at night to go to the bathroom? – Do you feel rested when you wake up? – Do you have enough energy to carry out your daily activities? – Do you take a nap? Describe.
Self-Perception / Self-Concept	– What makes you feel good about yourself? – Are you pleased with what you have accomplished? Are there things you would like to do in the future? – What would you describe as your strengths? – Are there things you would like to change about yourself?
Role – Relationship Pattern	– Who is your greatest support? – Are you satisfied with your current relationships? – Describe current roles and responsibilities within your family? Extended family? – Are you satisfied with your current work?
Sexuality – Reproductive Pattern	– Are you comfortable with your sexuality? Discuss. – Are you sexually active? – Are you involved in a relationship? – Do you have children?

Table 7.1 *(Continued)*

Pattern	Sample Questions
Coping / Stress Tolerance Pattern	– How would you describe your current level of stress? – Are there things in your life you would describe as stressful? Discuss. – How do you manage stressful situations? – Does stress interfere with your relationships/work?
Value – Belief Pattern	– What do you value most in life? – What gives your life meaning? – Is health a life value? What do you do to keep yourself healthy?

FHP assessment, they use purposeful questioning and branching (or expanded questions) to obtain an unfolding picture of functional health. As data are collected and considered, the information obtained provides an individual's perceptions of function, along with objective (measurable) data about her health. When the assessment is completed, information from all eleven patterns is then synthesized by the nurse, and risks, problems and strengths are identified (Jones, 2013).

Therefore, it is essential to assess all eleven health patterns before making a clinical judgment about the information under analysis. ▸ Table 7.1 can be used to capture critical data about the person's usual responses, as well as changes within patterns. In addition, it is important to remember that all assessment data within each pattern are open to revision. When data change, a re-synthesis of data and a reevaluation of the original nursing diagnoses identified is required.

Types of assessment formats within FHP. There are several types of data collection formats within in the FHP assessment framework. These include partial, screening, and in-depth assessments. A **partial assessment** refers to data collected within several patterns at a given point in time. For example, the nurse may collect data about the nutritional metabolic pattern or activity/exercise for a patient with obesity. Again, while assessment data about a pattern are collected, it is critical that no clinical judgment is finalized until data from all eleven patterns is obtained.

A **screening assessment** may be similar to a partial assessment, but could also contain limited information from all eleven functional patterns. A data collection form might require inclusion of vital signs, for example. The nurse obtains and inputs those data into the assessment form. The form requires that information is collected about the patient's various physiologic systems, and the nurse completes all the blank spaces on the form that deal with this system (heart rhythm, presence of a murmur, pedal pulses, lung sounds, bowel sounds, etc.), along with basic psychosocial and spiritual data. Until a more complete database involving the patient's story is included in the assessment, information needed to confirm the nursing diagnosis may not be sufficient (Jones & Lunney et al., 2011; Lunney, 2009).

A **full assessment** involves complete evaluation of all health patterns. The process usually takes between 30 minutes to an hour to complete. The nurse generates a series of initial questions, and then follow up questions, to explore patient perceptions of each pattern (Herdman & Kamitsuru, 2018; Gordon, 2004, 1994; Jones & Lepley, 1986). A complete assessment of all eleven health patterns can help the nurse determine if there are other human responses occurring that are of concern, indicate risks, or that suggest health promotion opportunities. A full assessment is critical to data synthesis, identification of a nursing diagnosis, and identification of the etiology or precipitating factors of these areas of concern that can guide interventions, and promote achievement of the desired outcome for the patient.

Instruments used to measure FHPs. A recent integrative literature review aimed to identify essential patient data used by nurses in research, education, and clinical practice, in order to update a standardized comprehensive nursing assessment screening tool. Taking into account the huge number of publications addressing different assessment tools, the search was narrowed to the tools based on the FHP, or on minimum data set (MDS) elements. This search strategy recalled 384 manuscripts in three databases, among which 14 were included in the final sample. Of these, 11 validated items or tools for nursing assessment were identified.

Eight studies that were selected focused on physiological and psychosocial functioning. Ranegger, Hackl and Ammenwerth (2014) identified that patient demographics, medical condition, problems (nursing assessment and diagnosis, risk assessment), nursing outcomes, nursing interventions, nursing intensity, and healthcare institutional data should be elements of the Austrian nursing MDS. Shimanouchi, Uchida, Kamei, Sasaki and Shinoda (2001) found that the refinement of the assessment form for home care, which included information on the family, caregiver, living situation, and nursing care significantly shortened documentation time and helped with the identification of client's needs.

Three tools used the FHP framework to assess patients with head and neck cancer and older adults, and to use in clinical and teaching settings. All tools had some modification of the FHPs, either with additions, removals, changing names, or combining of two FHP together. Beyea & Matzo (1989) and Fernández-Sola, Granero-Molina, Mollinedo-Mallea, Gonzales, Aguilera-Manrique & Ponce (2012) did not integrate physical assessment in the FHP assessment, so they added a physical examination section to their tools. In the tool developed by Rodrigues, Cunha, Aquino, Rocha, Mendes, Firmeza, et al. (2018) Activity/Exercise and Sleep/Rest were integrated into one pattern, called Activity/Rest, a Safety/protection section was added, and another FHP was renamed.

Standardized tools developed within Gordon's FHPs are available in the literature (Rodriquez, Cunha, et al., 2018, Zega, D'Agostino, 2014, Jones, Barrett, et al., 1997). In particular, the *Functional Health Pattern Assessment Screening Tool* (FHPAST) is a comprehensive, reliable, and valid tool aimed at screening patients' FHP (Jones & Foster, 1999).

The Functional Health Pattern Assessment Screening Tool (FHPAST). Screening assessment tools are often used in response to challenges with time and patient availability (Jones, 2013). Each item is presented in declarative sentence, based on the FHP definitions and relevant literature. The original tool has been adapted over the years, based on additional research, which resulted in the current tool having 57 items which are representative of the 11 FHPs (Jones, Foster, Flanagan & Duffy, 2012; Beyea & Matzo,1989). Current revisions are underway.

The FHPAST is useful in clinical practice to map health problems or risks and inform patients' responses to illness, or changes in health status over time. Additionally, it provides clinicians and researchers with information on patients' readiness for health promotion, describes responsiveness to nursing interventions, and provides data on patient outcomes (Jones, Foster, Flanagan & Duffy, 2012).

Responses to the screening questions are completed by the patient, or by someone designated by the patient (e.g., family member or a nurse). In practice, the nurse can review data from the FHPAST prior to seeing the patient, isolate patient problems or risks, and seek additional information and conduct pattern exploration during a more complete assessment. The FHPAST can serve as a guide for nursing assessment, as it allows the nurse to respond to patient concerns quickly, and provides information about his changing health status, or helps to identify risks of strengths.

Translation and the FHPAST. Over the years, the FHPAST has been translated into many languages. To enable clinicians and researchers to use the FHPAST in other cultures, the translation, cultural adaptation, and validation in a sample representative of that culture is required. For example, Barros,

Michel, & Nobrega (2003) validated the 58-item version of the FHPAST in Brazil. Although the tool that was translated into Portuguese had excellent reliability, the authors mentioned that further language adaptation was needed in order for the FHPAST to be sensitive to the Brazilian culture. A more recent tool is under review and has been revised for further validation of the FHPAST-revised Brazilian version (FHPAST-VBR).

7.4 References

Barros ALBL, Michel JLM, Nóbrega MML. Translation, utilization and psychometric properties of the functional health assessment screening tool with patients in Brazil. International Journal of Nursing Terminologies and Classifications 2002; 14: 17.

Banning M. Clinical reasoning and its application to nursing: concepts and research studies. Nurse Education in Practice 2008; 8(3): 177–183.

Beyea S, Matzo M. Assessing elders using the functional health pattern assessment model. Nurse Educator 1989; 14(5): 32–37.

Capovilla FC, Capovilla AGS, Macedo EC. Analisando as rotas lexical e perilexical na leitura em voz alta: efeitos da lexicalidade, familiaridade, extensão, regularidade, estrutura silábica e complexidade grafêmica do item e de escolaridade do leitor sobre o tempo de reação, duração e segmentação na pronúncia. In: Pasquali L. Instrumentação psicológica: fundamentos e práticas. Porto Alegre: Artmed, 2010.

Chase S. Response to the concept of nursing presence. State of the Science Scholarly Inquiry for Nursing Practcice: an International Journal 2001;15: 323–327.

Chase SK. Clinical judgment and communication in nurse practitioner practice. Philadelphia, PA: F.A. Davis, 2004.

Doona ME, Chase SK, Haggerty LA. Nursing presence: As real as a milky way, bar. Journal of Holistic Nursing 1999; 17(1): 54–70.

Dossey BM, Keegan L. Holistic nursing: A handbook for practice. 6th ed. Burlington, MA: Jones and Bartlett Learning, 2013.

Fernández-Sola C, Granero-Molina J, Mollinedo-Mallea J, de Gonzales MHP, Aguilera-Manrique G, Ponce, ML. Development and validation of an instrument for initial nursing assessment. Revista da Escola de Enfermagem da USP 2012; 46(6): 1415–1422. https://dx.doi.org/10.1590/S0080–62342012000600019.

Flanagan J. Patient and nurse experiences of theory-based care. Nursing Science Quarterly 2009; 22(2): 160–172.

Gordon M. Nursing diagnosis: Process and application. New York, NY: McGraw-Hill, 1982.

Gordon M. Nursing Diagnosis: Process and application. 3rd ed. St. Louis: Mosby, 1994.

Gordon M. Assess Notes: Nursing assessment and diagnostic reasoning. Philadelphia, PA: FA Davis, 2008.

Gordon M. Manual of nursing diagnosis. Philadelphia, PA: F. A. Davis, 2010.

Herdman TH. Manejo de casos empleando diagnósticos de enfermería de la NANDA Internacional. [Case management using NANDA International nursing diagnoses]. XXX CONGRESO FEMAFEE 2013. Monterrey, Mexico: 2013 (Spanish).

Ives Erickson J, Jones D, Ditomassi M. Fostering nurse-led care at the bedside. Indianapolis, Indiana: Sigma Theta Tau International, 2013.

Jones D, Baker B, Lepley M. Health assessment across the lifespan. New York, NY: McGraw Hill, 1984.

Jones D, Lepley M. Health assessment manual. New York, NY: McGraw-Hill, 1986.

Jones D, Barrett F. Development and testing of a functional health pattern assessment-screening tool. In: Rantz M, LeMone P. Classification of nursing diagnoses: proceedings of the twelfth conference. Glendale, CA: CINAHL Information Systems, 1997.

Jones D, Foster F. Further development and testing of a functional health pattern assessment-screening tool. In: Rantz M, LeMone P. Classification of nursing diagnoses: Proceedings of the thirteenth conference, North American Nursing Diagnosis Association. Celebrating the 25th anniversary of NANDA. Glendale, CA: CINAHL Information Systems, 1999.

Jones D. Health as expanding consciousness. Nursing Science Quarterly 2006; 19(4): 330–332.

Jones D. A synthesis of philosophical perspectives for knowledge development. In: Roy C, Jones DA (eds.). Nursing Knowledge Development and Clinical Practice. New York, NY: Springer Publishing, 2007, p. 163–176.

Jones D, Flanagan J. Guest editorial. International Journal of Nursing Terminologies and Classifications 2007; Winter-Feb/March.

Jones D, Lunney M, Keegan G, Moorhead S. Standardized nursing languages: Essential for nursing workforce. In: Debisette A, Vessey J (eds.). Annual Review of Nursing Research, Volume 28: Nursing Workforce Issues. New York, NY: Springer, 2010, p. 253–294.

Jones D, Duffy ME, Flanagan J, Foster F. Psychometric evaluation of the functional health pattern assessment-screening tool (FHPAST). Int J Nurs Terminol Knowledge 2012; 23: 140–145. https://doi.org/10.1111/j.2047–3095.2012.01224.x

Jones D. Nurse patient relationship: Knowledge transforming practice at the bedside, In: Ives Erickson J, Jones DA, Ditomassi M (eds.). Fostering nurse-led care at the bedside. Indianapolis, Indiana: Sigma Theta Tau International, 2013, Chapter 5, p. 55–121.

Lunney M. Critical thinking to achieve positive health outcomes: Nursing case studies and analysis. 2nd ed. Ames, lA.: Wiley Blackwell, 2009.

Koharchik L, Caputi L, Robb M, Culleiton AL. Fostering Clinical Reasoning in Nursing: How can instructors in practice settings impart this essential skill? American Journal of Nursing 2015; 115(1): 58–61.

MacLeod C. Understanding the experiences of spousal caregivers in health as expanding consciousness. Advances in Nursing Science 2011; 24(3): 245–255.

Newman MA. Health as expanding consciousness. 2nd ed. Sudbury, MA: NLN Press, 1994.

Newman MA. Transforming presence: The difference that nursing makes. Sudbury, MA: Jones and Bartlett, 2008.

Newman MA, Smith M, Pharris M, Jones D. Focus of the discipline revisited. Advances in Nursing Science 2008; 31(1): E16–27.

Picard C, Jones D. Giving voice to what we know: Margaret Newman's theory of health as expanding consciousness in nursing practice, education and research. Sudbury, MA: Jones and Bartlett, 2005.

Ranegger R, Hackl WO, Ammenwerth E. A Proposal for an Austrian Nursing Minimum Data Set (NMDS): A Delphi Study. Applied Clinical Informatics 2014; 5(2): 538–547. http://doi.org/10.4338/ACI-2014–04-RA-0027.

Rodrigues AB, Cunha GH, Aquino CBQ, Rocha SR, Mendes CRS, Firmeza MA, et al. Head and neck cancer: validation of a data collection instrument. Rev Bras Enferm 2018; 71: 1899–1906. http://dx.doi.org/10.1590/0034-7167-2017-0227.

Roy C, Jones DA. Nursing knowledge development and clinical practice. New York, NY: Springer, 2007.

Shimanouchi S, Uchida E, Kamei T, Sasaki A, Shinoda M. Development of an assessment sheet for home care. International Journal of Nursing Practice 2001; 7(3): 140–145.

Simmons, B. Clinical reasoning: concept analysis. Journal of Advanced Nursing 2009; 66(5): 1151–1158.

Smith M. Integrative review of research related to Margaret Newman's theory of health as expanding consciousness. Advances in Nursing Science 2011; 24(3): 256–272.

Somerville J. Development and psychometric testing of patient's perception of feeling known by their nurse scale. International Journal of Human Caring 2009; 13(4): 38–43.

Tanner C. Thinking like a nurse: a research-based model of clinical judgment in nursing. Journal of Nursing Education 2006; 45(6): 204–211.

Walker LO, Avant KC. Strategies for Theory Construction in Nursing. 6th ed. New York, NY: Pearson, Prentice Hall, 2019.

Watson J. Unitary caring science: The philosophy of praxis in nursing. Louisville, CO: Press of Colorado, 2018.

Willis DG, Grace PJ, Roy C. A central unifying focus for the discipline: facilitating humanization, meaning, choice, quality of life, and healing in living and dying. Advances in Nursing Science 2008; 31(1): E28–40.

Young AM, Kidston S, Banks MD, Mudge AM, Isenring EA. Malnutrition screening tools: comparison against two validated nutrition assessment methods in older medical inpatients. Nutrition 2013; 29(1): 101–106.

Zega M, D'Agostino F, Bowles KH, De Marinis MG, Rocco G, Vellone E, et al. Development and validation of a computerized assessment form. Int J Nurs Terminol Knowledge 2014; 25: 22–29. https://doi.org/10.1111/2047-3095.1200.

8 Clinical Application: Data Analysis to Determine Appropriate Nursing Diagnosis

T. Heather Herdman, Dorothy A. Jones, Camila Takáo Lopes

8.1 Clustering of Information/Seeing a Pattern

In the previous chapter, we discussed objective and subjective data collection. Once the nurse has collected data and transformed it into information, the next step is to begin to answer the question: what are my patient's human responses? This requires the substantive knowledge of a variety of theories and models from nursing, as well as several related disciplines. And, as previously noted, it requires knowledge about the concepts that underlie the nursing diagnoses themselves.

In other words, assessment techniques are meaningless if we do not know how to use the data we collect! ▶ Fig. 8.1 provides an example of how objective and subjective data can be converted to information through the application of nursing knowledge for a case study of Mrs. H, a 36-year-old woman with an HbA1c of 9.0% and an exudative ulcer on the medial malleolar region. If the nurse who assessed Mrs. H did not know the normal blood glucose level, he would not have been able to interpret that patient's HbA1c as being abnormal. If he did not understand theories related to tissue integrity, pain, and blood glucose level management, then he might not identify other susceptibilities or problem responses exhibited by this woman.

8.2 Identifying Potential Nursing Diagnoses (Diagnostic Hypotheses)

At this point in the decision-making, or problem-solving process, the nurse looks at the information that is coming together to form a pattern; it provides him with a way of seeing what human responses the patient may be experiencing. Initially, the nurse considers all potential diagnoses that may come to mind. In the expert nurse, this can happen in seconds – for novice or student nurses, it may take support from more expert nurses or faculty members to guide their thinking.

Seeing patterns in the data requires an understanding of the concept that supports each diagnosis. For example, you might find yourself providing care to Mr. K, who has been hospitalized for 14 days due to an infected ankle ulcer, which became septic. Mr. K used to live with his daughter and primary caregiver, Janine, his son-in-law, Don, and his two grandchildren (ages 3 and 6).

Janine and Don had agreed to separate two months before. While handling divorce arrangements, Janine started looking for a job and interviewing candidates to serve as caregivers to Mr. K, when his ankle wound infected and he had to be taken to the hospital with respiratory discomfort.

Mr. K is expected to be discharged the following week. During the visiting hours, Janine is clearly tired, and admits she has not been able to get much sleep because she has not been able to find a job yet and she does not want to place Mr. K in a nursing home, but she is afraid that she will not be able to afford a caregiver.

Throughout your conversation with Janine, you observe that she seems frustrated and nervous, and she frequently refers to not being sure if she has been doing the right thing for Mr. K and her children. She is sure that her lack of care during the divorce process caused his father to have the infection. She is clearly very concerned about her father, but also mentions that her younger daughter had almost been run over by a car the day before, because she dozed off while watching her play and nearly missed her running towards the traffic.

What does all of this tell you? Unless you have a good understanding of family dynamics, stress, coping, role strain and grief theories, it may not tell you very much at all! You may know that Mr. K has a severe infection. But would you know to also focus on the family, and look for a cause (related factors) or other data (defining characteristics) to determine an accurate diagnosis for Janine?

Although you might be assigned to Mr. K, if you aren't attentive to what is happening in the family, are you truly attending to Mr. K's needs? Such a situation can lead to the nurse simply focusing on the patient of record, rather than considering the family and its impact on patient outcomes. Or, if the nurse did realize the need to address what is happening with Janine, but did not have good baseline knowledge of the previously noted theories, she might simply "pick a diagnosis" from a list to describe her response. Conceptual knowledge of each nursing diagnosis allows the nurse to assign accurate meanings to the data collected from the patient, and prepares her to perform the in-depth assessment.

When you have this type of conceptual knowledge, you will begin to look at the data you collect in a different way. You will turn that data into information, and begin to observe how that information starts to group together to form patterns, or to "paint a picture" of what might be happening with your patient. Take another look at ▸ Fig. 8.1. With conceptual nursing knowledge of blood glucose level, tissue integrity, pain theories and pain management,

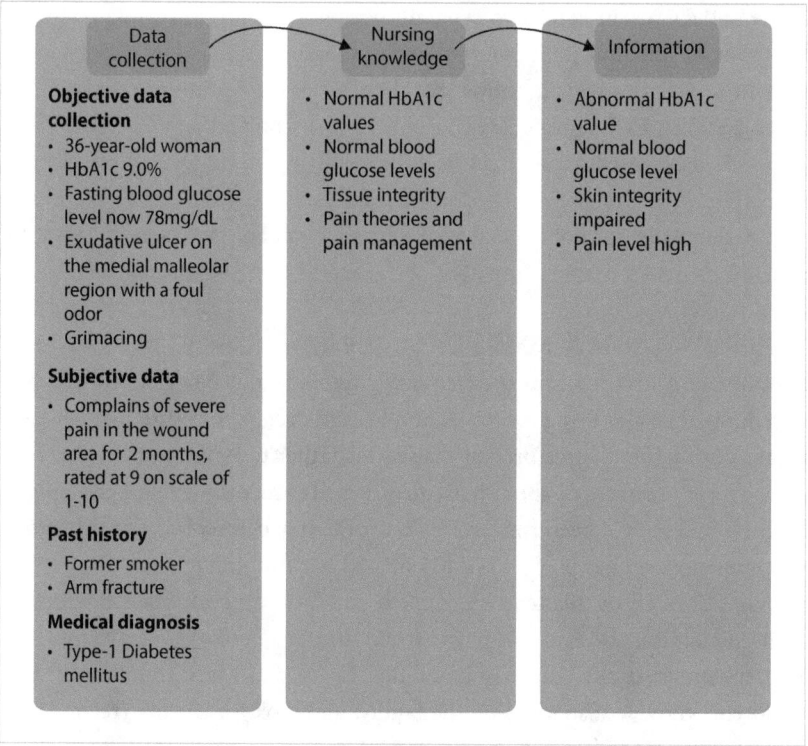

Data collection	Nursing knowledge	Information
Objective data collection	• Normal HbA1c values	• Abnormal HbA1c value
• 36-year-old woman	• Normal blood glucose levels	• Normal blood glucose level
• HbA1c 9.0%	• Tissue integrity	• Skin integrity impaired
• Fasting blood glucose level now 78mg/dL	• Pain theories and pain management	• Pain level high
• Exudative ulcer on the medial malleolar region with a foul odor		
• Grimacing		
Subjective data		
• Complains of severe pain in the wound area for 2 months, rated at 9 on scale of 1-10		
Past history		
• Former smoker		
• Arm fracture		
Medical diagnosis		
• Type-1 Diabetes mellitus		

Fig. 8.1 The case of Mrs. H: converting data to information

you might begin to see the information as possible tentative nursing diagnoses, such as:

– Risk for unstable blood glucose level (00179)
– Impaired tissue integrity (00044)
– Acute pain (00132)

It is not enough, however, to merely "select/choose/pick" a diagnosis label. Unfortunately, this step is often where nurses stop – they develop a list of diagnoses, and either launch directly into action (determining interventions) or they simply "pick" one of the nursing diagnoses that sounds most appropriate for a patient's medical condition, based on what they think the nursing diagnosis label represents, and then move on to selecting interventions for those diagnoses. Others may determine that they wish to obtain a certain outcome, and simply aim interventions at that outcome. These are not appropriate methods for diagnosing, and can lead to poor patient outcomes.

Determining a nursing diagnosis requires synthesizing all of the information available to determine what the real problem might be, based on objective and subjective data (defining characteristics), and what you think may be causing the response (related factors), in order to plan the best interventions and achieve the desired outcome. Unless we know the problem *and its cause* (etiology), the interventions selected may be completely inappropriate for this particular patient. For diagnoses to be accurate, they must be validated – and that requires additional, in-depth assessment based upon data unique to each patient to confirm or to refute, or "rule out", the possibility of a diagnosis. Only when we use nursing knowledge, and reflect on the patient's manifestation of his response to the health/illness experience, can a nursing diagnosis be generated: this is the essence of diagnosing the response of an individual, caregiver, family, group, or community.

8.3 Refining the Diagnosis

As you review information from your assessment it is important to determine if the responses (probabilities) are normal responses, abnormal (or unusual responses), represent a risk (susceptibility) or a strength. Those items that are not considered normal, or were seen as a susceptibility, should be considered in relation to a problem-focused or risk diagnosis. Areas in which the patient indicates a desire to improve something (for example, to enhance nutrition) should be considered as a potential health promotion diagnosis.

If some data are interpreted as abnormal, further in-depth assessment is crucial to accurately diagnose the patient. It is important to remember that if one simply collects data to complete a required form, without considering the importance of the data, this can lead to critical data being overlooked. Take another look at ▶ Fig. 8.1 which related to our first case in this chapter: Mrs. H. The nurse could have stopped his assessment here, and simply moved on to the diagnoses of *risk for unstable blood glucose level, impaired tissue integrity, acute pain*. He could have administered analgesics, applied a dressing, provided education about how to administer insulin correctly, how to apply dressings, and how to take the analgesics at home, for example. However, while all those things might be appropriate, he would have neglected to identify some major issues which are probably significant and which, if not addressed, will lead to continued issues with Mrs. H's status.

Mrs. H's nurse, however, understood the need for an in-depth assessment and was therefore able to identify her recent remarriage, potential areas of concern in her family processes, relationships, and personal identity (▶ Fig. 8.2). He

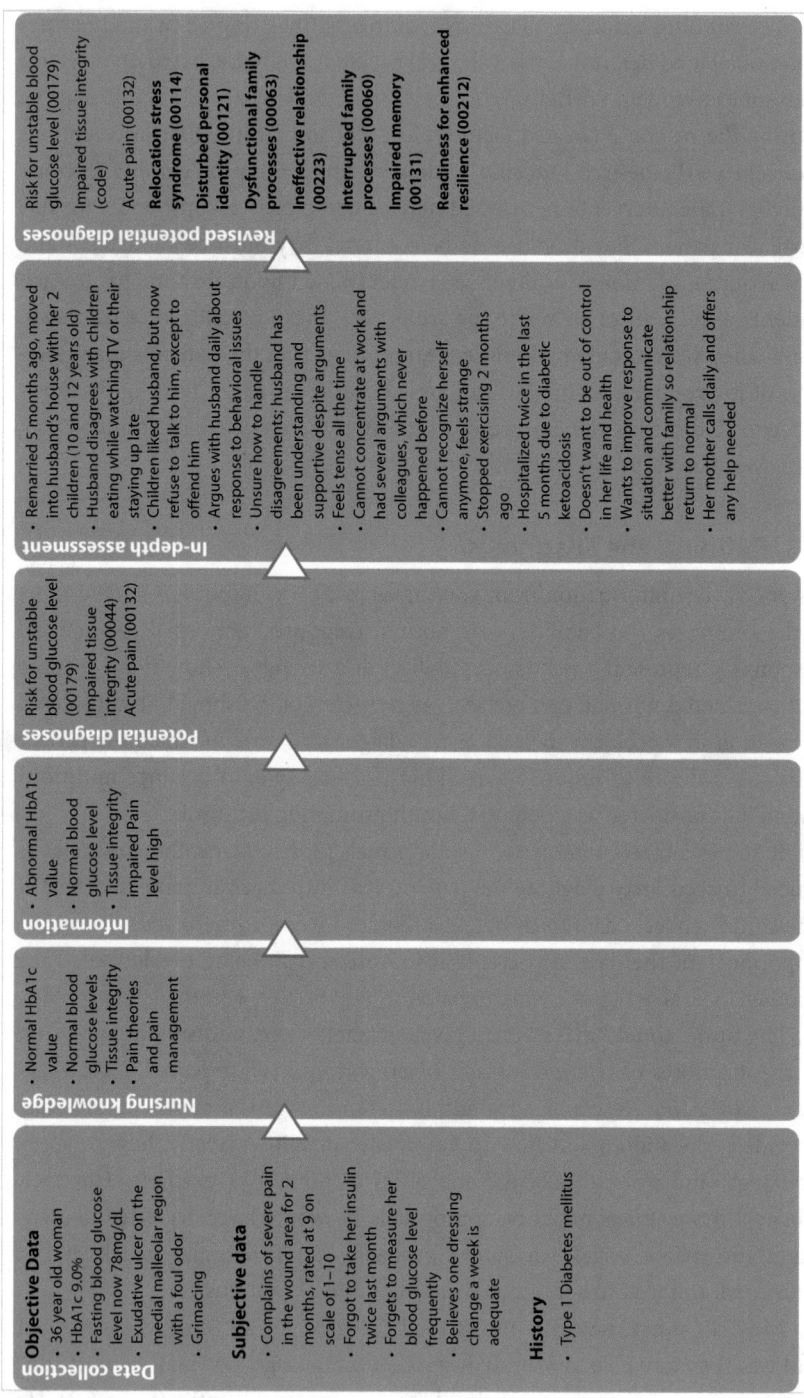

Fig. 8.2 The case of Mrs. H: in-depth assessment

learned that Mrs. H had problems consistent with a stressful new life situation (recent remarriage, moving to her husband's house, family conflicts, change in exercise pattern, forgetting to take her insulin, arguing at work). However, he also identified that Mrs. H had an important strength in the support she received from her mother, and her verbalized desire to improve the way she was responding to this situation: these are all very important things to build into any plan of care! So, with this additional in-depth assessment, the nurse could now revise his potential diagnoses:

- Risk for unstable blood glucose level (00179)
- Impaired tissue integrity (00044)
- Acute pain (00132)
- Relocation stress syndrome (00114)
- Disturbed personal identity (00121)
- Dysfunctional family processes (00063)
- Ineffective relationship (00223)
- Interrupted family processes (00060)
- Impaired memory (00131)
- Readiness for enhanced resilience (00212)

8.4 Confirming/Refuting Potential Nursing Diagnoses

Whenever new data is collected, and processed into information, it is time to reconsider our diagnostic hypotheses. During this period, there are three primary things to consider:

- Did the in-depth assessment provide new data that would rule out or eliminate one or more of your potential diagnoses?
- Did the in-depth assessment point toward new diagnoses that you had not previously considered?
- How can you differentiate between similar diagnoses?

It is essential that other nurses continue to validate the diagnosis, and to understand how you arrived at your diagnosis. It is for this reason that it is important to use standardized terms, such as the NANDA-I nursing diagnoses, which provide not only a label (e.g., *dysfunctional family processes*, Code 00063), but also a definition and assessment criteria (defining characteristics and related factors, or risk factors) so that other nursing professionals can continue to validate – or perhaps refute – the diagnosis as new data become available for the patient.

The nurse might create a term, such as *ineffective family communication*, to address the issues he identified when listening to Mrs. H talk about her communication with her new husband, and how her children and he relate to each other. But what does this diagnosis mean? How is it defined, and how would other nurses be able to recognize the diagnosis when they completed their assessments? Terms that are simply constructed by nurses at the bedside, without validated definitions and, most importantly, assessment criteria, have *no* consistent meaning and *cannot* be clinically validated or confirmed. When a NANDA-I nursing diagnosis does not exist that fits a pattern you identify in a patient, it is safer to *describe the condition in detail* rather than to "make up" a term that will have different meanings to different nurses. If you asked ten nurses to define the "created" diagnosis of *ineffective family communication*, and to identify defining characteristics and related factors, it is quite possible you would have ten different definitions, and a laundry list of potential diagnostic indicators. This is neither helpful nor safe when we are considering the health and well-being of the patients for whom we provide care.

8.5 Eliminating Possible Diagnoses

One of the goals of in-depth assessment is to eliminate, or "rule out", one or more of the potential diagnoses you were considering. You do this by synthesizing the information you have obtained, and comparing it to what you know about the diagnoses. It is critical that the assessment data support each diagnosis. Diagnoses that are not well supported through the assessment criteria provided by NANDA-I (defining characteristics, related/risk factors) and/or that are not supported by etiological factors (causes or contributors to the diagnoses) are not appropriate for a patient. It is important to remember that nurses must be able to independently address related (or risk) factors. In other words, medical diagnoses or physician-ordered treatments are not related (or risk) factors, although they may be associated conditions. If the nurse cannot independently resolve or diminish the effect of an etiological factor, then it is not a related (or risk) factor.

As we look at ▸ Fig. 8.2 and consider the potential diagnoses that Mrs. H's nurse identified, we can begin to eliminate some of these as valid diagnoses. Sometimes it is helpful to do a side-to-side comparison of the diagnoses, focusing on those defining characteristics and related factors that were identified throughout the assessment and patient history. An example of a comparison of diagnoses within one domain is provided in (▸ Table 8.1).

Table 8.1 The case of Mrs. H: comparing diagnoses in the same domain

Diagnosis	Dysfunctional family processes	Ineffective relationship	Interrupted family processes
Domain	7. Role relationship	7. Role relationship	7. Role relationship
Class	2. Family relationships	3. Role performance	2. Family relationships
Definition	Family functioning which fails to support the well-being of its members.	A pattern of mutual partnership that is insufficient to provide for each other's needs.	Break in the continuity of family functioning which fails to support the well-being of its members
Defining characteristics	– Contradictory communication pattern – Escalating conflict – Difficulty adapting to change – Verbal abuse of children – Expresses tension	– Imbalance in collaboration between partners – Dissatisfaction with complementary relationship between partners – Unsatisfying communication with partner	– Power alliance change – Ritual change – Changes in relationship pattern – Changes in participation for decision-making – Altered communication pattern – Altered family conflict resolution
Related/Risk factors	– Ineffective coping strategies – Inadequate problem-solving skills	– Inadequate communication skills – Excessive stress	– Difficulty dealing with power shift among family members

For example, Mrs. H's nurse quickly eliminates from consideration the diagnoses, *relocation stress syndrome* and *impaired memory*. Although Mrs. H does indicate she feels tense all the time, the nurse considers that this is more related to her *personal identity, family processes, and relationship,* than to a disturbance following the move from one environment to another, or a persistent inability to remember something.

8.6 Potential New Diagnoses

It is very possible, such as in the case of Mrs. H (► Fig. 8.2) that new data will lead to new information, and in turn, to new diagnoses. The same questions that you used to eliminate potential diagnoses should be used as you consider these diagnoses.

8.7 Differentiating Similar Diagnoses

It is helpful to narrow down your potential diagnoses by considering those that are very similar, but that have a distinctive feature which makes one more relevant to the patient than the other. Let's take another look at our patient, Mrs. H. After the in-depth assessment, the nurse had 11 potential diagnoses; two diagnoses were eliminated, leaving 9 potential diagnoses. One way to start the process of differentiation is to look at where the diagnoses are located within the NANDA-I taxonomy. This gives you a clue about how the diagnoses are grouped together into the broad area of nursing knowledge (domain) and the subcategories, or group of diagnoses with similar attributes (class).

After eliminating two diagnoses, her nurse is considering: three diagnoses in the role relationship domain (*dysfunctional family processes, ineffective relationship* and *interrupted family processes*), two diagnoses in the coping/stress tolerance domain (*ineffective coping* and *readiness for enhanced resilience*); one in the nutrition domain (*risk for unstable blood glucose level*), one in the self-perception domain (*disturbed personal identity*), and one in the safety/protection domain (*impaired tissue integrity*), and one in the comfort domain (*acute pain*). The nurse realizes that *dysfunctional family processes, ineffective relationship, interrupted family processes,* and *disturbed personal identity* cluster into *disturbed family identity syndrome* (00283).

When reviewing patient information in light of similar nursing diagnoses, consider the following questions:
- Do the diagnoses share a similar focus, or is it different?
- If the diagnoses share a similar focus, is one more focused/specific than the other?

– Does one diagnosis potentially lead to another that I have identified? That is, could it be the causative factor of that other diagnosis?

As the nurse considers what he knows about Mrs. H, he can look at the responses he identified as potential diagnoses in light of these questions. Mrs. H clearly has a diabetes-related injury (*impaired tissue integrity*), it appears that her susceptibility for a variation in serum levels of glucose from the normal range (*risk for unstable blood glucose level*) is actually a consequence of her excessive stress due to *disturbed family identity syndrome*. Therefore, although the nurse is concerned about her pain and will need to treat her injury, he believes he can best address these issues for the long-term by addressing her *disturbed family identity syndrome*, which he believes is the underlying causes of her current health status.

After talking with Mrs. H, it appears that using the health promotion diagnosis, *readiness for enhanced resilience*, will best support her in setting goals around her blood glucose level management and family identity, while reinforcing her ability to regain control over her life and improving her resilience.

The nurse recognizes that she has verbalized a desire to improve her resilience, and feels that working with her on this issue from a health promotion perspective (*readiness for enhanced resilience*) could be more positive for her. This, coupled with the previously mentioned belief that goal setting could be used within this diagnosis to address *risk for unstable blood glucose level*, makes this diagnosis more appropriate for Mrs. H. He feels it is imperative to acknowledge her family identity, and to work with her on this response.

Finally, it is important to manage the *acute pain* that Mrs. H is experiencing. Because one of the goals is to get her more active to improve blood glucose levels, and to assist with overall wellbeing, it is important to increase her comfort so that her pain does not prohibit her from increasing her level of activity.

8.8 Diagnosing/Prioritizing

After completing your assessment, identifying response patterns, generating, refining and finalizing the nursing diagnosis(es) along with an etiology, nursing interventions can be planned mutually with your patient. After reviewing everything he learned about his patient, Mrs. H, the nurse may have determined five key diagnoses:

– Risk for unstable blood glucose level (00179)
– Impaired tissue integrity (00044)

- Acute pain (00132)
- Disturbed family identity syndrome (00283)
- Readiness for enhanced resilience (00212)

Remember that the nursing process, which includes continuous re-evaluation of the diagnosis, is an ongoing process. This means that as more data becomes available, or as the patient's condition changes, the diagnoses may also change – or the prioritization may change. Think back for a moment to the initial screening assessment the nurse performed on Mrs. H. Do you see that, without further follow up, he would have missed the very important diagnosis of *disturbed family identity syndrome*, along with the health promotion opportunity for Mrs. E (*readiness for enhanced resilience*), and he might have designed a plan to address issues that would not have resolved her underlying issues?

Can you see why the idea of just "picking" a nursing diagnosis to go along with the medical diagnosis simply isn't the way to go? The in-depth, ongoing assessment provided so much more information about Mrs. H, that can be used to determine not only the appropriate diagnoses, but realistic outcomes and interventions that will best meet her individual needs.

8.9 Summary

Assessment is a critical role of professional nurses, and requires disciplinary knowledge of nursing theories, concepts, and foci of concern to the discipline upon on which nursing diagnoses are developed. Collecting data only for the sake of completing some mandatory form or computer screen is a waste of time, and it certainly does not support individualized care for our patients. Establishing an effective nurse-patient relationship enables the nurse to come to know the person and his/her experiences with health and illness. Having an organized approach to a nursing assessment, such as Gordon's Functional Health Pattern assessment, provides the nurse with an assessment framework that can guide data collection to appropriately diagnose, and to identify causative factors which will be responsive to nursing interventions and evidence–driven outcomes. Developing, refining, and prioritizing nursing diagnoses based upon data analysis and synthesis, is the hallmark of professional nursing.

Assessing, followed by synthesizing of data, is essential for diagnosing. Selecting nursing diagnoses without assessment can result in inaccurate diagnoses, inappropriate outcomes, and ineffective and/or unnecessary interventions for diagnoses that are not relevant to the patient – and may lead to completely missing the most important clinical judgment about your patient!

8.10 References

Bellinger G, Casstro D, Mills A. Date, Information, Knowledge, and Wisdom. http://otec.uoregon.edu/data-wisdom.htm.

Bergstrom N, Braden BJ, Laguzza A, Holman V. (1987). The Braden Scale for predicting pressure sore risk. Nursing Research 1987; 36(4): 205–210.

Cambridge University Press. Cambridge Dictionary Online. 2020. Available from: https://dictionary.cambridge.org/us/. Accessed 2020 Aug 29.

Centers for Disease Control & Prevention. About adult BMI. 2015. Accessed: https://www.cdc.gov/healthyweight/assessing/bmi/adult_bmi/.

Gordon M. Nursing diagnosis: Process and application. 3rd ed. St. Louis, MO: Mosby, 1994.

Gordon M. Assess Notes: Nursing assessment and diagnostic reasoning. Philadelphia, PA: FA Davis, 2008.

Herdman TH. (2013). Manejo de casos empleando diagnósticos de enfermería de la NANDA Internacional. [Case management using NANDA International nursing diagnoses]. XXX CONGRESO FEMAFEE 2013. Monterrey, Mexico, 2013. (Spanish).

Koharchik L, Caputi L, Robb M, Culleiton AL. Fostering Clinical Reasoning in Nursing: How can instructors in practice settings impart this essential skill? American Journal of Nursing 2015; 115(1): 58–61.

Oliver D, Britton M, Seed P, Martin FC, Hopper AH. Development and evaluation of evidence based risk assessment tool (STRATIFY) to predict which elderly inpatients will fall: case-control and cohort studies. BMJ 1997; 315: 1049–1053.

Rencic J. Twelve tips for teaching expertise in clinical reasoning. Medical Teacher 2011; 33(11): 887–892.

Tanner C. Thinking like a nurse: a research-based model of clinical judgment in nursing. Journal of Nursing Education 2006; 45(6): 204–211.

9 Introduction to the NANDA International Taxonomy of Nursing Diagnoses

T. Heather Herdman, Shigemi Kamitsuru

9.1 Introduction to Taxonomy

NANDA International, Inc. provides a standardized *terminology* of nursing diagnoses, and it presents its diagnoses in a classifications scheme, more specifically a *taxonomy*. It is important to understand a little bit about a taxonomy, and how taxonomy differs from terminology. So, let us take a moment to talk about what taxonomy actually represents.

A *terminology* is the body of terms used with a particular technical application in a subject of study, profession, etc. (English Oxford Living Dictionary Online 2020).

With regard to nursing, the NANDA-I nursing diagnosis *terminology* includes the defined terms (labels) that are used to describe clinical judgments made by professional nurses: the diagnoses themselves. A definition of the NANDA-I *taxonomy* might be "a systematic ordering of phenomena/clinical judgments that define the knowledge of the nursing discipline". More simply put, the NANDA –I taxonomy of nursing diagnoses is a classification schema to help us organize the concepts of concern (nursing judgments or nursing diagnoses) for nursing practice. A classification is the arrangement of related phenomena in taxonomic groups according to their observed similarities; a category into which something is put (English Oxford Living Dictionary Online 2020).

A *taxonomy* is the branch of science concerned with classification, especially of organisms; systematics (English Oxford Living Dictionary Online 2020). A *taxonomy* can be compared to a filing cabinet – in a drawer (domain) you may file all information you have related to your bills/debts. Within that drawer, you may have individual file folders (classes) for different types of bills/debt: household, automobile, health care, child care, animal care, etc. Within each file folder (class), you would then have individual bills representing each type of debt (nursing diagnoses). The current biological taxonomy originated with Carl Linnaeus in 1735. He originally identified three kingdoms (animal, plant, and mineral), which were then divided into classes, orders, families, genera, and species (Quammen 2007). You probably learned about the revised biological taxonomy in a basic science class in your high school or university setting.

Terminology, on the other hand, is the language that is used to describe a specific thing; it is the language used in a particular discipline to describe its knowledge. Therefore, the nursing diagnoses form a discipline-specific language, so when we want to talk about the diagnoses themselves, we are talking about the *terminology* of nursing knowledge. When we want to talk about the way that we structure or categorize the NANDA-I diagnoses, then we are talking about the *taxonomy.*

Classification systems in health care denote disciplinary knowledge and demonstrate how a specific group of professionals perceive what are the significant areas of knowledge of the discipline. Therefore, a classification system in health care has multiple functions, including to

- provide a view of the knowledge and practice area of a specific profession.
- organize phenomena in a way that refers to changes in health, processes, and mechanisms that are of concern to the professional.
- show the logical connection between factors that can be controlled or manipulated by professionals in the discipline (von Krogh 2011).

Let us think about taxonomy as it relates to something we all deal with in our daily lives. When you need to buy food, you go to the grocery store. Suppose that there is a new store in your neighborhood, *Classified Groceries, Inc.,* so you decide to go there to do your shopping. When you enter the store, you notice that the layout seems very different from your regular store, but the person greeting you at the door hands you a diagram to help you learn your way around (► Fig. 9.1).

You can see that this store has organized the grocery items into eight main categories or grocery store aisles: proteins, grain products, vegetables, fruits, processed foods, snack foods, deli foods, and beverages. These categories/aisles could also be called "domains" – they are broad levels of classification that divide phenomena into main groups. In this case, the phenomena represent "groceries".

You may also have noticed that the diagram does not just show the eight aisles; each aisle has a few key phrases identified that further help us to understand what types of foods would be found in each aisle. For example, in the aisle (domain) entitled "Beverages", we see six subcategories: "Coffee", "Tea", "Soda", "Water", "Beer/hard cider", and "Wine/sake". Another way of saying this would be that these subcategories are "Classes" of products that are found under the "Domain" of beverages.

One of the rules people try to follow when they develop a taxonomy is that the classes should be mutually exclusive – in other words, one type of grocery

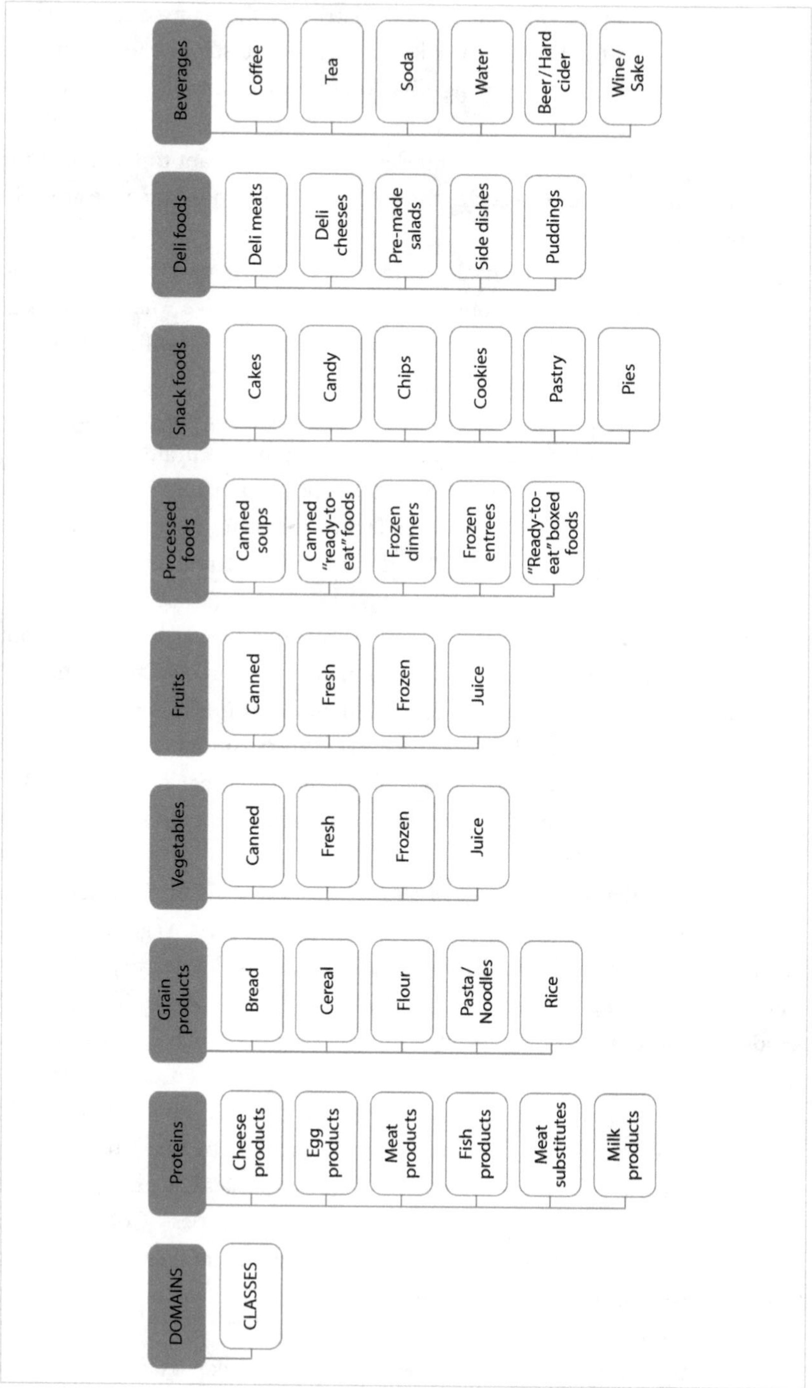

Fig. 9.1 Domains and classes of Classified Groceries, Inc.

product should not be found in multiple classes. This is not always possible, but this should still be the goal, because it makes it much clearer for people who want to use the structure. If you find cheddar cheese in the protein aisle, but find cheddar cheese spread in the snack foods aisle, it makes it hard for people to understand the classification system that is being used.

Looking back at our store diagram, there is additional information to be added (▶ Fig. 9.1). Each of the grocery aisles is further explained, providing a more detailed level of information about the groceries that are found in the various aisles. As an example, ▶ Fig. 9.2 shows the detailed information provided on the "Beverages" aisle. You will note the six "classes" along with additional detail for each of those classes. These represent various types (or concepts) of beverage products, all of which share similar properties that cluster them together into one group.

Given the information with which we have been provided, we could easily manage our shopping list. If we wanted to find some herbal soda, we would quickly be able to find the aisle marked "Beverages", the shelf marked "Sodas", and we could confirm that herbal sodas would be found there. Likewise, if we wanted some loose leaf green tea, we would again look at the aisle marked "Beverages", find the shelf marked "Tea", and then we would find "Green loose leaf teas".

The purpose of this grocery taxonomy is to help the shopper quickly determine what section of the store contains the grocery supplies that he/she wants to buy. Without this information, the shopper would have to walk up and down each aisle and try to make sense of what products were in which aisle; depending on the size of the store, this could be a very frustrating and confusing experience! Thus, the diagram being provided by the store personnel provides a "concept map", or a guide for shoppers to quickly understand how the groceries have been classified into locations within the store, with the goal of improving the shopping experience.

By now, you are probably getting a good idea of the difficulty of developing a taxonomy that reflects the concepts it is trying to classify in a clear, concise, and consistent manner. Thinking about our grocery store example, can you imagine different ways that items in the store could be grouped together?

This example of a grocery taxonomy may not meet the goal of avoiding overlap between concepts and classes in a way that is logical for all shoppers. For example, tomato juice is found in the domain *Vegetables* (vegetable juices), but *not* in the domain *Beverages*. Although one group of individuals might find this categorization logical and clear, others might suggest that all beverages should be together. What is important is that the distinction

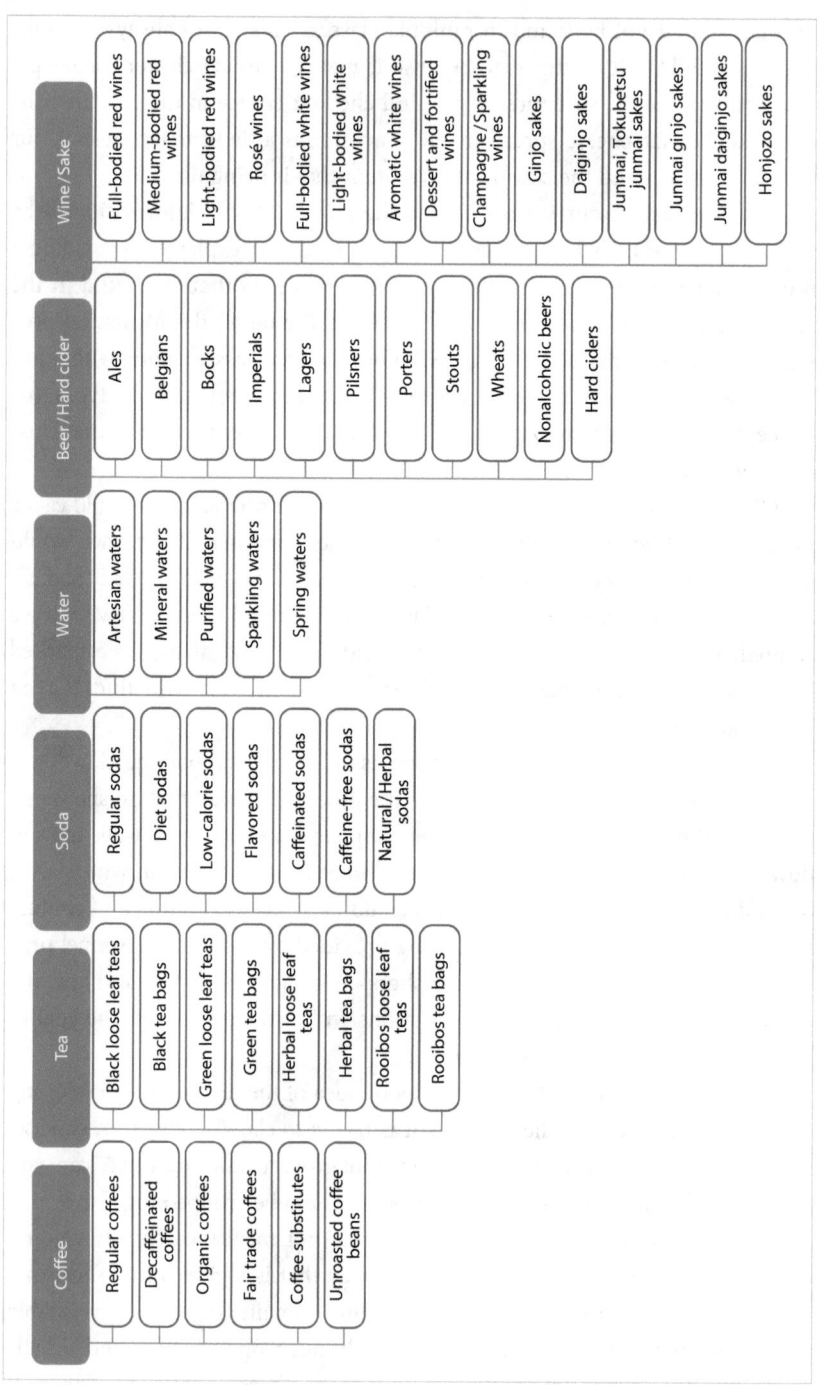

Fig. 9.2 Classes and types (concepts) of beverages at Classified Groceries, Inc.

between the domains is well-defined, i.e., all vegetables and vegetable products are found within the vegetable domain, whereas the beverage domain contains beverages that are not vegetable-based. The problem with this distinction might be that we could then argue that wine and hard cider should be in the fruit aisle, and beer and sake should be in the grain aisle!

Taxonomies are works in progress – they continue to grow, evolve, and even dramatically change as more knowledge is developed about the area of study. There is often significant debate about what structure is best for categorizing phenomena of concern to different disciplines. There are many ways of categorizing things, and truly, there is no "absolutely right" way. The goal is to find a logical, consistent way to categorize similar things while avoiding overlap between the concepts and the classes. For users of taxonomies, the goal is to understand how it classifies similar concepts into its domains and classes to quickly identify specific concepts as needed.

9.2 Organizing Nursing Knowledge

Professions organize their formal knowledge into consistent, logical, conceptualized dimensions so that it reflects the professional domain and makes it relevant for clinical practice. For professionals in health care, the knowledge of diagnosis is a significant part of professional knowledge and is essential for clinical practice. Knowledge of nursing diagnoses must therefore be organized in a way that legitimizes professional nursing practice and consolidates the nursing profession's jurisdiction (Abbott 1988).

Within the NANDA-I nursing diagnostic taxonomy, we use a hierarchical graphic to show our domains and classes (▶ Fig. 9.3). The diagnoses themselves are not depicted in this graphic, although they could be. The primary reason we do not include the diagnoses is that there are 267 of them, and that would make the graphic very large – and very hard to read!

In nursing, it is most important that the diagnoses are classified in a way that makes sense clinically, so that when a nurse is trying to identify a diagnosis that he/she may not see very often in practice, he/she can logically use the taxonomy to find the appropriate information on possible related diagnoses. Although the NANDA-I Taxonomy II (▶ Fig. 9.3) is *not* intended to function as a nursing assessment framework, it does provide structure for classifying nursing diagnoses into domains and classes, each of which is clearly defined.

To provide an example of what it would look like if we included the nursing diagnoses in the graphic representation of the taxonomy, ▶ Fig. 9.4 shows

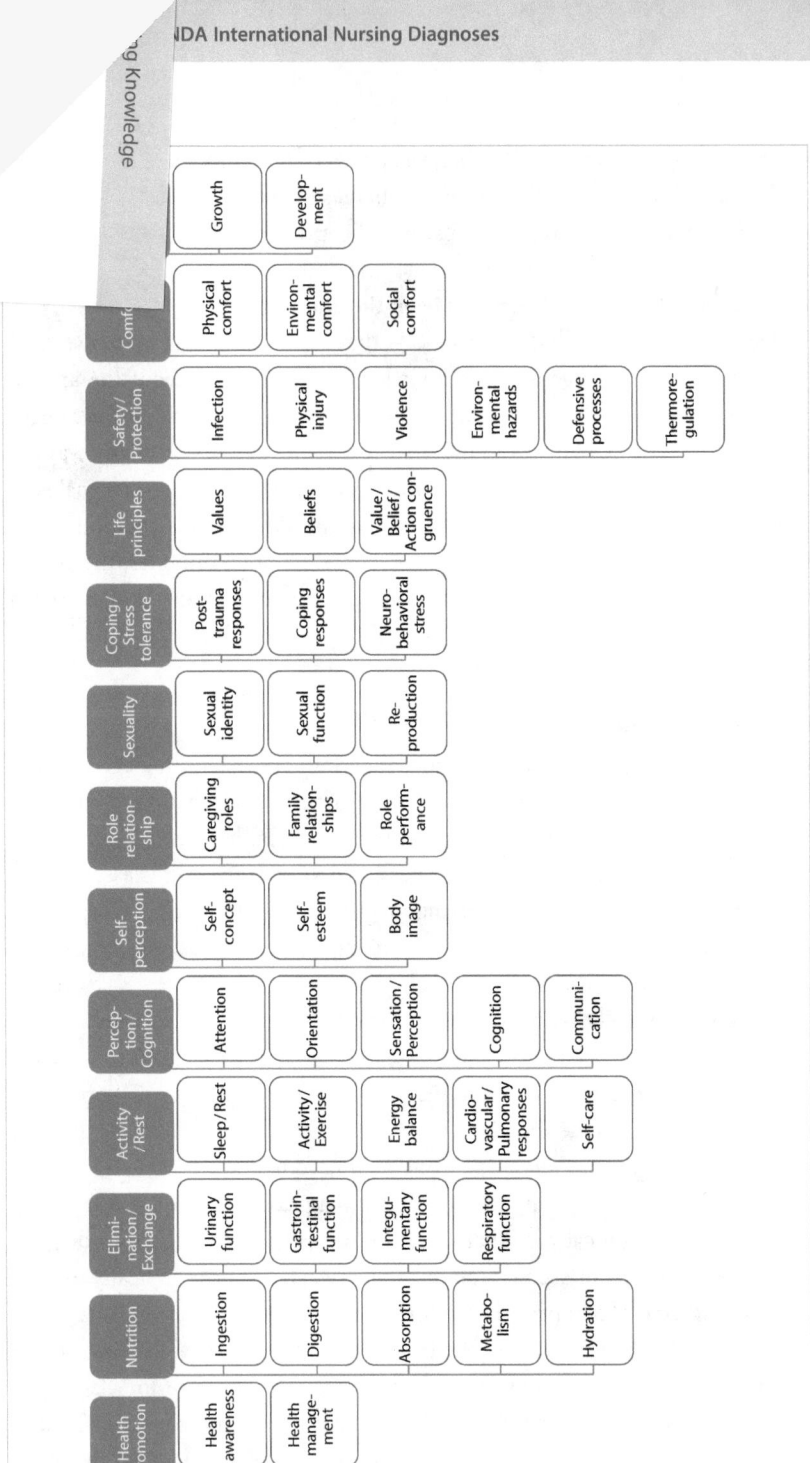

Fig. 9.3 NANDA-I Taxonomy II domains and classes

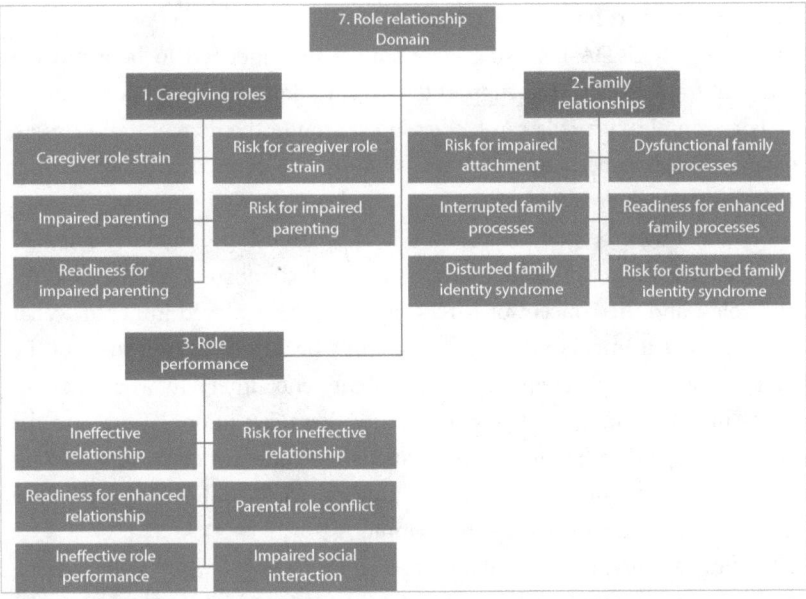

Fig. 9.4 NANDA-I Domain 7, Role relationship, with classes and nursing diagnoses

only one domain with its classes and nursing diagnoses. As you can see, this is a lot of information to depict in graphic form.

Nursing knowledge includes individual, family, group, and community responses, risks, and strengths. According to von Krogh (2011), the NANDA-I taxonomy is meant to function in the following ways; it should

- provide a model, or cognitive map, of the knowledge of the nursing discipline.
- communicate that knowledge, and those perspectives and theories.
- provide structure and order for that knowledge.
- serve as a support tool for clinical reasoning.
- provide a way to organize nursing diagnoses within an electronic health record.

9.3 Using NANDA-I Taxonomy

Although the taxonomy provides a way of categorizing nursing phenomena, it can also serve other functions. It can help faculty to develop a nursing curriculum, for example, and it can help a nurse identify a diagnosis, perhaps one that he/she may not use frequently, but that he/she needs for a specific patient. Let us look at both situations.

9.3.1 Structuring Nursing Curricula

Although the NANDA-I nursing taxonomy is not intended to be a nursing assessment framework, it can support the organization of undergraduate education. For example, curricula can be developed around the domains and classes, allowing courses to be taught that are based on the core concepts of nursing practice, and which are categorized in each of the NANDA-I domains.

A course might be built around the Role relationship domain (▶ Fig. 9.4) with units based on each of the classes. In Unit 1, the focus could be on caregiving roles, and the concept of parenting would be explored in depth. What is it? How does it impact individual and family health? What are some of the common parenting problems that our patients encounter? In what types of patients might we be most likely to identify these conditions? What are the primary etiologies? What are the consequences if these conditions go undiagnosed and/or untreated? How can we prevent, treat, and/or improve these conditions? How can we manage the symptoms?

Building a nursing curriculum around these key concepts of nursing knowledge enables students to truly understand and build expertise in the knowledge of nursing science, while also learning about and understanding related medical diagnoses and conditions which they will encounter in everyday practice.

Designing nursing courses in this way enables students to learn a lot about the disciplinary knowledge of nursing. Attachment, family processes, relationship, role conflict, role performance, and social interaction are some of the key concepts of Domain 7, Role relationship (▶ Fig. 9.4) – they are the "neutral states" that we must understand before we can identify potential or actual problems with these responses.

Understanding *role performance*, for example, as a core concept of nursing practice, requires a strong understanding of anatomy, physiology, pathophysiology (including related medical diagnoses), and responses from other domains that might coincide with problems in balanced nutrition. Once you truly understand the concept of balanced nutrition (the "normal" or neutral state), identifying the abnormal state is much easier because you know what you should be seeing if nutrition was balanced, and if you don't see those data, you start to suspect that there might be a problem (or a risk may exist for a problem to develop). So, developing nursing courses around these core concepts enables nursing faculty to focus on the knowledge of the nursing discipline and then to incorporate related medical diagnoses and/or interdisciplinary concerns in a way that allows nurses to focus first on nursing phenomena and then to bring their specific knowledge to an interdisciplinary view of the patient to improve patient care. This then moves into content on realistic patient outcomes and evidence-based interventions that nurses will utilize (dependent and independent nursing interventions) to provide the best possible care for the patient to achieve outcomes for which nurses have accountability.

9.3.2 Identifying Nursing Diagnoses Outside Area of Expertise

Nurses gain expertise in those nursing diagnoses that they most commonly see in their clinical practice. If your area of interest is reproductive health nursing practice, then your expertise may include such key concepts as *sexual function, childbearing process, breastfeeding,* and *parenting,* just to name a few! But you will deal with patients who, despite being primarily in your care because of a complication of pregnancy, will also have other issues that require your attention. The NANDA-I taxonomy can help you to identify potential diagnoses for these patients and support your clinical reasoning skills by clarifying what assessment data/diagnostic indicators are necessary for quickly, but accurately, diagnosing your patients.

Perhaps, as you are admitting a 36-year old patient, Miss K, with a 34-week pregnancy for the treatment of severe pre-eclampsia, you notice that she is restless and tense. Your patient tells you that she did not receive prenatal care, due to her former partner's domestic violence and stalking; she has been staying at a shelter with her 3-year-old daughter for the last three months. Her parents died from a large mudslide when she was 12, and she grew up in an orphanage. Despite having no relatives or close friends to rely upon for help, Miss K has overcome many difficulties. Her body mass index (BMI) is 38.6. She has chronic hypertension, but has not taken her antihypertensive medication for one year, because she has not been able to afford the prescription. Her current blood pressure is 168/110. She is anxious about the possible emergency delivery.

You have not cared for many patients with a complex background such as you are now encountering with Miss K. You want to reflect her risk and/or problems, but you are not sure which nursing diagnosis is the most accurate for this patient in this situation. By looking at the taxonomy, you can quickly form a "cognitive map" that can help you to find more information on diagnoses of relevance to this patient (▶ Fig. 9.5).

You are concerned about Miss K's response related to her resilience, and a quick review of the taxonomy leads you to Domain 9 (coping/stress tolerance), Class 2 (coping responses). You then see that there are three diagnoses specifically related to resilience, and you can review the definitions and diagnostic indicators to clarify the most appropriate diagnosis for this patient.

Using the taxonomy in this way supports clinical reasoning and helps you to navigate a large volume of information/knowledge (267 diagnoses!) in an effective and efficient manner. A review of the risk factors or the related factors and defining characteristics of these three diagnoses can: (1) provide you with additional data that you need to obtain in order to make an informed decision and/or (2) enable you to compare your assessment with those diagnostic indicators to accurately diagnose your patient.

Think about a recent patient – did you struggle to diagnose his/her human response? Did you find it difficult to know how to identify potential diagnoses? Using the taxonomy can support you in identifying possible diagnoses because of the way the diagnoses are grouped together in classes and domains that represent specific areas of knowledge. Do not forget, however, that *simply looking at the diagnosis label and "picking a diagnosis" is not safe care!* You need to review the definition and diagnostic indicators (defining characteristics, related factors, or risk factors) for each of the potential diagnoses you identify, which will help you to identify what additional data you should collect or if you have enough data to accurately diagnose the patient's human response.

Let us review the case study of Mr. S to understand how you might use the taxonomy to help you to identify potential diagnoses.

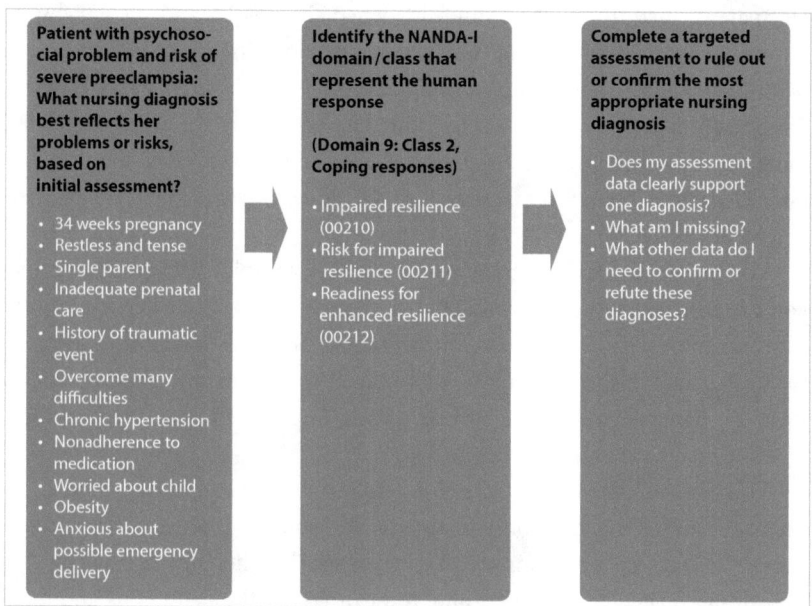

Fig. 9.5 Use of the NANDA-I Taxonomy to identify and validate a nursing diagnosis outside the nurse's area of expertise

Case Study: Mr. S

Let us suppose that your patient, Mr. S, an 87-year-old widower, presents with complaints of severe, shooting pain in his right hip area. He has been living in an assisted living facility for two years, since his wife died, and the staff members there have noticed that he is very agitated and shows signs of severe pain whenever they try to help him walk. They have brought him in to rule out any possible fracture or need for a hip replacement. They note that he had his other hip replaced three years ago, due to osteoporosis. Apparently, the surgery was very successful.

Mr. S has no noticeable edema or bruising to his right hip area, but clearly complains of pain when you palpate the area. He has good lower extremity bilateral peripheral pulses and a lower extremity capillary refill time of 4 seconds. His medical history includes a cerebrovascular attack (stroke) at age 80. According to his medical records, he had initial paralysis on the right side and lost all speech function. He received alteplase IV r-tPA, a tissue plasminogen activator (TPA), and recovered full mobility and speech. He was in an inpatient rehabilitation center for 26 days, received speech, physical and occupational therapy, and cared for himself independently after he was discharged home. He has moderate coronary artery disease, but otherwise no significant medical history. According to the staff member accompanying him, Mr. S has been active until a few weeks ago when he started to complain of pain. He enjoyed ballroom dancing, exercised at the facility on a regular basis, and was frequently seen walking around the complex speaking to people, or taking walks outdoors on the grounds of the complex when the weather was nice. She also indicates he has become less social recently, and has not attended different activities that he normally enjoys. She indicates the staff members have attributed this to his level of discomfort.

What you notice most about Mr. S, however, is that he seems withdrawn, he barely speaks, and rarely makes eye contact. He struggles to answer your questions, and the staff member often jumps in to provide answers rather than allowing him to answer for himself. Although his speech does not appear to be impaired, he seems to be struggling to find answers to even basic questions, such as his age or the year that his wife died.

After completing your assessment and reviewing his history, you believe that Mr. S may be dealing with an issue related to cognition, but this is an area of nursing in which you have little experience; you need some review of potential diagnoses. Since you are considering a cognition issue, you look at the NANDA-I taxonomy to identify the logical location of these diagnoses. You identify that Domain 5, Perception/cognition, deals with the human information processing system including attention, orientation, sensation, perception, cognition, and communication. Because you are considering issues related to cognition, you think this domain will contain diagnoses of relevance to Mr. S.

You then quickly identify Class 4, Cognition. A review of this class leads to the identification of three potential diagnoses: acute confusion, chronic confusion, and impaired memory.

Questions you should ask yourself include: What other human responses should I rule out or consider? What other signs/symptoms, or etiologies, should I look for to confirm this diagnosis?

Once you review the definitions and diagnostic indicators (related factors, defining characteristics, and risk factors), you diagnose Mr. S with chronic confusion (00129).

Some final questions should include: Am I missing anything? Am I diagnosing without sufficient evidence? If you believe you are correct in your diagnosis, your questions move on to: What outcomes can I realistically expect to achieve with Mr. S? What are the evidence-based nursing interventions that I should consider? How will I evaluate whether or not they were effective?

9.4 The NANDA-I Nursing Diagnosis Taxonomy II: A Short History

In 1987, NANDA-I published Taxonomy I, which was structured to reflect nursing theoretical models from North America. In 2002, Taxonomy II was adopted, which was adapted from the Functional Health Patterns assessment framework of Dr. Marjory Gordon. This assessment framework is probably the most used nursing assessment framework around the world.

▶ Table 9.1 demonstrates the domains, classes, and nursing diagnoses and how they are currently located within the NANDA-I Taxonomy II.

Table 9.1   Domains, classes, and nursing diagnoses in the NANDA-I Taxonomy II

Domain / Class / Diagnosis code	Focus of diagnosis	Domain / Class definition; Diagnosis
Domain 1. Health promotion		**The awareness of well-being or normality of function and the strategies used to maintain control of and enhance that well-being or normality of function**
Class 1. Health awareness		**Recognition of normal function and well-being**
00097	Diversional activity engagement	Decreased diversional activity engagement
00262	Health literacy	Readiness for enhanced health literacy
00168	Lifestyle	Sedentary lifestyle

Table 9.1 *(Continued)*

Domain / Class / Diagnosis code	Focus of diagnosis	Domain / Class definition; Diagnosis
Class 2. **Health** **management**		**Identifying, controlling, performing, and integrating activities to maintain health and well-being**
00290	Elopement attempt	Risk for elopement attempt
00257	Frail elderly syndrome	Frail elderly syndrome
00231	Frail elderly syndrome	Risk for frail elderly syndrome
00307	Exercise engagement	Readiness for enhanced exercise engagement
00215	Health	Deficient community health
00188	Health behavior	Risk-prone health behavior
00292	Health maintenance behaviors	Ineffective health maintenance behaviors
00276	Health self-management	Ineffective health self-management
00293	Health self-management	Readiness for enhanced health self-management
00294	Health self-management	Ineffective family health self-management
00300	Home maintenance behaviors	Ineffective home maintenance behaviors
00308	Home maintenance behaviors	Risk for ineffective home maintenance behaviors
00309	Home maintenance behaviors	Readiness for enhanced home maintenance behaviors
00043	Protection	Ineffective protection
Domain 2. **Nutrition**		**The activities of taking in, assimilating, and using nutrients for the purposes of tissue maintenance, tissue repair, and the production of energy**
Class 1. **Ingestion**		**Taking food or nutrients into the body**
00002	Balanced nutrition	Imbalanced nutrition: less than body requirements
00163	Nutrition	Readiness for enhanced nutrition[a]
00216	Breast milk production	Insufficient breast milk production
00104	Breastfeeding	Ineffective breastfeeding
00105	Breastfeeding	Interrupted breastfeeding
00106	Breastfeeding	Readiness for enhanced breastfeeding
00269	Eating dynamics	Ineffective adolescent eating dynamics
00270	Eating dynamics	Ineffective child eating dynamics
00271	Feeding dynamics	Ineffective infant feeding dynamics

Table 9.1 *(Continued)*

Domain / Class / Diagnosis code	Focus of diagnosis	Domain / Class definition; Diagnosis
00232	Obesity	Obesity
00233	Overweight	Overweight
00234	Overweight	Risk for overweight
00295	Suck-swallow response	Ineffective infant suck-swallow response
00103	Swallowing	Impaired swallowing
Class 2. **Digestion**		**The physical and chemical activities that convert foodstuffs into substances suitable for absorption and assimilation**
		None at present time
Class 3. **Absorption**		**The act of taking up nutrients through body tissues**
		None at present time
Class 4. **Metabolism**		**The chemical and physical processes occurring in living organisms and cells for the development and use of protoplasm, the production of waste and energy, with the release of energy for all vital processes**
00179	Blood glucose level	Risk for unstable blood glucose level
00194	Hyperbilirubinemia	Neonatal hyperbilirubinemia
00230	Hyperbilirubinemia	Risk for neonatal hyperbilirubinemia
00178	Liver function	Risk for impaired liver function
00296	Metabolic syndrome	Risk for metabolic syndrome
Class 5. **Hydration**		**The taking in and absorption of fluids and electrolytes**
00195	Electrolyte balance	Risk for electrolyte imbalance
00025	Balanced fluid volume	Risk for imbalanced fluid volume[b]
00027	Fluid volume	Deficient fluid volume
00028	Fluid volume	Risk for deficient fluid volume
00026	Fluid volume	Excess fluid volume
Domain 3. **Elimination and exchange**		**Secretion and excretion of waste products from the body**
Class 1. **Urinary function**		**The process of secretion, reabsorption, and excretion of urine**
00297	Disability-associated incontinence	Disability-associated urinary incontinence
00016	Elimination	Impaired urinary elimination
00310	Incontinence	Mixed urinary incontinence

Table 9.1 *(Continued)*

Domain / Class / Diagnosis code	Focus of diagnosis	Domain / Class definition; Diagnosis
00017	Incontinence	Stress urinary incontinence
00019	Incontinence	Urge urinary incontinence
00022	Incontinence	Risk for urge urinary incontinence
00023	Retention	Urinary retention
00322	Retention	Risk for urinary retention
Class 2. Gastrointestinal function		**The process of absorption and excretion of the end products of digestion**
00011	Constipation	Constipation
00015	Constipation	Risk for constipation
00012	Constipation	Perceived constipation
00235	Functional constipation	Chronic functional constipation
00236	Functional constipation	Risk for chronic functional constipation
00319	Continence	Impaired bowel continence
00013	Diarrhea	Diarrhea
00196	Gastrointestinal motility	Dysfunctional gastrointestinal motility
00197	Gastrointestinal motility	Risk for dysfunctional gastrointestinal motility
Class 3. Integumentary function		**The process of secretion and excretion through the skin**
		None at present time
Class 4. Respiratory function		**The process of exchange of gases and removal of the end products of metabolism**
00030	Gas exchange	Impaired gas exchange
Domain 4. Activity/rest		**The production, conservation, expenditure, or balance of energy resources**
Class 1. Sleep/rest		**Slumber, repose, ease, relaxation, or inactivity**
00095	Insomnia	Insomnia
00096	Sleep	Sleep deprivation
00165	Sleep	Readiness for enhanced sleep
00198	Sleep pattern	Disturbed sleep pattern
Class 2. Activity/exercise		**Moving parts of the body (mobility), doing work, or performing actions often (but not always) against resistance**
00298	Activity tolerance	Decreased activity tolerance
00299	Activity tolerance	Risk for decreased activity tolerance

Table 9.1 (Continued)

Domain / Class / Diagnosis code	Focus of diagnosis	Domain / Class definition; Diagnosis
00040	Disuse syndrome	Risk for disuse syndrome
00091	Mobility	Impaired bed mobility
00085	Mobility	Impaired physical mobility
00089	Mobility	Impaired wheelchair mobility
00237	Sitting	Impaired sitting
00238	Standing	Impaired standing
00090	Transfer ability	Impaired transfer ability
00088	Walking	Impaired walking
Class 3. **Energy balance**		**A dynamic state of harmony between intake and expenditure of resources**
00273	Balanced energy field	Imbalanced energy field
00093	Fatigue	Fatigue
00154	Wandering	Wandering
Class 4. **Cardiovascular/pulmonary responses**		**Cardiopulmonary mechanisms that support activity/rest**
00032	Breathing pattern	Ineffective breathing pattern
00029	Cardiac output	Decreased cardiac output
00240	Cardiac output	Risk for decreased cardiac output
00311	Cardiovascular function	Risk for impaired cardiovascular function
00278	Lymphedema self-management	Ineffective lymphedema self-management
00281	Lymphedema self-management	Risk for ineffective lymphedema self-management
00033	Spontaneous ventilation	Impaired spontaneous ventilation
00267	Stable blood pressure	Risk for unstable blood pressure
00291	Thrombosis	Risk for thrombosis
00200	Tissue perfusion	Risk for decreased cardiac tissue perfusion
00201	Tissue perfusion	Risk for ineffective cerebral tissue perfusion
00204	Tissue perfusion	Ineffective peripheral tissue perfusion
00228	Tissue perfusion	Risk for ineffective peripheral tissue perfusion
00034	Ventilatory weaning response	Dysfunctional ventilatory weaning response
00318	Ventilatory weaning response	Dysfunctional adult ventilatory weaning response

Table 9.1 *(Continued)*

Domain / Class / Diagnosis code	Focus of diagnosis	Domain / Class definition; Diagnosis
Class 5. **Self-care**		**Ability to perform activities to care for one's body and bodily functions**
00108	Bathing self-care	Bathing self-care deficit
00109	Dressing self-care	Dressing self-care deficit
00102	Feeding self-care	Feeding self-care deficit
00110	Toileting self-care	Toileting self-care deficit
00182	Self-care	Readiness for enhanced self-care
00193	Self-neglect	Self-neglect
Domain 5. **Perception/** **cognition**		**The human processing system including attention, orientation, sensation, perception, cognition, and communication**
Class 1. **Attention**		**Mental readiness to notice or observe**
00123	Unilateral neglect	Unilateral neglect
Class 2. **Orientation**		**Awareness of time, place, and person**
		None at present time
Class 3. **Sensation/** **perception**		**Receiving information through the senses of touch, taste, smell, vision, hearing, and kinesthesia, and the comprehension of sensory data resulting in naming, associating, and/or pattern recognition**
		None at present time
Class 4. **Cognition**		**Use of memory, learning, thinking, problem-solving, abstraction, judgment, insight, intellectual capacity, calculation, and language**
00128	Confusion	Acute confusion
00173	Confusion	Risk for acute confusion
00129	Confusion	Chronic confusion
00251	Emotional control	Labile emotional control
00222	Impulse control	Ineffective impulse control
00126	Knowledge	Deficient knowledge
00161	Knowledge	Readiness for enhanced knowledge
00131	Memory	Impaired memory
00279	Thought process	Disturbed thought process
Class 5. **Communication**		**Sending and receiving verbal and non-verbal information**
00157	Communication	Readiness for enhanced communication
00051	Verbal communication	Impaired verbal communication

Table 9.1 *(Continued)*

Domain / Class / Diagnosis code	Focus of diagnosis	Domain / Class definition; Diagnosis
Domain 6. Self-perception		Awareness about the self
Class 1. Self-concept		The perception(s) about the total self
00124	Hope	Hopelessness
00185	Hope	Readiness for enhanced hope
00174	Human dignity	Risk for compromised human dignity
00121	Personal identity	Disturbed personal identity
00225	Personal identity	Risk for disturbed personal identity
00167	Self-concept	Readiness for enhanced self-concept
Class 2. Self-esteem		Assessment of one's own worth, capability, significance, and success
00119	Self-esteem	Chronic low self-esteem
00224	Self-esteem	Risk for chronic low self-esteem
00120	Self-esteem	Situational low self-esteem
00153	Self-esteem	Risk for situational low self-esteem
Class 3. Body image		A mental image of one's own body
00118	Body image	Disturbed body image
Domain 7. Role relationship		The positive and negative connections or associations between people or groups of people and the means by which those connections are demonstrated
Class 1. Caregiving roles		Socially expected behavior patterns by people providing care who are not health care professionals
00056	Parenting	Impaired parenting
00057	Parenting	Risk for impaired parenting
00164	Parenting	Readiness for enhanced parenting
00061	Role strain	Caregiver role strain
00062	Role strain	Risk for caregiver role strain
Class 2. Family relationships		Associations of people who are biologically related or related by choice
00058	Attachment	Risk for impaired attachment
00283	Disturbed family identity syndrome	Disturbed family identity syndrome
00284	Disturbed family identity syndrome	Risk for disturbed family identity syndrome

Table 9.1 *(Continued)*

Domain / Class / Diagnosis code	Focus of diagnosis	Domain / Class definition; Diagnosis
00063	Family processes	Dysfunctional family processes
00060	Family processes	Interrupted family processes
00159	Family processes	Readiness for enhanced family processes
Class 3. Role performance		**Quality of functioning in socially expected behavior patterns**
00223	Relationship	Ineffective relationship
00229	Relationship	Risk for ineffective relationship
00207	Relationship	Readiness for enhanced relationship
00064	Role conflict	Parental role conflict
00055	Role performance	Ineffective role performance
00052	Social interaction	Impaired social interaction
Domain 8. Sexuality		**Sexual identity, sexual function, and reproduction**
Class 1. Sexual identity		**The state of being a specific person in regard to sexuality and/or gender**
		None at present time
Class 2. Sexual function		**The capacity or ability to participate in sexual activities**
00059	Sexual function	Sexual dysfunction
00065	Sexuality pattern	Ineffective sexuality pattern
Class 3. Reproduction		**Any process by which human beings are produced**
00221	Childbearing process	Ineffective childbearing process
00227	Childbearing process	Risk for ineffective childbearing process
00208	Childbearing process	Readiness for enhanced childbearing process
00209	Maternal-fetal dyad	Risk for disturbed maternal-fetal dyad
Domain 9. Coping/stress tolerance		**Contending with life events/life processes**
Class 1. Post-trauma responses		**Reactions occurring after physical or psychological trauma**
00260	Immigration transition	Risk for complicated immigration transition
00141	Post-trauma syndrome	Post-trauma syndrome
00145	Post-trauma syndrome	Risk for post-trauma syndrome
00142	Rape-trauma syndrome	Rape-trauma syndrome
00114	Relocation stress syndrome	Relocation stress syndrome

Table 9.1 *(Continued)*

Domain / Class / Diagnosis code	Focus of diagnosis	Domain / Class definition; Diagnosis
00149	Relocation stress syndrome	Risk for relocation stress syndrome
Class 2. Coping responses		**The process of managing environmental stress**
00199	Activity planning	Ineffective activity planning
00226	Activity planning	Risk for ineffective activity planning
00146	Anxiety	Anxiety
00071	Coping	Defensive coping
00069	Coping	Ineffective coping
00158	Coping	Readiness for enhanced coping
00077	Coping	Ineffective community coping
00076	Coping	Readiness for enhanced community coping
00074	Coping	Compromised family coping
00073	Coping	Disabled family coping
00075	Coping	Readiness for enhanced family coping
00147	Death anxiety	Death anxiety
00072	Denial	Ineffective denial
00148	Fear	Fear
00301	Grieving	Maladaptive grieving
00302	Grieving	Risk for maladaptive grieving
00285	Grieving	Readiness for enhanced grieving
00241	Mood regulation	Impaired mood regulation
00125	Power	Powerlessness
00152	Power	Risk for powerlessness
00187	Power	Readiness for enhanced power
00210	Resilience	Impaired resilience
00211	Resilience	Risk for impaired resilience
00212	Resilience	Readiness for enhanced resilience
00137	Sorrow	Chronic sorrow
00177	Stress	Stress overload
Class 3. Neurobehavioral stress		**Behavioral responses reflecting nerve and brain function**
00258	Acute substance withdrawal syndrome	Acute substance withdrawal syndrome
00259	Acute substance withdrawal syndrome	Risk for acute substance withdrawal syndrome

Table 9.1 *(Continued)*

Domain / Class / Diagnosis code	Focus of diagnosis	Domain / Class definition; Diagnosis
00009	Autonomic dysreflexia	Autonomic dysreflexia
00010	Autonomic dysreflexia	Risk for autonomic dysreflexia
00264	Neonatal abstinence syndrome	Neonatal abstinence syndrome
00116	Organized behavior	Disorganized infant behavior
00115	Organized behavior	Risk for disorganized infant behavior
00117	Organized behavior	Readiness for enhanced organized infant behavior
Domain 10. Life principles		**Principles underlying conduct, thought, and behavior about acts, customs, or institutions viewed as being true or having intrinsic worth**
Class 1. Values		**The identification and ranking of preferred modes of conduct or end states**
		None at present time
Class 2. Beliefs		**Opinions, expectations, or judgments about acts, customs, or institutions viewed as being true or having intrinsic worth**
00068	Spiritual well-being	Readiness for enhanced spiritual well-being
Class 3. Value/belief/action congruence		**The correspondence or balance achieved among values, beliefs, and actions**
00184	Decision-making	Readiness for enhanced decision-making
00083	Decisional conflict	Decisional conflict
00242	Emancipated decision-making	Impaired emancipated decision-making
00244	Emancipated decision-making	Risk for impaired emancipated decision-making
00243	Emancipated decision-making	Readiness for enhanced emancipated decision-making
00175	Moral distress	Moral distress
00169	Religiosity	Impaired religiosity
00170	Religiosity	Risk for impaired religiosity
00171	Religiosity	Readiness for enhanced religiosity
00066	Spiritual distress	Spiritual distress
00067	Spiritual distress	Risk for spiritual distress

Table 9.1 *(Continued)*

Domain / Class / Diagnosis code	Focus of diagnosis	Domain / Class definition; Diagnosis
Domain 11. Safety/protection		**Freedom from danger, physical injury, or immune system damage; preservation from loss; and protection of safety and security**
Class 1. Infection		**Host responses following pathogenic invasion**
00004	Infection	Risk for infection
00266	Surgical site infection	Risk for surgical site infection
Class 2. Physical injury		**Bodily harm or hurt**
00031	Airway clearance	Ineffective airway clearance
00039	Aspiration	Risk for aspiration
00206	Bleeding	Risk for bleeding
00048	Dentition	Impaired dentition
00219	Dry eye	Risk for dry eye
00277	Dry eye self-management	Ineffective dry eye self-management
00261	Dry mouth	Risk for dry mouth
00303	Falls	Risk for adult falls
00306	Falls	Risk for child falls
00035	Injury	Risk for injury[c]
00245	Injury	Risk for corneal injury
00320	Injury	Nipple-areolar complex injury
00321	Injury	Risk for nipple-areolar complex injury
00250	Injury	Risk for urinary tract injury
00087	Perioperative positioning injury	Risk for perioperative positioning injury[c]
00220	Thermal injury	Risk for thermal injury[c]
00045	Mucous membrane integrity	Impaired oral mucous membrane integrity
00247	Mucous membrane integrity	Risk for impaired oral mucous membrane integrity
00086	Neurovascular function	Risk for peripheral neurovascular dysfunction
00038	Physical trauma	Risk for physical trauma
00213	Trauma	Risk for vascular trauma
00312	Pressure injury	Adult pressure injury
00304	Pressure injury	Risk for adult pressure injury
00313	Pressure injury	Child pressure injury

Table 9.1 *(Continued)*

Domain / Class / Diagnosis code	Focus of diagnosis	Domain / Class definition; Diagnosis
00286	Pressure injury	Risk for child pressure injury
00287	Pressure injury	Neonatal pressure injury
00288	Pressure injury	Risk for neonatal pressure injury
00205	Shock	Risk for shock
00046	Skin integrity	Impaired skin integrity
00047	Skin integrity	Risk for impaired skin integrity
00156	Sudden death	Risk for sudden infant death
00036	Suffocation	Risk for suffocation
00100	Surgical recovery	Delayed surgical recovery
00246	Surgical recovery	Risk for delayed surgical recovery
00044	Tissue integrity	Impaired tissue integrity
00248	Tissue integrity	Risk for impaired tissue integrity
Class 3. Violence		**The exertion of excessive force or power to cause injury or abuse**
00272	Female genital mutilation	Risk for female genital mutilation
00138	Other-directed violence	Risk for other-directed violence
00140	Self-directed violence	Risk for self-directed violence
00151	Self-mutilation	Self-mutilation
00139	Self-mutilation	Risk for self-mutilation
00289	Suicidal behavior	Risk for suicidal behavior
Class 4. Environmental hazards		**Sources of danger in the surroundings**
00181	Contamination	Contamination
00180	Contamination	Risk for contamination
00265	Occupational injury	Risk for occupational injury
00037	Poisoning	Risk for poisoning
Class 5. Defensive processes		**The processes by which the self protects itself from the nonself**
00218	Adverse reaction to iodinated contrast media	Risk for adverse reaction to iodinated contrast media
00217	Allergy reaction	Risk for allergy reaction
00042	Latex allergy reaction	Risk for latex allergy reaction
Class 6. Thermoregulation		**The physiological process of regulating heat and energy within the body for purposes of protecting the organism**
00007	Hyperthermia	Hyperthermia
00006	Hypothermia	Hypothermia

Table 9.1 (Continued)

Domain / Class / Diagnosis code	Focus of diagnosis	Domain / Class definition; Diagnosis
00253	Hypothermia	Risk for hypothermia
00280	Hypothermia	Neonatal hypothermia
00282	Hypothermia	Risk for neonatal hypothermia
00254	Perioperative hypothermia	Risk for perioperative hypothermia
00008	Thermoregulation	Ineffective thermoregulation
00274	Thermoregulation	Risk for ineffective thermoregulation
Domain 12. Comfort		**Sense of mental, physical, or social well-being or ease**
Class 1. Physical comfort		**Sense of well-being or ease and/or freedom from pain**
00214	Comfort	Impaired comfort
00183	Comfort	Readiness for enhanced comfort
00134	Nausea	Nausea
00132	Pain	Acute pain
00133	Pain	Chronic pain
00255	Chronic pain syndrome	Chronic pain syndrome[d]
00256	Labor pain	Labor pain[d]
Class 2. Environmental comfort		**Sense of well-being or ease in/with one's environment**
00214	Comfort	Impaired comfort
00183	Comfort	Readiness for enhanced comfort
Class 3. Social comfort		**Sense of well-being or ease with one's social situation**
00214	Comfort	Impaired comfort
00183	Comfort	Readiness for enhanced comfort
00054	Loneliness	Risk for loneliness
00053	Social isolation	Social isolation
Domain 13. Growth/ development		**Age-appropriate increases in physical dimensions, maturation of organ systems, and/or progression through the developmental milestones**
Class 1. Growth		**Increase in physical dimensions or maturity of organ systems**
		None at present time

Table 9.1 *(Continued)*

Domain / Class / Diagnosis code	Focus of diagnosis	Domain / Class definition; Diagnosis
Class 2. Development		**Progress or regression through a sequence of recognized milestones in life**
00314	Development	Delayed child development
00305	Development	Risk for delayed child development
00315	Motor development	Delayed infant motor development
00316	Motor development	Risk for delayed infant motor development

[a] The editors acknowledge this concept is not in alphabetical order; a decision was made to maintain all "nutrition" diagnoses in sequential order.

[b] The editors acknowledge this concept is not in alphabetical order; a decision was made to maintain all "fluid volume" diagnoses in sequential order.

[c] The editors acknowledge this concept is not in alphabetical order; a decision was made to maintain all "injury" diagnoses in sequential order.

[d] The editors acknowledge this concept is not in alphabetical order; a decision was made to maintain all "pain" diagnoses in sequential order.

9.5 References

Abbott A. The Systems of Professions. Chicago, IL: The University of Chicago Press, 1988.

Quammen D. A passion for order. National Geographic Magazine. 2007. Available at: ngm.nationalgeographic.com/print/2007/06/Linnaeus-name-giver/david-quammen-text (retrieved November 1, 2013).

Von Krogh G. Taxonomy III Proposal. NANDA International Latin American Symposium. Sao Paulo, Brazil. May, 2011.

10 Specifications and Definitions Within the NANDA International Taxonomy of Nursing Diagnoses

T. Heather Herdman, Silvia Caldeira

10.1 Structure of Taxonomy II

Taxonomy is defined as the "system for naming and organizing things … into groups that share similar qualities" (Cambridge Dictionary Online, 2017). Within the taxonomy, the domains are "an area of interest or an area over which one has control"; and the classes are "a group … with similar structure" (Cambridge Dictionary Online, 2017).

We can adapt the definition for a nursing diagnosis taxonomy; specifically, we are concerned with the orderly classification of diagnostic foci of concern to nursing, according to their presumed natural relationships. Taxonomy II has three levels: domains, classes, and nursing diagnoses. ▶ Fig. 9.3 depicts the organization of domains and classes in Taxonomy II; ▶ Table 9.1 shows Taxonomy II with its 13 domains, 47 classes, and 267 current diagnoses.

The Taxonomy II code structure is a 32-bit integer (or if the user's database uses another notation, the code structure is a five-digit code). This structure provides for the stability, or growth and development, of the classification structure by avoiding the need to change codes when new diagnoses, refinements, and revisions are added. New codes are assigned to newly approved diagnoses.

Taxonomy II has a code structure that is compliant with recommendations from the National Library of Medicine (NLM) concerning health care terminology codes. The NLM recommends that codes do not contain information about the classified concept, as did the Taxonomy I code structure, which included information about the location and the level of the diagnosis.

The NANDA-I terminology is a recognized nursing language that meets the criteria established by the Committee for Nursing Practice Information Infrastructure (CNPII) of the American Nurses Association (ANA) (Lundberg et al., 2008). The benefit of a recognized nursing language is the indication that the classification system is accepted as supporting nursing practice by providing clinically useful terminology. The terminology is also registered with Health Level Seven International (HL7), a health care informatics standard, as a terminology to be used in identifying nursing diagnoses in electronic messages among clinical information systems (www.HL7.org).

10.2 NANDA-I Taxonomy II: A Multiaxial System

The NANDA-I diagnoses are concepts constructed by means of a multiaxial system. An axis, for the purpose of the NANDA-I Taxonomy II, is operationally defined as a dimension of the human response that is considered in the diagnostic process. There are seven axes. The *NANDA-I Model of a Nursing Diagnosis* displays the seven axes and their relationship to each other.

- Axis 1: the focus of the diagnosis
- Axis 2: subject of the diagnosis (individual, family, group, caregiver, community, etc.)
- Axis 3: judgment (impaired, ineffective, etc.)
- Axis 4: location (oral, peripheral, cerebral, etc.)
- Axis 5: age (neonate, infant, child, adult, etc.)
- Axis 6: time (chronic, acute, intermittent)
- Axis 7: the status of the diagnosis.

The axes are represented in the labels of the nursing diagnoses through their values. In some cases they are named explicitly, such as with the diagnoses *ineffective community coping* and *dysfunctional family processes*, in which the subject of the diagnosis is named using the two values "community" and "family" taken from Axis 2 (subject of the diagnosis). "Ineffective" and "dysfunctional" are two of the values contained in Axis 3 (judgment).

In some cases, the axis is implicit, as is the case with the diagnosis *ineffective sexuality pattern*, in which the subject of the diagnosis (Axis 2) is always the patient. In some instances, an axis may not be pertinent to a diagnosis, and therefore is not part of the nursing diagnostic label. For example, the time axis may not be relevant to every diagnosis. In the case of diagnoses without explicit identification of the subject of the diagnosis, it may be helpful to remember that NANDA-I defines a patient as "an individual, family, caregiver, group, or community".

Axis 1 (the focus of the diagnosis) and Axis 3 (judgment) are essential components of a nursing diagnosis. In some cases, however, the focus of the diagnosis contains the judgment (e.g., *fear*); in these cases, the judgment is not explicitly separated from the focus of the diagnosis in the diagnostic label. Axis 2 (subject of the diagnosis) is also essential, although, as described earlier, it may be implied and therefore not included in the label. The Diagnosis Development Committee requires these axes for submission; the other axes may be used where relevant for clarity.

A recent basic statistical analysis of diagnostic labels demonstrated that the 2018–2020 NANDA-I nursing diagnoses (ND) used Axis 1 (focus) in association with different terms from the other axes, except in situations in which the ND label was a single word (e.g., anxiety, fear, obesity). Axis 3 (judgment) was the second most used axis, contributing to the construction of 82% of the ND. The remaining axes were used to a lesser extent, in 18% of the ND (Miguel, Romeiro, Martins, Casaleiro, Caldeira, & Herdman, 2019).

Although there were some additions in the 2021–2023 release of the NANDA-I terminology, there remain few ND which address the elderly ($n = 2$), child and adolescent ($n = 9$), and neonatal ($n=4$) populations within the ND label. Therefore, it seems the adequacy of ND to such populations, whose specificities make them unique when comparing them to the general population, may remain limited. The absence of a clinical picture consistent with those clients' reality – including differentiated defining characteristics, related and/or risk factors – and the complexity of decisions nurses undertake in caring for them, leads us to think that ND labels are far from being thoroughly developed (Miguel, Romeiro, Martins, Casaleiro, Caldeira, & Herdman, 2019).

The adjustments of ND labels to particular contexts, environments, and populations – implicitly including the rights of clinical reasoning advocated by Levett-Jones et al. (2010) – could raise the quality of nursing care. In addition, it would provide the necessary evidence base for the NANDA-I terminology, corroborating the ND hierarchy within taxonomy II, or lead to an appeal for more adequate and clear domains and classes (Miguel, Romeiro, Martins, Casaleiro, Caldeira, & Herdman, 2019).

NANDA-I supports developments in the specificity of ND labels, specifically regarding its multiaxial aspects, to increase the specificity and accuracy of the diagnostic process, which is known to be the core of clinical reasoning and practice.

10.3 Definitions of the Axes

10.3.1 Axis 1: The Focus of the Diagnosis

The focus of the diagnosis is the principal element or the fundamental and essential part, the root, of the diagnostic concept. It describes the "human response" that is the core of the diagnosis.

The focus of the diagnosis may consist of one or more nouns. When more than one noun is used (e.g., *mood regulation*), each one contributes a unique meaning to the focus of the diagnosis, as if the two were a single noun; the meaning of the combined term, however, is different from when the nouns are stated separately. Frequently, a noun (*conflict*) may be used with an adjective (*decisional*) to denote the focus of the diagnosis *decisional conflict*.

In some cases, the focus of the diagnosis and the diagnostic concept are one and the same, as is seen with the diagnosis of *hyperthermia (00007)*. This occurs when the nursing diagnosis is stated at its most clinically useful level and the separation of the focus of the diagnosis adds no meaningful level of abstraction. It can be very difficult to determine exactly what should be considered the focus of the diagnosis. For example, using the diagnoses of *impaired bowel continence* (00319) and *stress urinary incontinence* (00017), the question becomes: Is the focus of the diagnosis *incontinence* alone, or are there two foci – *bowel incontinence* and *urinary incontinence*? In this instance, *incontinence* is the focus and the location terms (Axis 4) of *bowel* and *urinary* provide more clarification about the focus. However, *incontinence* in and of itself is a judgment term that can stand alone, and so it becomes the focus of the diagnosis regardless of location.

In some cases, however, removing the location (Axis 4) from the diagnostic focus would prevent it from providing meaning to nursing practice. For example, if we look at the focus of the diagnosis *risk for female genital mutilation*, is the focus of the diagnosis *genital mutilation* or simply *mutilation*? Or if you look at the diagnosis *impaired skin integrity*, is the focus *integrity* or *skin integrity*? Decisions about what constitutes the essence of the focus of the diagnosis, then, are made on the basis of what helps to identify the nursing practice implication and whether or not the term indicates a human response. *Mutilation* could refer to an act or instance of destroying, removing, or severely damaging a limb – so it is important to identify *female genital mutilation* as the diagnostic focus. Similarly, *integrity* can mean the quality of being honest and having strong moral principles – again, these are characteristics but not human responses, and are completely unrelated to the diagnosis of impaired skin integrity; *skin integrity*, however, refers to the health of the skin, and is a human response. In some cases, the focus may seem similar, but is in fact quite distinct: *other-directed violence* and *self-directed violence* are two different human responses, and therefore must be identified separately in terms of diagnostic foci within Taxonomy II. The diagnostic foci of the NANDA-I nursing diagnoses are shown in ▶ Table 10.1.

10.3.2 Axis 2: Subject of the Diagnosis

The subject of the diagnosis is defined as the person(s) for whom a nursing diagnosis is determined. The terms in Axis 2 are individual, caregiver, family, group, and community, representing the NANDA-I definition of "patient":

- *Individual*: A single human being distinct from others, a person.

of the Axes

Diagnostic foci of the NANDA-I nursing diagnoses

- ...nning
- ...rance
- ...ance withdrawal syndrome
- Adverse reaction to iodinated contrast media
- Airway clearance
- Allergy reaction
- Anxiety
- Aspiration
- Attachment
- Autonomic dysreflexia
- Balanced energy field
- Balanced fluid volume
- Balanced nutrition
- Bathing self-care
- Bleeding
- Blood glucose level
- Body image
- Breast milk production
- Breastfeeding
- Breathing pattern
- Cardiac output
- Cardiovascular function
- Childbearing process
- Chronic pain syndrome
- Comfort
- Communication
- Confusion
- Constipation
- Contamination
- Continence
- Coping
- Death anxiety
- Decision-making
- Decisional conflict
- Denial
- Dentition
- Development
- Diarrhea
- Disability-associated incontinence
- Disturbed family identity syndrome
- Disuse syndrome
- Diversional activity engagement
- Dressing self-care
- Dry eye
- Dry eye self-management
- Dry mouth
- Eating dynamics
- Electrolyte balance
- Elimination
- Elopement attempt
- Emancipated decision-making
- Emotional control
- Exercise engagement
- Falls
- Family processes

- Fatigue
- Fear
- Feeding dynamics
- Feeding self-care
- Female genital mutilation
- Fluid volume
- Frail elderly syndrome
- Functional constipation
- Gas exchange
- Gastrointestinal motility
- Grieving
- Health
- Health behavior
- Health literacy
- Health maintenance behaviors
- Health self-management
- Home maintenance behaviors
- Hope
- Human dignity
- Hyperbilirubinemia
- Hyperthermia
- Hypothermia
- Immigration transition
- Impulse control
- Incontinence
- Infection
- Injury
- Insomnia
- Knowledge
- Labor pain
- Latex allergy reaction
- Lifestyle
- Liver function
- Loneliness
- Lymphedema self-management
- Maternal-fetal dyad
- Memory
- Metabolic syndrome
- Mobility
- Mood regulation
- Moral distress
- Motor development
- Mucous membrane integrity
- Nausea
- Neonatal abstinence syndrome
- Neurovascular function
- Nutrition
- Obesity
- Occupational injury
- Organized behavior
- Other-directed violence
- Overweight
- Pain
- Parenting
- Perioperative hypothermia
- Perioperative positioning injury
- Personal identity
- Physical trauma

- Poisoning
- Post-trauma syndrome
- Power
- Pressure injury
- Protection
- Rape-trauma syndrome
- Relationship
- Religiosity
- Relocation stress syndrome
- Resilience
- Retention
- Role conflict
- Role performance
- Role strain
- Self-care
- Self-concept
- Self-directed violence
- Self-esteem
- Self-mutilation
- Self-neglect
- Sexual function
- Sexuality pattern
- Shock
- Sitting
- Skin integrity
- Sleep
- Sleep pattern
- Social interaction
- Social isolation
- Sorrow
- Spiritual distress
- Spiritual well-being
- Spontaneous ventilation
- Stable blood pressure
- Standing
- Stress
- Suck-swallow response
- Sudden death
- Suffocation
- Suicidal behavior
- Surgical recovery
- Surgical site infection
- Swallowing
- Thermal injury
- Thermoregulation
- Thought process
- Thrombosis
- Tissue integrity
- Tissue perfusion
- Toileting self-care
- Transfer ability
- Trauma
- Unilateral neglect
- Ventilatory weaning response
- Verbal communication
- Walking
- Wandering

- *Caregiver*: A family member or helper who regularly looks after a child or a sick, elderly, or disabled person.
- *Family*: Two or more people having continuous or sustained relationships, perceiving reciprocal obligations, sensing common meaning, and sharing certain obligations toward others; related by blood and/or choice.
- *Group*: A number of people with shared characteristics.
- *Community*: A group of people living in the same locale under the same governance. Examples include neighborhoods and cities.

When the subject of the diagnosis is not explicitly stated, it becomes the individual by default. However, it is perfectly appropriate to consider such diagnoses for the other subjects of the diagnosis as well. The diagnosis *fear* (00148) could be applied to an individual who has a learned response to threat and is in an unfamiliar setting, separated from her support system, which is evidenced by her experiencing feelings of dread, panic, and terror, and suffers from fatigue, change in physiological response, and anorexia. It could also be appropriate for a community that has experienced consistent violence (e.g., ongoing war, gang violence, etc.), and whose members have insufficient control over their environment and insufficient resources to combat the issues within the community, and whose residents are experiencing distressing symptoms such as apprehensiveness, decrease in productivity, avoidance behaviors, increase in alertness, and focus narrowed to the source of fear.

10.3.3 Axis 3: Judgment
A judgment is a descriptor or modifier that limits or specifies the meaning of the focus of the diagnosis. The focus of the diagnosis, together with the nurse's judgment about it, forms the diagnosis. All the definitions used are found in the Oxford Lexico (Oxford University Press, 2019), unless otherwise specified. The values in Axis 3 are found in ▸ Table 10.2.

10.3.4 Axis 4: Location
Location describes the parts/regions of the body and/or their related functions – all tissues, organs, anatomical sites, or structures. All the definitions used are found in the *Oxford* Lexico (Oxford University Press, 2019), unless otherwise stated. The terms in Axis 4 are shown in ▸ Table 10.3.

10.3.5 Axis 5: Age
Age refers to the age group of the person who is the subject of the diagnosis (Axis 2). The terms in Axis 5 are noted below, with all definitions, *except* that

Table 10.2 Definitions of judgment terms for Axis 3, NANDA-I Taxonomy II

Judgment	Definition
Complicated	Consisting of many interconnecting parts or elements; intricate; involving many different and confusing aspects; involving complications
Compromised	Cause to become vulnerable or function less effectively
Decreased	Make or become smaller or fewer in size, amount, intensity, or degree
Defensive	Used or intended to defend or protect; anxious to challenge or avoid criticism
Deficient/deficit	Not having enough of a specified quality or ingredient; lacking some elements or characteristics
Delayed	Late, slow, deferred, or postponed
Deprivation	Damaging lack of material benefits considered to be basic necessities in a society; lack or denial of something considered to be a necessity
Disabled	Limited in movements, senses, or activities
Disorganized	Not properly planned and controlled; unable to plan one's activities efficiently
Disturbed	Having had its normal pattern or function disrupted; suffering or resulting from emotion and mental health problems
Dysfunctional	Not operating normally or properly; deviating from the norms of social behavior in a way regarded as bad
Emancipated	Free from legal, social, or political restrictions
Enhanced	Intensified, increased, or further improved the quality, value, or extent of
Excess	An amount of something that is more than necessary, permitted, or desirable
Functional	Of or having a special activity, purpose, or task; relating to the way in which something works or operates
Imbalanced	Lack of proportion or relation between corresponding things
Impaired	Weakened or damaged (something, especially a faculty or function)
Inadequate	Not having enough of a specified quality or ingredient; lacking some elements or characteristics
Ineffective	Not producing any significant or desired effect
Insufficient	Lacking quantity; not enough
Interrupted	To stop something from happening for a short period (Cambridge Dictionary Online)
Labile	Liable to change; easily altered; of or characterized by emotions that are easily aroused or freely expressed, and that tend to alter quickly and spontaneously; emotionally unstable

Table 10.2 (Continued)

Judgment	Definition
Low	Below average in amount, extent, or intensity; small; containing smaller quantities than usual of a specified ingredient; ranking below other people or things in importance or class
Maladaptive	Not adjusting adequately or appropriately to the environment or situation
Mixed	Consisting of different qualities or elements
Overload	Give too much of something, typically something undesirable; put too great a demand on
Perceived	Became aware or conscious (of something); came to realize or understand; became aware (of something) by the use of one of the senses, especially that of sight; interpret or look on (someone or something) in a particular way
Readiness for	The state of being fully prepared for something; willingness to do something; immediacy, quickness, or promptness
Risk for	Situation involving exposure to danger; possibility that something unpleasant or unwelcome will happen
Risk-prone	Propensity to be attracted to, or the willingness to tolerate, options that entail a potentially high risk of loss (Dictionary of the American Psychological Association, 2020)
Sedentary	Tending to spend much time seated; somewhat inactive; characterized by much sitting and little physical exercise
Situational	Related to or dependent on a set of circumstances or state of affairs; relating to the location and surroundings of a place
Unstable	Prone to change, fail, or give way; not stable; prone to psychiatric problems or sudden changes of mood
Urge	A strong desire or impulse.

of older adult and aged adult, being drawn from the World Health Organization (2013).

- *Fetus*: unborn human more than 8 weeks after conception, until birth
- *Neonate*: person < 28 days of age
- *Infant*: child < 1 year of age
- *Child*: person ≤ 19 years unless national law defines a person to be an adult at an earlier age
- *Adolescent*: person 10 to 19 years of age, inclusive
- *Adult*: person > 19 years of age unless national law defines a person as being an adult at an earlier age
- *Older adult*: person 65–84 years of age
- *Aged adult*: person ≥ 85 years of age.

Table 10.3 Locations and their definitions in Axis 4, NANDA-I Taxonomy II

Term	Definition
Body	Physical structure, including the bones, flesh, and organs, of a person; the physical and mortal aspect of a person as opposed to the soul or spirit
Bowel	Part of the alimentary canal below the stomach; the intestine
Breast	Either of the two soft, protruding organs on the upper front of a woman's body which secrete milk after childbirth; the less-developed part of a man's body corresponding with a woman's breast; a person's chest
Cardiac	Relating to the heart; relating to the part of the stomach nearest the esophagus.
Cardiovascular	Relating to the heart and blood vessels
Cerebral	Of the cerebrum of the brain; intellectual rather than emotional or physical
Eye	One of a pair of globular organs of sight in the human head through which people see
Gastrointestinal	Relating to the stomach and the intestines
Genital	A person's external organs of reproduction
Liver	Large lobed glandular organ in the abdomen, involved in many metabolic processes
Lymph	A colourless fluid containing white blood cells, which bathes the tissues and drains through the lymphatic system into the bloodstream
Mouth	Opening and cavity in the lower part of the human face, surrounded by the lips, through which food is taken in and from which speech and other vocal sounds are emitted
Mucous membranes	Epithelial tissues which secrete mucus and line many body cavities and tubular organs including the gut and respiratory passages
Neurovascular	Containing neural and vascular structures; of or relating to the nervous system and the vascular systems, or their interactions
Nipple-areolar complex	A pigmented area on the breast mound with an elevated structure in the center; the primary landmark of the breast (Nimboriboonporn & Chuthapisith, 2014)
Oral	Relating to the mouth
Peripheral	Near the surface of the body, with special reference to the circulation and nervous system
Skin	The thin layer of tissue forming the natural outer covering of the body
Tissue	Any of the distinct types of material of which humans are made, consisting of specialized cells and their products
Tract	A major passage in the body, large bundle of nerve fibers, or other continuous elongated anatomical structure or region

Table 10.3 *(Continued)*

Term	Definition
Urinary	Relating to or denoting the system of organs, structures, and ducts by which urine is produced and discharged, in mammals comprising the kidneys, ureters, bladder, and urethra
Vascular	Relating to, affecting, or consisting of a vessel or vessels, especially those which carry blood
Venous	Relating to a vein or the veins; relating to the dark red, oxygen-poor blood in the veins and pulmonary artery

10.3.6 Axis 6: Time

Time describes the duration of the focus of the diagnosis (Axis 1). The terms in Axis 6 are:

– *Acute*: lasting < 3 months
– *Chronic*: lasting ≥ 3 months
– *Intermittent*: stopping or starting again at intervals, periodic, cyclic
– *Continuous*: uninterrupted, going on without stop

10.3.7 Axis 7: Status of the Diagnosis

The status of the diagnosis refers to the actuality or potentiality of the problem/syndrome or to the categorization of the diagnosis as a health promotion diagnosis. The terms in Axis 7 are:

– *(Problem-focused)*: undesirable human response to a health condition/life process that exists in the current moment (includes syndrome diagnoses) *Note:* In problem-focused diagnoses this status is assumed in the label itself, there are not standardized terms used for every problem-focused diagnosis
– *Readiness for*: motivation and desire to increase well-being and to actualize human health potential that exists in the current moment (Pender et al 2006)
– *Risk for*: susceptibility for developing, in the future, an undesirable human response to health conditions/life processes.

The terms in Axis 7 (status) are not currently expressed, explicitly, in any of the NANDA-I ND labels (Miguel, Romeiro, Martins, Casaleiro, Caldeira, & Herdman, T.H., 2019). However, the axis is implicit in every diagnosis as this relates to the type of diagnosis that is represented by the label. The DDC plans to move forward a discussion during the next cycle as to whether or not Axis 7 should remain within our multiaxial system.

10.4 Developing and Submitting a Nursing Diagnosis

A nursing diagnosis is constructed by combining the terms from Axis 1 (the focus of the diagnosis), Axis 2 (subject of the diagnosis), and Axis 3 (judgment), and adding terms from the other axes for relevant clarity. Researchers or interested professional nurses would begin with the focus of the diagnosis (Axis 1) and add the appropriate judgment term (Axis 3).

Remember that these two axes are sometimes combined into a single diagnostic concept, as can be seen with the nursing diagnosis *fear* (00148). Next, they would specify the subject of the diagnosis (Axis 2). If the subject is an "individual", they need not make it explicit. Finally, as previously stated, NANDA-I supports developments in ND labels with regard to their multiaxial aspects, to increase the specificity and accuracy of the diagnostic process, which is known to be the core of clinical reasoning and practice. Thus, submitters are encouraged to consider whether the distinction possible by use of additional axes could lead to a more precise diagnosis, which could then aid diagnostic reasoning. For example, a review of the diagnoses, *Neonatal hypothermia* (00280) and *Hypothermia* (00006) demonstrates a significant difference in defining characteristics and related factors based on the incorporation of the axis 5 term (neonate).

NANDA-I does not support the *random construction* of diagnostic concepts that would occur by simply matching terms from one axis to another to create a diagnosis label to represent judgments based on a patient assessment. Clinical problems/areas of nursing foci that are identified and which do not have a NANDA-I label should be carefully described in documentation to ensure accuracy of other nurses'/health care professionals' interpretation of the clinical judgment.

Creating a diagnosis to be used in clinical practice and/or documentation by matching terms from different axes, without development of the definition and other component parts of a diagnosis (defining characteristics, related factors, and risk factors, associated conditions, and at risk populations, as appropriate) in an evidence-based manner, negates the purpose of a standardized language as a method to truly represent, inform, and direct clinical judgment and practice.

This is a serious concern with regard to patient safety, because the lack of the knowledge inherent within the component diagnostic parts makes it impossible to ensure diagnostic accuracy. Nursing terms arbitrarily created at the point of care could result in misinterpretation of the clinical problem/area of focus, and subsequently lead to inappropriate outcome setting and intervention choice. It also makes it impossible to accurately research incidence of nursing diagnoses or to conduct outcome or intervention studies related to diagnoses since, without clear component parts of a diagnosis (definitions, defining characteristics, related factors, or risk factors), it is impossible to know if the concept being studied truly represents the same phenomena.

Therefore, when discussing construction of diagnostic concepts in this chapter, the intent is to inform clinicians as to how diagnostic concepts are developed and to provide clarity for individuals who are developing diagnoses, for submission into the NANDA-I Taxonomy; it *should not* be **misinterpreted to suggest that NANDA-I supports the creation of diagnosis labels by clinicians at the point of patient care.**

10.5 Further Development: Using Axes

NANDA International will be focusing on revision of diagnoses that are currently included in the terminology, but which were "grandfathered" in after the level of evidence criteria was adopted in 2002. There are over 50 such diagnoses, which will be removed from the terminology during the next edition should this revision not occur. Therefore, we strongly discourage the development of new diagnoses at this time, with the focus instead on bringing diagnoses to a minimum level of evidence of 2.1., and raising the level of evidence of other diagnoses.

The other focus for NANDA-I will be to strengthen the clinical usefulness of diagnostic indicators (defining characteristics and related/risk factors). Our desire is to be able to identify, through clinical research and meta-analysis/meta-synthesis, those defining characteristics that are required for a diagnosis to be made ("critical defining characteristics") and to remove those that are not clinically useful. This will strengthen our ability to provide decision support for nurses at the bedside.

If individuals are moving forward with developing new diagnoses, or are clinically validating diagnoses in specific patient populations, we encourage them to review the new guidelines prior to submission. Finally, research is needed to provide evidence-based support for interventions that are most effective when addressing specific related factors of our ND. Unfortunately, much of the literature to date on intervention is aimed at symptom control (addressing defining characteristics) which, although important, does not enable us to fully resolve the diagnosis.

10.6 References

American Psychological Association. Dictionary. 2020. Available from: https://dictionary.apa.org/. Access 2020 Aug 29.

Caldeira SMA, Chaves ECL, Carvalho EC, Vieira MMS. Validation of nursing diagnoses: the differential diagnostic validation model as a strategy. Revista de Enfermagem UFPE 2012; 6(6): 1441–1445.

Cambridge University Press. Cambridge Dictionary Online. 2020. Available from: https://dictionary.cambridge.org/us/. Access 2020 Aug 29.

Levett-Jones T, Hoffman K, Dempsey J, Jeong S, Noble D, Norton CA, Roche J, Hickey, N. The 'five rights' of clinical reasoning: An educational model to enhance nursing students' ability to identify and manage clinically 'at risk' patients. Nurse Education Today 2010; 30(6): 515–520.

Lundberg C, Warren J, Brokel J, et al. Selecting a standardized terminology for the electronic health record that reveals the impact of nursing on patient care. Online J Nurs Inform 2008; 12(2). Available at: http://ojni.org/12_2/lundberg.pdf

Matos FGOA, Cruz DALM. Development of an instrument to evaluate diagnosis accuracy. Rev Esc Enferm USP 2009; 43: 1087–1095.

Miguel S, Romeiro J, Martins H, Casaleiro T, Caldeira S, Herdman TH. "Call for the Use of Axial Terms": Toward Completeness of NANDA-I Nursing Diagnoses Labels. Int J Nurs Knowl 2019; 30(3): 131–136.

Nimboriboonporn A, Chuthapisith S. Nipple-areola complex reconstruction. Gland Surg 2014; 3(1): 35-42. https://doi.org/10.3978/j.issn.2227-684X.2014.02.06.

Oxford University Press. Oxford English Living Dictionary Online. Oxford University Press: Oxford, 2019. Available at: https://en.oxforddictionaries.com.

Paans W, Nieweg RMB, van der Schans CP, Sermeus W. What factors influence the prevalence and accuracy of nursing diagnoses documentation in clinical practice? A systematic literature review. J Clin Nurs 2011; 20(17–18): 2386–2403. https://pubmed.ncbi.nlm.nih.gov/21676043/.

Pender NJ, Murdaugh CL, Parsons MA. Health Promotion in Nursing Practice. 5th ed. Upper Saddle River, NJ: Pearson Prentice-Hall, 2006.

World Health Organization. Definition of key terms. 2013. Available at: http://www.who.int/hiv/pub/guidelines/arv2013/intro/keyterms/en/.

World Health Organization. Health topics: Infant, newborn. 2013. Available at: http://www.who.int/topics/infant_newborn/en/.

11 Glossary of Terms

T. Heather Herdman, Shigemi Kamitsuru, Camila Takáo Lopes

11.1 Nursing Diagnosis

A nursing diagnosis is a clinical judgment concerning a human response to health conditions/life processes, or a susceptibility to that response, that is recognized in an individual, caregiver, family, group, or community. A nursing diagnosis provides the basis for selection of nursing interventions to achieve outcomes for which the nurse has accountability (approved at the Ninth NANDA Conference; amended in 2009, 2013, and 2019).

11.1.1 Problem-Focused Nursing Diagnosis

A clinical judgment concerning an undesirable human response to health conditions/life processes that is recognized in an individual, caregiver, family, group, or community.

To diagnose a human response a problem-focused diagnosis, the following must be present: defining characteristics that cluster in patterns of related cues or inferences, and related factors.

11.1.2 Health Promotion Nursing Diagnosis

A clinical judgment concerning motivation and desire to increase well-being and to actualize health potential that is recognized in an individual, caregiver, family, group, or community.

These responses are expressed by a readiness to enhance specific health behaviors, and can be used in any health state. In individuals who are unable to express their own readiness to enhance health behaviors, the nurse may determine a condition for health promotion exists and act on the client's behalf. Health promotion responses may exist in an individual, caregiver, family, group, or community.

To diagnose a human response as a health promotion diagnosis, the following must be present: defining characteristics that cluster in patterns of related cues or inferences which reflect a desire to enhance a current behavior or response, or that represent such a possibility in patients who cannot express their own readiness.

11.1.3 Risk Nursing Diagnosis

A clinical judgment concerning the susceptibility for developing an undesirable human response to health conditions/life processes that is recognized in an individual, caregiver, family, group, or community.

To diagnose a risk diagnosis, the following must be present: risk factors that contribute to increased susceptibility.

11.1.4 Syndrome

A clinical judgment concerning a specific cluster of nursing diagnoses that occur together, and are best addressed together and through similar interventions.

To diagnose a syndrome diagnosis, the following must be present: defining characteristics, which must be two or more nursing diagnoses, and related factors. Other defining characteristics that are not nursing diagnoses may be used, so long as similar interventions may be used to address them.

11.2 Diagnostic Axes

11.2.1 Axis

An axis is operationally defined as a dimension of the human response that is considered in the diagnostic process. There are seven axes that parallel the International Standards Reference Model for a Nursing Diagnosis.

- Axis 1: the focus of the diagnosis
- Axis 2: subject of the diagnosis (individual, family, group, caregiver, community)
- Axis 3: judgment (impaired, ineffective, etc.)
- Axis 4: location (bladder, auditory, cerebral, etc.)
- Axis 5: age (neonate, infant, child, adult, etc.)
- Axis 6: time (chronic, acute, intermittent)
- Axis 7: status of the diagnosis (problem-focused, risk, health promotion).

The axes are represented in the labels of the nursing diagnoses through their terms. In some cases, they are named explicitly, such as with the diagnoses *ineffective community coping* and *compromised family coping*, in which the subject of the diagnosis is named using the two terms "community" and "family" taken from Axis 2 (subject of the diagnosis). "Ineffective" and "compromised" are two of the terms contained in Axis 3 (judgment).

In some cases, the axis is implicit, as is the case with the diagnosis *decreased activity tolerance*, in which the subject of the diagnosis (Axis 2) is always the patient. In some instances, an axis may not be pertinent to a particular diagnosis and therefore is not part of the nursing diagnostic label. For example, the time axis may not be relevant to every diagnosis. In the case of diagnoses without explicit identification of the subject of the diagnosis, it may be helpful to remember that NANDA-I defines patient as "an individual, caregiver, family, group, or community".

Axis 1 (the focus of the diagnosis) and Axis 3 (judgment) are essential components of a nursing diagnosis. In some cases, however, the focus of the diagnosis contains the judgment (e.g., nausea); in these cases, the judgment is not explicitly separated out in the diagnostic label. Axis 2 (subject of the diagnosis) is also essential, although, as described above, it may be implied and therefore not included in the label. The DDC requires these axes for submission; the other axes may be used where relevant for clarity.

11.2.2 Definitions of the Axes

Axis 1: Focus of the Diagnosis

The focus of the diagnosis is the principal element or the fundamental and essential part, the root, of the diagnostic concept. It describes the "human response" that is the core of the diagnosis.

The focus of the diagnosis may consist of one or more nouns. When more than one noun is used (e.g., mood regulation), each one contributes a unique meaning to the focus of the diagnosis, as if the two were a single noun; the meaning of the combined term, however, is different from when the nouns are stated separately. Frequently, an adjective (spiritual) may be used with a noun (distress) to denote the focus of the diagnosis *spiritual distress* (see ▶ Table 10.1).

Axis 2: Subject of the Diagnosis

The person(s) for whom a nursing diagnosis is determined. The terms in Axis 2 that represent the NANDA-I definition of "patient" are the following:

- *Individual*: a single human being distinct from others, a person
- *Caregiver*: a family member or helper who regularly looks after a child or a sick, elderly, or disabled person
- *Family*: two or more people having continuous or sustained relationships, perceiving reciprocal obligations, sensing common meaning, and sharing certain obligations toward others; related by blood and/or choice
- *Group*: a number of people with shared characteristics
- *Community*: a group of people living in the same locale under the same governance; examples include neighborhoods and cities.

Axis 3: Judgment

A descriptor or modifier that limits or specifies the meaning of the focus of the diagnosis. The focus of the diagnosis together with the nurse's judgment about it forms the diagnosis. The terms in Axis 3 are found in ▶ Table 10.2.

Axis 4: Location

Describes the parts/regions of the body and/or their related functions – all tissues, organs, anatomical sites, or structures. For the locations in Axis 4, see ► Table 10.3.

Axis 5: Age

Refers to the age group of the person who is the subject of the diagnosis (Axis 2). The terms in Axis 5 are noted below, with all definitions except that of older adult being drawn from the World Health Organization (2013):

- *Fetus*: unborn human more than 8 weeks after conception, until birth
- *Neonate*: person < 28 days of age
- *Infant*: child < 1 year of age
- *Child*: person ≤ 19 years of age unless national law defines a person to be an adult at an earlier age
- *Adolescent*: person 10 to 19 years of age, inclusive
- *Adult*: person > 19 years of age unless national law defines a person as being an adult at an earlier age
- *Older adult*: person 65–84 years of age
- *Aged adult*: person ≥ years of age.

Axis 6: Time

Describes the duration of the diagnostic concept (Axis 1). The terms in Axis 6 are as follows:

- *Acute*: lasting < 3 months
- *Chronic*: lasting > 3 months
- *Intermittent*: stopping or starting again at intervals, periodic, cyclic
- *Continuous*: uninterrupted, going on without stop

Axis 7: Status of the Diagnosis

Refers to the actuality or potentiality of the problem/syndrome or health promotion opportunity to the categorization of the diagnosis as a health promotion diagnosis. The terms in Axis 7 are problem-focused, health promotion, risk.

11.3 Components of a Nursing Diagnosis

11.3.1 Diagnosis Label

Provides a name for a diagnosis that reflects, at a minimum, the focus of the diagnosis (from Axis 1) and the nursing judgment (from Axis 3). It is a concise term or phrase that represents a pattern of related cues. It may include modifiers.

11.3.2 Definition

Provides a clear, precise description; delineates its meaning and helps differentiate it from similar diagnoses.

11.3.3 Defining Characteristics

Observable cues/inferences that cluster as manifestations of a problem-focused, health promotion diagnosis or syndrome. This implies not only those things that the nurse can see, but also things that are seen, heard (e.g., the patient/family tells us), touched, or smelled.

11.3.4 Risk Factors

Antecedent factors that increase the susceptibility of an individual, caregiver, family, group, or community to an undesirable human response. These factors must be modifiable by independent nursing interventions, and whenever possible, interventions should be aimed at these factors.

11.3.5 Related Factors

Antecedent factors shown to have a patterned relationship with the human response. Such factors may be described as associated with, related to, or contributing to that response. These factors must be modifiable by independent nursing interventions, and whenever possible, interventions should be aimed at these etiological factors. Problem-focused nursing diagnoses and syndromes must have related factors; health promotion diagnoses may have related factors, if they help clarify the diagnosis.

11.3.6 At Risk Populations

Groups of people who share sociodemographic characteristics, health/family history, stages of growth/development, exposure to certain events/experiences that cause each member to be susceptible to a particular human response. These characteristics are not modifiable by independent nursing interventions.

11.3.7 Associated Conditions

Medical diagnoses, diagnostic/surgical procedures, medical/surgical devices, or pharmaceutical preparations; these conditions are not modifiable by independent nursing interventions.

11.4 Definitions for Terms Associated with Nursing Diagnoses

11.4.1 Independent Nursing Interventions

Interventions that can be initiated by the professional nurse that go beyond basic monitoring, referral to other professionals, compliance with organizational protocol, and/or that do not require orders from other health professionals. They are sanctioned by professional nurse practice acts or regulations.

11.4.2 Nursing-Sensitive Outcomes

Measurable individual, caregiver, group, family, or community state, behaviors or perceptions in response to nursing interventions.

11.4.3 Nursing Plan of Care

Includes nursing diagnoses, the outcomes, and individualized nursing interventions, based on a complete nursing assessment and understanding of the goals and desires of the individual, caregiver, group, family, or community receiving care.

11.5 Definitions for Classification of Nursing Diagnoses

11.5.1 Classification

The arrangement of related phenomena in taxonomic groups according to their observed similarities; a category into which something is put (English Oxford Living Dictionary Online 2020).

11.5.2 Level of Abstraction

Describes the concreteness/abstractness of a concept:

- Very abstract concepts are theoretical, may not be directly measurable, are defined by concrete concepts, are inclusive of concrete concepts, are disassociated from any specific instance, are independent of time and space, have more general descriptors, and may not be clinically useful for planning treatment.
- Concrete concepts are observable and measurable, limited by time and space, constitute a specific category, are more exclusive, name a real thing or class of things, are restricted by nature, and may be clinically useful for planning treatment.

11.5.3 Terminology

The body of terms used with a particular technical application in a subject of study, profession, etc. (English Oxford Living Dictionary Online 2020).

11.5.4 Taxonomy

The branch of science concerned with classification, especially of organisms; systematics (English Oxford Living Dictionary Online 2020).

11.6 References

Oxford University Press. English Oxford Living Dictionary Online, British and World Version. 2020. Available at: https://en.oxforddictionaries.com.

Pender NJ, Murdaugh CL, Parsons MA. Health Promotion in Nursing Practice. 5th ed. Upper Saddle River, NJ: Pearson Prentice-Hall, 2006.

World Health Organization. Definition of key terms. 2013. Available at: https://www.who.int/hiv/pub/guidelines/arv2013/intro/keyterms/en/

World Health Organization. Health topics: infant, newborn. 2013. Available at: https://www.who.int/infant-newborn/en/.

Part 4
The NANDA International Nursing Diagnoses

NANDA International, Inc. Nursing Diagnoses: Definitions and Classification 2021–2023, 12th Edition.
Edited by T. Heather Herdman, Shigemi Kamitsuru, and Camila Takáo Lopes.
© 2021 NANDA International, Inc. Published 2021 by Thieme Medical Publishers, Inc., New York.
Companion website: www.thieme.com/nanda-i.

Domain 1.
Health promotion

The awareness of well-being or normality of function and the strategies used to maintain control of and enhance that well-being or normality of function

Class 1. Health awareness
Recognition of normal function and well-being

Code	Diagnosis	Page
00097	Decreased diversional activity engagement	188
00262	Readiness for enhanced health literacy	189
00168	Sedentary lifestyle	190

Class 2. Health management
Identifying, controlling, performing, and integrating activities to maintain health and well-being

Code	Diagnosis	Page
00290	Risk for elopement attempt	192
00257	Frail elderly syndrome	193
00231	Risk for frail elderly syndrome	195
00307	Readiness for enhanced exercise engagement	196
00215	Deficient community health	197
00188	Risk-prone health behavior	198
00292	Ineffective health maintenance behaviors	199
00276	Ineffective health self-management	201
00293	Readiness for enhanced health self-management	203
00294	Ineffective family health self-management	204
00300	Ineffective home maintenance behaviors	206
00308	Risk for ineffective home maintenance behaviors	207
00309	Readiness for enhanced home maintenance behaviors	208
00043	Ineffective protection	209

Domain 1 • Class 1 • Diagnosis Code 00097

Decreased diversional activity engagement

Focus of the diagnosis: diversional activity engagement
Approved 1980 • Revised 2017 • Level of Evidence 2.1

Definition
Reduced stimulation, interest, or participation in recreational or leisure activities.

Defining characteristics
- Altered mood
- Boredom
- Expresses discontentment with situation
- Flat affect
- Frequent naps
- Physical deconditioning

Related factors
- Current setting does not allow engagement in activities
- Environmental constraints
- Impaired physical mobility
- Inadequate available activities
- Inadequate motivation
- Insufficient physical endurance
- Physical discomfort
- Psychological distress

At risk population
- Individuals at extremes of age
- Individuals experiencing prolonged hospitalization
- Individuals experiencing prolonged institutionalization

Associated conditions
- Prescribed movement restrictions
- Therapeutic isolation

Original literature support available at www.thieme.com/nanda-i.

NANDA International, Inc. Nursing Diagnoses: Definitions and Classification 2021–2023, 12th Edition.
Edited by T. Heather Herdman, Shigemi Kamitsuru, and Camila Takáo Lopes.
© 2021 NANDA International, Inc. Published 2021 by Thieme Medical Publishers, Inc., New York.
Companion website: www.thieme.com/nanda-i.

Domain 1 • Class 1 • Diagnosis Code 00262

Readiness for enhanced health literacy

Focus of the diagnosis: health literacy
Approved 2016 • Level of Evidence 2.1

Definition

A pattern of using and developing a set of skills and competencies (literacy, knowledge, motivation, culture and language) to find, comprehend, evaluate and use health information and concepts to make daily health decisions to promote and maintain health, decrease health risks and improve overall quality of life, which can be strengthened.

Defining characteristics

- Expresses desire to enhance ability to read, write, speak and interpret numbers for everyday health needs
- Expresses desire to enhance awareness of civic and/or government processes that impact public health
- Expresses desire to enhance health communication with health care providers
- Expresses desire to enhance knowledge of current determinants of health on social and physical environments

- Expresses desire to enhance personal health care decision-making
- Expresses desire to enhance social support for health
- Expresses desire to enhance understanding of customs and beliefs to make health care decisions
- Expresses desire to enhance understanding of health information to make health care choices
- Expresses desire to obtain sufficient information to navigate the health care system

Original literature support available at www.thieme.com/nanda-i.

Domain 1 • Class 1 • Diagnosis Code 00168

Sedentary lifestyle

Focus of the diagnosis: lifestyle
Approved 2004 • Revised 2020 • Level of Evidence 3.2

> **Definition**
> An acquired mode of behavior that is characterized by waking hour activities that require low energy expenditure.

Defining characteristics

- Average daily physical activity is less than recommended for age and gender
- Chooses a daily routine lacking physical exercise
- Does not exercise during leisure time
- Expresses preference for low physical activity
- Performs majority of tasks in a reclining posture
- Performs majority of tasks in a sitting posture
- Physical deconditioning

Related factors

- Conflict between cultural beliefs and health practices
- Decreased activity tolerance
- Difficulty adapting areas for physical activity
- Exceeds screen time recommendations for age
- Impaired physical mobility
- Inadequate interest in physical activity
- Inadequate knowledge of consequences of sedentarism
- Inadequate knowledge of health benefits associated with physical activity
- Inadequate motivation for physical activity
- Inadequate resources for physical activity
- Inadequate role models
- Inadequate social support
- Inadequate time management skills
- Inadequate training for physical exercise
- Low self efficacy
- Low self-esteem
- Negative affect toward physical activity
- Pain
- Parenting practices that inhibit child's physical activity
- Perceived physical disability
- Perceived safety risk

At risk population

- Adolescents
- Individuals aged ≥ 60 years
- Individuals living in urban areas
- Individuals living with a partner
- Individuals with high educational level
- Individuals with high socioeconomic status

- Individuals with significant time constraints
- Married individuals
- Women

Original literature support available at www.thieme.com/nanda-i.

191

Domain 1 • Class 2 • Diagnosis Code 00290

Risk for elopement attempt

Focus of the diagnosis: elopement attempt
Approved 2020 • Level of Evidence 2.1

Definition
Susceptible to leaving a health care facility or a designated area against recommendation or without communicating to health care professionals or caregivers, which may compromise safety and/or health.

Risk factors

- Anger behaviors
- Dissatisfaction with current situation
- Exit-seeking behavior
- Frustration about delay in treatment regimen
- Inadequate caregiver vigilance
- Inadequate interest in improving health
- Inadequate social support
- Perceived complexity of treatment regimen
- Perceived excessive family responsibilities
- Perceived excessive responsibilities in interpersonal relations
- Perceived lack of safety in surrounding environment
- Persistent wandering
- Psychomotor agitation
- Self-harm intent
- Substance misuse

At risk population

- Economically disadvantaged individuals
- Homeless individuals
- Individuals brought to designated area against own wishes
- Individuals frequently requesting discharge
- Individuals hospitalized < three weeks
- Individuals with history of elopement
- Individuals with history of non-adherence to treatment regimen
- Individuals with history of self-harm
- Individuals with impaired judgment
- Men
- Older adults with cognitive disorders
- Unemployed individuals
- Young adults

Associated conditions

- Autism spectrum disorder
- Developmental disabilities
- Mental disorders

Original literature support available at www.thieme.com/nanda-i.

Domain 1 • Class 2 • Diagnosis Code 00257

Frail elderly syndrome

Focus of the diagnosis: frail elderly syndrome
Approved 2013 • Revised 2017 • Level of Evidence 2.1

Definition
Dynamic state of unstable equilibrium that affects the older individual experiencing deterioration in one or more domain of health (physical, functional, psychological, or social) and leads to increased susceptibility to adverse health effects, in particular disability.

Defining characteristics
- Bathing self-care deficit (00108)
- Decreased activity tolerance (00298)
- Decreased cardiac output (00029)
- Dressing self-care deficit (00109)
- Fatigue (00093)
- Feeding self-care deficit (00102)
- Hopelessness (00124)
- Imbalanced nutrition: less than body requirements (00002)
- Impaired memory (00131)
- Impaired physical mobility (00085)
- Impaired walking (00088)
- Social isolation (00053)
- Toileting self-care deficit (00110)

Related factors
- Anxiety
- Cognitive dysfunction
- Decreased energy
- Decreased muscle strength
- Exhaustion
- Fear of falling
- Impaired postural balance
- Inadequate knowledge of modifiable factors
- Inadequate social support
- Malnutrition
- Neurobehavioral manifestations
- Obesity
- Sadness
- Sedentary lifestyle

At risk population
- Economically disadvantaged individuals
- Individuals aged > 70 years
- Individuals experiencing prolonged hospitalization
- Individuals for whom walking 15 feet requires > 6 seconds (4 meters > 5 seconds)
- Individuals living alone
- Individuals living in constricted spaces
- Individuals with history of falls
- Individuals with low educational level

- dividuals with unintentional loss of 25% of body weight over one year
- Individuals with unintentional weight loss > 10 pounds (> 4.5 kg) in one year
- Socially vulnerable individuals
- Women

Associated conditions

- Anorexia
- Blood coagulation disorders
- Chronic disease
- Decreased serum 25-hydroxyvitamin D concentration
- Depression
- Endocrine regulatory dysfunction
- Mental disorders
- Sarcopenia
- Sarcopenic obesity
- Sensation disorders
- Suppressed inflammatory response

Original literature support available at www.thieme.com/nanda-i.

Domain 1 • Class 2 • Diagnosis Code 00231

Risk for frail elderly syndrome

Focus of the diagnosis: frail elderly syndrome
Approved 2013 • Revised 2017 • Level of Evidence 2.1

Definition
Susceptible to a dynamic state of unstable equilibrium that affects the older individual experiencing deterioration in one or more domain of health (physical, functional, psychological, or social) and leads to increased susceptibility to adverse health effects, in particular disability.

Risk factors

- Anxiety
- Cognitive dysfunction
- Decreased energy
- Decreased muscle strength
- Exhaustion
- Fear of falling
- Impaired postural balance
- Inadequate knowledge of modifiable factors
- Inadequate social support
- Malnutrition
- Neurobehavioral manifestations
- Obesity
- Sadness
- Sedentary lifestyle

At risk population

- Economically disadvantaged individuals
- Individuals aged > 70 years
- Individuals experiencing prolonged hospitalization
- Individuals for whom walking 15 feet requires > 6 seconds (4 meters > 5 seconds)
- Individuals living alone
- Individuals living in constricted spaces
- Individuals with history of falls
- Individuals with low educational level
- Individuals with unintentional loss of 25% of body weight over one year
- Individuals with unintentional weight loss > 10 pounds (> 4.5 kg) in one year
- Socially vulnerable individuals
- Women

Associated conditions

- Anorexia
- Blood coagulation disorders
- Chronic disease
- Decreased serum 25-hydroxyvitamin D concentration
- Depression
- Endocrine regulatory dysfunction
- Mental disorders
- Sarcopenia
- Sarcopenic obesity
- Sensation disorders
- Suppressed inflamma\tory response

Original literature support available at www.thieme.com/nanda-i.

Domain 1 • Class 2 • Diagnosis Code 00307

Readiness for enhanced exercise engagement

Focus of the diagnosis: exercise engagement
Approved 2020 • Level of Evidence 2.1

Definition
A pattern of attention to physical activity characterized by planned, structured, repetitive body movements, which can be strengthened.

Defining characteristics

- Expresses desire to enhance autonomy for activities of daily living
- Expresses desire to enhance competence to interact with physical and social environments
- Expresses desire to enhance knowledge about environmental conditions for participation in physical activity
- Expresses desire to enhance knowledge about group opportunities for participation in physical activity
- Expresses desire to enhance knowledge about physical settings for participation in physical activity
- Expresses desire to enhance knowledge about the need for physical activity
- Expresses desire to enhance physical abilities
- Expresses desire to enhance physical appearance
- Expresses desire to enhance physical conditioning
- Expresses desire to maintain motivation to participate in a physical activity plan
- Expresses desire to maintain physical abilities
- Expresses desire to maintain physical well-being through physical activity
- Expresses desire to meet others' expectations about physical activity plans

Original literature support available at www.thieme.com/nanda-i.

Domain 1 • Class 2 • Diagnosis Code 00215

Deficient community health

Focus of the diagnosis: health
Approved 2010 • Level of Evidence 2.1

Definition
Presence of one or more health problems or factors that deter wellness or increase the risk of health problems experienced by a group or population.

Defining characteristics
- Health problem experienced by groups or populations
- Program unavailable to enhance wellness of a group or population
- Programs unavailable to eliminate health problems of a group or population
- Programs unavailable to prevent health problems of a group or population
- Programs unavailable to reduce health problems of a group or population
- Risk of hospitalization to a group or population
- Risk of physiological manifestations to a group or population
- Risk of psychological manifestations to a group or population

Related factors
- Inadequate access to health care provider
- Inadequate consumer satisfaction with programs
- Inadequate expertise within the community
- Inadequate health resources
- Inadequate program budget
- Inadequate program evaluation plan
- Inadequate program outcome data
- Inadequate social support for programs
- Programs incompletely address health problems

Original literature support available at www.thieme.com/nanda-i.

Domain 1 • Class 2 • Diagnosis Code 00188

Risk-prone health behavior

Focus of the diagnosis: health behavior
Approved 1986 • Revised 1998, 2006, 2008, 2017 • Level of Evidence 2.1

Definition
Impaired ability to modify lifestyle and/or actions in a manner that improves the level of wellness.

Defining characteristics
– Failure to achieve optimal sense of control
– Failure to take action that prevents health problem
– Minimizes health status change
– Nonacceptance of health status change
– Smoking
– Substance misuse

Related factors
– Inadequate social support
– Inadequate understanding of health information
– Low self efficacy
– Negative perception of health care provider
– Negative perception of recommended health care strategy
– Social anxiety
– Stressors

At risk population
– Economically disadvantaged individuals
– Individuals with family history of alcoholism

Original literature support available at www.thieme.com/nanda-i.

Domain 1 • Class 2 • Diagnosis Code 00292

Ineffective health maintenance behaviors

Focus of the diagnosis: health maintenance behaviors
Approved 2020 • Level of Evidence 2.1

Definition
Management of health knowledge, attitudes, and practices underlying health actions that is unsatisfactory for maintaining or improving well-being, or preventing illness and injury.

Defining characteristics
- Failure to take action that prevents health problem
- Failure to take action that reduces risk factor
- Inadequate commitment to a plan of action
- Inadequate health literacy
- Inadequate interest in improving health
- Inadequate knowledge about basic health practices
- Ineffective choices in daily living for meeting health goal
- Pattern of lack of health-seeking behavior

Related factors
- Cognitive dysfunction
- Competing demands
- Competing lifestyle preferences
- Conflict between cultural beliefs and health practices
- Conflict between health behaviors and social norms
- Conflicts between spiritual beliefs and health practices
- Depressive symptoms
- Difficulty accessing community resources
- Difficulty navigating complex health care systems
- Difficulty with decision-making
- Inadequate health resources
- Inadequate social support
- Inadequate trust in health care professional
- Individuals with limited decision-making experience
- Ineffective communication skills
- Ineffective coping strategies
- Ineffective family coping
- Low self efficacy
- Maladaptive grieving
- Neurobehavioral manifestations
- Perceived prejudice
- Perceived victimization
- Spiritual distress

At risk population
- Economically disadvantaged individuals
- Individuals from families with ineffective family coping
- Individuals with history of violence
- Men
- Older adults
- Young adults

Associated conditions

- Chronic disease
- Developmental disabilities
- Mental disorders
- Motor skills disorders

Original literature support available at www.thieme.com/nanda-i.

Domain 1 • Class 2 • Diagnosis Code 00276

Ineffective health self-management

Focus of the diagnosis: health self-management
Approved 2020 • Level of Evidence 3.3

Definition
Unsatisfactory management of symptoms, treatment regimen, physical, psychosocial, and spiritual consequences and lifestyle changes inherent in living with a chronic condition.

Defining characteristics

- Exacerbation of disease signs
- Exacerbation of disease symptoms
- Exhibits disease sequelae
- Expresses dissatisfaction with quality of life
- Failure to attend appointments with health care provider
- Failure to include treatment regimen into daily living
- Failure to take action that reduces risk factor
- Inattentive to disease signs
- Inattentive to disease symptoms
- Ineffective choices in daily living for meeting health goal

Related factors

- Cognitive dysfunction
- Competing demands
- Competing lifestyle preferences
- Conflict between cultural beliefs and health practices
- Conflict between health behaviors and social norms
- Conflict between spiritual beliefs and treatment regimen
- Decreased perceived quality of life
- Depressive symptoms
- Difficulty accessing community resources
- Difficulty managing complex treatment regimen
- Difficulty navigating complex health care systems
- Difficulty with decision-making
- Inadequate commitment to a plan of action
- Inadequate health literacy
- Inadequate knowledge of treatment regimen
- Inadequate number of cues to action
- Inadequate role models
- Inadequate social support
- Individuals with limited decision-making experience
- Limited ability to perform aspects of treatment regimen
- Low self efficacy
- Negative feelings toward treatment regimen
- Neurobehavioral manifestations
- Nonacceptance of condition
- Perceived barrier to treatment regimen
- Perceived social stigma associated with condition
- Substance misuse

- Unrealistic perception of seriousness of condition
- Unrealistic perception of susceptibility to sequelae
- Unrealistic perception of treatment benefit

At risk population

- Children
- Economically disadvantaged individuals
- Individuals experiencing adverse reactions to medications
- Individuals with caregiving responsibilities
- Individuals with history of ineffective health self-management
- Individuals with low educational level
- Older adults

Associated conditions

- Asymptomatic disease
- Developmental disabilities
- High acuity illness
- Neurocognitive disorders
- Polypharmacy
- Significant comorbidity

Original literature support available at www.thieme.com/nanda-i.

Domain 1 • Class 2 • Diagnosis Code 00293

Readiness for enhanced health self-management

Focus of the diagnosis: health self-management
Approved 2020 • Level of Evidence 2.1

Definition
A pattern of satisfactory management of symptoms, treatment regimen, physical, psychosocial, and spiritual consequences and lifestyle changes inherent in living with a chronic condition, which can be strengthened.

Defining characteristics
- Expresses desire to enhance acceptance of the condition
- Expresses desire to enhance choices of daily living for meeting health goals
- Expresses desire to enhance commitment to follow-up care
- Expresses desire to enhance decision making
- Expresses desire to enhance inclusion of treatment regimen into daily living
- Expresses desire to enhance management of risk factors
- Expresses desire to enhance management of signs
- Expresses desire to enhance management of symptoms
- Expresses desire to enhance recognition of disease signs
- Expresses desire to enhance recognition of disease symptoms
- Expresses desire to enhance satisfaction with quality of life

Original literature support available at www.thieme.com/nanda-i.

Domain 1 · Class 2 · Diagnosis Code 00294

Ineffective family health self-management

Focus of the diagnosis: health self-management
Approved 2020 · Level of Evidence 2.1

Definition

Unsatisfactory management of symptoms, treatment regimen, physical, psychosocial and spiritual consequences and lifestyle changes inherent in living with one or more family members' chronic condition.

Defining characteristics

- Caregiver strain
- Decrease in attention to illness in one or more family members
- Depressive symptoms of caregiver
- Exacerbation of disease signs of one or more family members
- Exacerbation of disease symptoms of one or more family members
- Failure to take action to reduce risk factor in one or more family members
- Ineffective choices in daily living for meeting health goal of family unit
- One or more family members report dissatisfaction with quality of life

Related factors

- Cognitive dysfunction
- Cognitive dysfunction of one or more caregivers
- Competing demands on family unit
- Competing lifestyle preferences within family unit
- Conflict between health behaviors and social norms
- Conflict between spiritual beliefs and treatment regimen
- Difficulty accessing community resources
- Difficulty dealing with role changes associated with condition
- Difficulty managing complex treatment regimen
- Difficulty navigating complex health care systems
- Difficulty with decision-making
- Family conflict
- Inadequate commitment to a plan of action
- Inadequate health literacy of caregiver
- Inadequate knowledge of treatment regimen
- Inadequate number of cues to action
- Inadequate social support
- Ineffective communication skills
- Ineffective coping skills
- Limited ability to perform aspects of treatment regimen
- Low self efficacy
- Negative feelings toward treatment regimen
- Nonacceptance of condition
- Perceived barrier to treatment regimen
- Perceived social stigma associated with condition

- Substance misuse
- Unrealistic perception of seriousness of condition
- Unrealistic perception of susceptibility to sequelae

- Unrealistic perception of treatment benefit
- Unsupportive family relations

At risk population
- Economically disadvantaged families
- Families with member experiencing delayed diagnosis
- Families with members experiencing low educational level

- Families with members who have limited decision-making experience
- Families with premature infant

Associated conditions
- Chronic disease
- Mental disorders

- Neurocognitive disorders
- Terminal illness

Original literature support available at www.thieme.com/nanda-i.

Domain 1 • Class 2 • Diagnosis Code 00300

Ineffective home maintenance behaviors

Focus of the diagnosis: home maintenance behaviors
Approved 2020 • Level of Evidence 2.1

Definition
An unsatisfactory pattern of knowledge and activities for the safe upkeep of one's residence.

Defining characteristics

- Cluttered environment
- Difficulty maintaining a comfortable environment
- Failure to request assistance with home maintenance
- Home task-related anxiety
- Home task-related stress
- Impaired ability to regulate finances
- Negative affect toward home maintenance
- Neglected laundry
- Pattern of hygiene-related diseases
- Trash accumulation
- Unsafe cooking equipment
- Unsanitary environment

Related factors

- Cognitive dysfunction
- Competing demands
- Depressive symptoms
- Difficulty with decision-making
- Environmental constraints
- Impaired physical mobility
- Impaired postural balance
- Inadequate knowledge of home maintenance
- Inadequate knowledge of social resources
- Inadequate organizing skills
- Inadequate role models
- Inadequate social support
- Insufficient physical endurance
- Neurobehavioral manifestations
- Powerlessness
- Psychological distress

At risk population

- Economically disadvantaged individuals
- Individuals living alone
- Older adults

Associated conditions

- Depression
- Mental disorders
- Neoplasms
- Neurocognitive disorders
- Sensation disorders
- Vascular diseases

Original literature support available at www.thieme.com/nanda-i.

Domain 1 • Class 2 • Diagnosis Code 00308

Risk for ineffective home maintenance behaviors

Focus of the diagnosis: home maintenance behaviors
Approved 2020 • Level of Evidence 2.1

1. Health promotion

Definition
Susceptible to an unsatisfactory pattern of knowledge and activities for the safe upkeep of one's residence, which may compromise health.

Risk factors
- Cognitive dysfunction
- Competing demands
- Depressive symptoms
- Difficulty with decision-making
- Environmental constraints
- Impaired physical mobility
- Impaired postural balance
- Inadequate knowledge of home maintenance
- Inadequate knowledge of social resources
- Inadequate organizing skills
- Inadequate role models
- Inadequate social support
- Insufficient physical endurance
- Neurobehavioral manifestations
- Powerlessness
- Psychological distress

At risk population
- Economically disadvantaged individuals
- Individuals living alone
- Older adults

Associated conditions
- Depression
- Mental disorders
- Neoplasms
- Neurocognitive disorders
- Sensation disorders
- Vascular diseases

Original literature support available at www.thieme.com/nanda-i.

Domain 1 • Class 2 • Diagnosis Code 00309

Readiness for enhanced home maintenance behaviors

Focus of the diagnosis: home maintenance behaviors
Approved 2020 • Level of Evidence 2.1

Definition
A pattern of knowledge and activities for the safe upkeep of one's residence, which can be strengthened.

Defining characteristics

- Expresses desire to enhance affect toward home tasks
- Expresses desire to enhance attitude toward home maintenance
- Expresses desire to enhance comfort of the environment
- Expresses desire to enhance home safety
- Expresses desire to enhance household hygiene
- Expresses desire to enhance laundry management skills
- Expresses desire to enhance organizational skills
- Expresses desire to enhance regulation of finances
- Expresses desire to enhance trash management

Original literature support available at www.thieme.com/nanda-i.

Domain 1 • Class 2 • Diagnosis Code 00043

Ineffective protection

Focus of the diagnosis: protection
Approved 1990 • Revised 2017, 2020 • Level of Evidence 3.2

Definition
Decrease in the ability to guard self from internal or external threats such as illness or injury.

Defining characteristics

- Altered sweating
- Anorexia
- Chilling
- Coughing
- Disorientation
- Dyspnea
- Expresses itching
- Fatigue
- Impaired physical mobility
- Impaired tissue healing
- Insomnia
- Leukopenia
- Low serum hemoglobin level
- Maladaptive stress response
- Neurosensory impairment
- Pressure injury
- Psychomotor agitation
- Thrombocytopenia
- Weakness

Related factors

- Depressive symptoms
- Difficulty managing complex treatment regimen
- Hopelessness
- Inadequate vaccination
- Ineffective health self-management
- Low self efficacy
- Malnutrition
- Physical deconditioning
- Substance misuse

Associated conditions

- Blood coagulation disorders
- Immune system diseases
- Neoplasms
- Pharmaceutical preparations
- Treatment regimen

Domain 2. Nutrition

The activities of taking in, assimilating, and using nutrients for the purposes of tissue maintenance, tissue repair, and the production of energy

Class 1. Ingestion
Taking food or nutrients into the body

Code	Diagnosis	Page
00002	Imbalanced nutrition: less than body requirements	213
00163	Readiness for enhanced nutrition	215
00216	Insufficient breast milk production	216
00104	Ineffective breastfeeding	217
00105	Interrupted breastfeeding	219
00106	Readiness for enhanced breastfeeding	220
00269	Ineffective adolescent eating dynamics	221
00270	Ineffective child eating dynamics	222
00271	Ineffective infant feeding dynamics	224
00232	Obesity	226
00233	Overweight	228
00234	Risk for overweight	230
00295	Ineffective infant suck-swallow response	232
00103	Impaired swallowing	234

Class 2. Digestion
The physical and chemical activities that convert foodstuffs into substances suitable for absorption and assimilation

Code	Diagnosis	Page
This class does not currently contain any diagnoses		

Class 3. Absorption
The act of taking up nutrients through body tissues

Code	Diagnosis	Page
	This class does not currently contain any diagnoses	

Class 4. Metabolism
The chemical and physical processes occurring in living organisms and cells for the development and use of protoplasm, the production of waste and energy, with the release of energy for all vital processes

Code	Diagnosis	Page
00179	Risk for unstable blood glucose level	236
00194	Neonatal hyperbilirubinemia	238
00230	Risk for neonatal hyperbilirubinemia	239
00178	Risk for impaired liver function	240
00296	Risk for metabolic syndrome	241

Class 5. Hydration
The taking in and absorption of fluids and electrolytes

Code	Diagnosis	Page
00195	Risk for electrolyte imbalance	242
00025	Risk for imbalanced fluid volume	243
00027	Deficient fluid volume	244
00028	Risk for deficient fluid volume	245
00026	Excess fluid volume	246

NANDA International, Inc. Nursing Diagnoses: Definitions and Classification 2021–2023, 12th Edition.
Edited by T. Heather Herdman, Shigemi Kamitsuru, and Camila Takáo Lopes.
© 2021 NANDA International, Inc. Published 2021 by Thieme Medical Publishers, Inc., New York.
Companion website: www.thieme.com/nanda-i.

Domain 2 • Class 1 • Diagnosis Code 00002

Imbalanced nutrition: less than body requirements

Focus of the diagnosis: balanced nutrition
Approved 1975 • Revised 2000, 2017, 2020 • Level of Evidence 2.1

Definition
Intake of nutrients insufficient to meet metabolic needs.

Defining characteristics

- Abdominal cramping
- Abdominal pain
- Body weight below ideal weight range for age and gender
- Capillary fragility
- Constipation
- Delayed wound healing
- Diarrhea
- Excessive hair loss
- Food intake less than recommended daily allowance (RDA)
- Hyperactive bowel sounds
- Hypoglycemia
- Inadequate head circumference growth for age and gender
- Inadequate height increase for age and gender
- Lethargy
- Muscle hypotonia
- Neonatal weight gain < 30 g per day
- Pale mucous membranes
- Weight loss with adequate food intake

Related factors

- Altered taste perception
- Depressive symptoms
- Difficulty swallowing
- Food aversion
- Inaccurate information
- Inadequate food supply
- Inadequate interest in food
- Inadequate knowledge of nutrient requirements
- Injured buccal cavity
- Insufficient breast milk production
- Interrupted breastfeeding
- Misperception about ability to ingest food
- Satiety immediately upon ingesting food
- Sore buccal cavity
- Weakened muscles required for swallowing
- Weakened of muscles required for mastication

At risk population

- Competitive athletes
- Displaced individuals
- Economically disadvantaged individuals
- Individuals with low educational level
- Premature infants

Associated conditions

- Body dysmorphic disorders
- Digestive system diseases
- Immunosuppression
- Kwashiorkor
- Malabsorption syndromes
- Mental disorders
- Neoplasms
- Neurocognitive disorders
- Parasitic disorders

Domain 2 • Class 1 • Diagnosis Code 00163

Readiness for enhanced nutrition

Focus of the diagnosis: nutrition
Approved 2002 • Revised 2013 • Level of Evidence 2.1

Definition
A pattern of nutrient intake, which can be strengthened.

Defining characteristics
- Expresses desire to enhance
  nutrition

Domain 2 • Class 1 • Diagnosis Code 00216

Insufficient breast milk production

Focus of the diagnosis: breast milk production
Approved 2010 • Revised 2017 • Level of Evidence 3.1

Definition
Inadequate supply of maternal breast milk to support nutritional state of an infant or child.

Defining characteristics

- Absence of milk production with nipple stimulation
- Breast milk expressed is less than prescribed volume for infant
- Delayed milk production
- Infant constipation
- Infant frequently crying
- Infant frequently seeks to suckle at breast
- Infant refuses to suckle at breast
- Infant voids small amounts of concentrated urine
- Infant weight gain < 500 g in a month
- Prolonged breastfeeding time
- Unsustained suckling at breast

Related factors

- Ineffective latching on to breast
- Ineffective sucking reflex
- Infant's refusal to breastfeed
- Insufficient maternal fluid volume
- Insufficient opportunity for suckling at breast
- Insufficient suckling time at breast
- Maternal alcohol consumption
- Maternal malnutrition
- Maternal smoking
- Maternal treatment regimen

At risk population

- Women who become pregnant while breastfeeding

Original literature support available at www.thieme.com/nanda-i.

Domain 2 • Class 1 • Diagnosis Code 00104

Ineffective breastfeeding

Focus of the diagnosis: breastfeeding
Approved 1988 • Revised 2010, 2013, 2017 • Level of Evidence 3.1

Definition
Difficulty providing milk from the breast, which may compromise nutritional status of the infant/child.

Defining characteristics

Infant or Child

- Arching at breast
- Crying at breast
- Crying within one hour after breastfeeding
- Fussing within one hour after breastfeeding
- Inability to latch on to maternal breast correctly
- Inadequate stooling
- Inadequate weight gain
- Resisting latching on to breast
- Sustained weight loss
- Unresponsive to other comfort measures
- Unsustained suckling at breast

Mother

- Insufficient emptying of each breast during feeding
- Insufficient signs of oxytocin release
- Perceived inadequate milk supply
- Sore nipples persisting beyond first week

Related factors

- Delayed stage II lactogenesis
- Inadequate family support
- Inadequate parental knowledge regarding breastfeeding techniques
- Inadequate parental knowledge regarding importance of breastfeeding
- Ineffective infant suck-swallow response
- Insufficient breast milk production
- Insufficient opportunity for suckling at breast
- Interrupted breastfeeding
- Maternal ambivalence
- Maternal anxiety
- Maternal breast anomaly
- Maternal fatigue
- Maternal obesity
- Maternal pain
- Pacifier use
- Supplemental feedings with artificial nipple

At risk population

- Individuals with history of breast surgery
- Individuals with history of breast-feeding failure
- Mothers of premature infants
- Premature infants
- Women with short maternity leave

Associated conditions

- Oropharyngeal defect

Original literature support available at www.thieme.com/nanda-i.

Domain 2 • Class 1 • Diagnosis Code 00105

Interrupted breastfeeding

Focus of the diagnosis: breastfeeding
Approved 1992 • Revised 2013, 2017 • Level of Evidence 2.2

2. Nutrition

Definition
Break in the continuity of feeding milk from the breasts, which may compromise breastfeeding success and/or nutritional status of the infant/child.

Defining characteristics
- Nonexclusive breastfeeding

Related factors
- Abrupt weaning of infant
- Maternal-infant separation

At risk population
- Employed mothers
- Hospitalized children
- Hospitalized infants
- Premature infants

Associated conditions
- Contraindications to breastfeeding
- Infant illness
- Maternal illness

Original literature support available at www.thieme.com/nanda-i.

Domain 2 • Class 1 • Diagnosis Code 00106

Readiness for enhanced breastfeeding

Focus of the diagnosis: breastfeeding
Approved 1990 • Revised 2010, 2013, 2017 • Level of Evidence 2.2

Definition
A pattern of providing milk from the breasts to an infant or child, which can be strengthened.

Defining characteristics
- Expresses desire to enhance ability to exclusively breastfeed
- Expresses desire to enhance ability to provide breast milk for child's nutritional needs

Original literature support available at www.thieme.com/nanda-i.

Domain 2 • Class 1 • Diagnosis Code 00269

Ineffective adolescent eating dynamics

Focus of the diagnosis: eating dynamics
Approved 2016 • Level of Evidence 2.1

2. Nutrition

Definition
Altered attitudes and behaviors resulting in over or under eating patterns that compromise nutritional health.

Defining characteristics
- Avoids participation in regular mealtimes
- Complains of hunger between meals
- Depressive symptoms
- Food refusal
- Frequent snacking
- Frequently consumes fast food
- Frequently eating processed food
- Frequently eats low quality food
- Inadequate appetite
- Overeating
- Undereating

Related factors
- Altered family relations
- Anxiety
- Changes to self-esteem upon entering puberty
- Eating disorder
- Eating in isolation
- Excessive family mealtime control
- Excessive stress
- Inadequate dietary habits
- Irregular mealtime
- Media influence on eating behaviors of high caloric unhealthy foods
- Media influence on knowledge of high caloric unhealthy foods
- Negative parental influences on eating behaviors
- Psychological neglect
- Stressful mealtimes
- Unaddressed abuse

Associated conditions
- Depression
- Parental psychiatric disorder
- Physical challenge with eating
- Physical challenge with feeding
- Physical health issue of parent
- Psychological health issue of parent

Original literature support available at www.thieme.com/nanda-i.

Domain 2 • Class 1 • Diagnosis Code 00270

Ineffective child eating dynamics

Focus of the diagnosis: eating dynamics
Approved 2016 • Level of Evidence 2.1

Definition
Altered attitudes, behaviors, and influences on eating patterns resulting in compromised nutritional health.

Defining characteristics
- Avoids participation in regular mealtimes
- Complains of hunger between meals
- Food refusal
- Frequent snacking
- Frequently consumes fast food
- Frequently eating processed food
- Frequently eats low quality food
- Inadequate appetite
- Overeating
- Undereating

Related factors
Eating Habit

- Abnormal eating habit patterns
- Bribing child to eat
- Consumption of large volumes of food in a short period of time
- Eating in isolation
- Excessive parental control over child's eating experience
- Excessive parental control over family mealtime
- Forcing child to eat
- Inadequate dietary habits
- Lack of regular mealtimes
- Limiting child's eating
- Rewarding child to eat
- Stressful mealtimes
- Unpredictable eating patterns
- Unstructured eating of snacks between meals

Family Process

- Abusive interpersonal relations
- Anxious parent-child relations
- Disengaged parenting
- Hostile parent-child relations
- Insecure parent-child relations
- Intrusive parenting
- Tense parent-child relations
- Uninvolved parenting

Parental

- Anorexia
- Inability to divide eating responsibility between parent and child

- Inability to divide feeding responsibility between parent and child
- Inability to support healthy eating patterns
- Ineffective coping strategies

Unmodified Environmental Factors

- Media influence on eating behaviors of high caloric unhealthy foods

- Lack of confidence in child to develop healthy eating habits
- Lack of confidence in child to grow appropriately
- Substance misuse

- Media influence on knowledge of high caloric unhealthy foods

At risk population

- Children born to economically disadvantaged families
- Children experiencing homelessness

- Children experiencing life transition
- Children living in foster care
- Children whose parents are obese

Associated conditions

- Depression
- Parental psychiatric disorder
- Physical challenge with eating
- Physical challenge with feeding

- Physical health issue of parent
- Psychological health issue of parent

2. Nutrition

Original literature support available at www.thieme.com/nanda-i.

Domain 2 • Class 1 • Diagnosis Code 00271

Ineffective infant feeding dynamics

Focus of the diagnosis: feeding dynamics
Approved 2016 • Level of Evidence 2.1

Definition
Altered parental feeding behaviors resulting in over or under eating patterns.

Defining characteristics
- Food refusal
- Inadequate appetite
- Inappropriate transition to solid foods
- Overeating
- Undereating

Related factors
- Abusive interpersonal relations
- Attachment issues
- Disengaged parenting
- Intrusive parenting
- Lack of confidence in child to develop healthy eating habits
- Lack of confidence in child to grow appropriately
- Lack of knowledge of appropriate methods of feeding infant for each stage of development
- Lack of knowledge of infant's developmental stages
- Lack of knowledge of parent's responsibility in infant feeding
- Media influence on feeding infant high caloric unhealthy foods
- Media influence on knowledge of high caloric unhealthy foods
- Multiple caregivers
- Uninvolved parenting

At risk population
- Abandoned infants
- Infants born to economically disadvantaged families
- Infants experiencing homelessness
- Infants experiencing life transition
- Infants experiencing prolonged hospitalization
- Infants living in foster care
- Infants who are small for gestational age
- Infants with history of hospitalization in neonatal intensive care
- Infants with history of unsafe eating and feeding experiences
- Premature infants

Associated conditions
- Chromosomal disorders
- Cleft lip
- Cleft palate
- Congenital heart disease
- Inborn genetic diseases
- Neural tube defects

- Parental psychiatric disorder
- Physical challenge with eating
- Physical challenge with feeding
- Physical health issue of parent
- Prolonged enteral nutrition
- Psychological health issue of parent
- Sensory integration dysfunction

2. Nutrition

Original literature support available at www.thieme.com/nanda-i.

225

Domain 2 · Class 1 · Diagnosis Code 00232

Obesity

Focus of the diagnosis: obesity
Approved 2013 · Revised 2017 · Level of Evidence 3.2

> **Definition**
> A condition in which an individual accumulates excessive fat for age and gender that exceeds overweight.

Defining characteristics

- ADULT: Body mass index > 30 kg/m^2
- CHILD 2-18 years: Body mass index > 95th percentile or 30 kg/m^2 for age and gender
- CHILD < 2 years: Term not used with children at this age

Related factors

- Abnormal eating behavior patterns
- Abnormal eating perception patterns
- Average daily physical activity is less than recommended for age and gender
- Consumption of sugar-sweetened beverages
- Dysomnias
- Energy expenditure below energy intake based on standard assessment
- Excessive alcohol consumption
- Fear regarding lack of food supply
- Frequent snacking
- High frequency of restaurant or fried food
- Insufficient dietary calcium intake by children
- Portion sizes larger than recommended
- Sedentary behavior occurring for ≥ 2 hours/day
- Shortened sleep time
- Solid foods as major food source at < 5 months of age

At risk population

- Economically disadvantaged individuals
- Individuals who experienced premature pubarche
- Individuals who experienced rapid weight gain during childhood
- Individuals who experienced rapid weight gain during infancy
- Individuals who inherit interrelated factors
- Individuals who were not exclusively breastfed
- Individuals who were overweight during infancy
- Individuals whose mothers had gestational diabetes
- Individuals whose mothers have diabetes
- Individuals whose mothers smoke during childhood

- Individuals whose mothers smoke during pregnancy
- Individuals with high disinhibition and restraint eating behavior score
- Individuals with parents who are obese
- Neonates whose mothers had gestational diabetes

Associated conditions

- Inborn genetic diseases

2. Nutrition

Original literature support available at www.thieme.com/nanda-i.

Domain 2 • Class 1 • Diagnosis Code 00233

Overweight

Focus of the diagnosis: overweight
Approved 2013 • Revised 2017 • Level of Evidence 3.2

Definition
A condition in which an individual accumulates excessive fat for age and gender.

Defining characteristics
- ADULT: Body mass index > 25 kg/m²
- CHILD 2-18 years: Body mass index > 85th percentile or 25 kg/m² but < 95th percentile or 30 kg/m² for age and gender
- CHILD < 2 years: Weight-for-length > 95th percentile

Related factors
- Abnormal eating behavior patterns
- Abnormal eating perception patterns
- Average daily physical activity is less than recommended for age and gender
- Consumption of sugar-sweetened beverages
- Dysomnias
- Energy expenditure below energy intake based on standard assessment
- Excessive alcohol consumption
- Fear regarding lack of food supply
- Frequent snacking
- High frequency of restaurant or fried food
- Inadequate knowledge of modifiable factors
- Insufficient dietary calcium intake by children
- Portion sizes larger than recommended
- Sedentary behavior occurring for ≥ 2 hours/day
- Shortened sleep time
- Solid foods as major food source at < 5 months of age

At risk population
- ADULT: Body mass index approaching 25 kg/m²
- CHILD 2-18 years: Body mass index approaching 85th percentile or 25 kg/m²
- CHILD < 2 years: Weight-for-length approaching 95th percentile
- Children with body mass index crossing percentiles upward
- Children with high body mass index percentiles for age and gender
- Economically disadvantaged individuals

- Individuals who experienced premature pubarche
- Individuals who experienced rapid weight gain during childhood
- Individuals who experienced rapid weight gain during infancy
- Individuals who inherit interrelated factors
- Individuals who were not exclusively breastfed
- Individuals who were obese during childhood
- Individuals whose mothers have diabetes
- Individuals whose mothers smoke during childhood
- Individuals whose mothers smoke during pregnancy
- Individuals with high disinhibition and restraint eating behavior score
- Individuals with parents who are obese

Associated conditions

- Inborn genetic diseases

2. Nutrition

2. Nutrition

Domain 2 · Class 1 · Diagnosis Code 00234

Risk for overweight

Focus of the diagnosis: overweight
Approved 2013 · Revised 2017 · Level of Evidence 3.2

Definition
Susceptible to excessive fat accumulation for age and gender, which may compromise health.

Risk factors

- Abnormal eating behavior patterns
- Abnormal eating perception patterns
- Average daily physical activity is less than recommended for age and gender
- Consumption of sugar-sweetened beverages
- Dysomnias
- Energy expenditure below energy intake based on standard assessment
- Excessive alcohol consumption
- Fear regarding lack of food supply
- Frequent snacking
- High frequency of restaurant or fried food
- Inadequate knowledge of modifiable factors
- Insufficient dietary calcium intake by children
- Portion sizes larger than recommended
- Sedentary behavior occurring for ≥ 2 hours/day
- Shortened sleep time
- Solid foods as major food source at < 5 months of age

At risk population

- ADULT: Body mass index approaching 25 kg/m^2
- CHILD 2-18 years: Body mass index approaching 85th percentile or 25 kg/m^2
- CHILD < 2 years: Weight-for-length approaching 95th percentile
- Children with body mass index crossing percentiles upward
- Children with high body mass index percentiles for age and gender
- Economically disadvantaged individuals
- Individuals who experienced premature pubarche
- Individuals who experienced rapid weight gain during childhood
- Individuals who experienced rapid weight gain during infancy
- Individuals who inherit interrelated factors
- Individuals who were not exclusively breastfed
- Individuals who were obese during childhood
- Individuals whose mothers have diabetes
- Individuals whose mothers smoke during childhood
- Individuals whose mothers smoke during pregnancy

- Individuals with high disinhibition and restraint eating behavior score
- Individuals with parents who are obese

Associated conditions
- Inborn genetic diseases

Original literature support available at www.thieme.com/nanda-i.

Domain 2 • Class 1 • Diagnosis Code 00295

Ineffective infant suck-swallow response

Focus of the diagnosis: suck-swallow response
Approved 2020 • Level of Evidence 2.1

Definition
Impaired ability of an infant to suck or to coordinate the suck-swallow response .

Defining characteristics
- Arrhythmia
- Bradycardic events
- Choking
- Circumoral cyanosis
- Excessive coughing
- Finger splaying
- Flaccidity
- Gagging
- Hiccups
- Hyperextension of extremities
- Impaired ability to initiate an effective suck
- Impaired ability to sustain an effective suck
- Impaired motor tone
- Inability to coordinate sucking, swallowing, and breathing
- Irritability
- Nasal flaring
- Oxygen desaturation
- Pallor
- Subcostal retraction
- Time-out signals
- Use of accessory muscles of respiration

Related factors
- Hypoglycemia
- Hypothermia
- Hypotonia
- Inappropriate positioning
- Unsatisfactory sucking behavior

At risk population
- Infants born to mothers with substance misuse
- Infants delivered using obstetrical forceps
- Infants delivered using obstetrical vacuum extraction
- Infants experiencing prolonged hospitalization
- Premature infants

Associated conditions
- Convulsive episodes
- Gastroesophageal reflux
- High flow oxygen by nasal cannula
- Lacerations during delivery
- Low Appearance, Pulse, Grimace, Activity, & Respiration (APGAR) scores
- Neurological delay

- – Neurological impairment
- – Oral hypersensitivity

- – Oropharyngeal deformity
- – Prolonged enteral nutrition

Original literature support available at www.thieme.com/nanda-i.

Domain 2 • Class 1 • Diagnosis Code 00103

Impaired swallowing

Focus of the diagnosis: swallowing
Approved 1986 • Revised 1998, 2017, 2020 • Level of Evidence 3.2

Definition
Abnormal functioning of the swallowing mechanism associated with deficits in oral, pharyngeal, or esophageal structure or function.

Defining characteristics

First Stage: Oral

- Abnormal oral phase of swallow study
- Bruxism
- Choking prior to swallowing
- Choking when swallowing cold water
- Coughing prior to swallowing
- Drooling
- Food falls from mouth
- Food pushed out of mouth
- Gagging prior to swallowing
- Impaired ability to clear oral cavity
- Inadequate consumption during prolonged meal time
- Inadequate lip closure
- Inadequate mastication
- Incidence of wet hoarseness twice within 30 seconds
- Inefficient nippling
- Inefficient suck
- Nasal reflux
- Piecemeal deglutition
- Pooling of bolus in lateral sulci
- Premature entry of bolus
- Prolonged bolus formation
- Tongue action ineffective in forming bolus

Second Stage: Pharyngeal

- Abnormal pharyngeal phase of swallow study
- Altered head position
- Choking
- Coughing
- Delayed swallowing
- Fevers of unknown etiology
- Food refusal
- Gagging sensation
- Gurgly voice quality
- Inadequate laryngeal elevation
- Nasal reflux
- Recurrent pulmonary infection
- Repetitive swallowing

Third Stage: Esophageal

- Abnormal esophageal phase of swallow study
- Acidic-smelling breath
- Difficulty swallowing
- Epigastric pain
- Food refusal
- Heartburn
- Hematemesis

2. Nutrition

- Hyperextension of head
- Nighttime awakening
- Nighttime coughing
- Odynophagia
- Regurgitation
- Repetitive swallowing

- Reports "something stuck"
- Unexplained irritability surrounding mealtimes
- Volume limiting
- Vomiting
- Vomitus on pillow

Related factors

- Altered attention
- Behavioral feeding problem

- Protein-energy malnutrition
- Self-injurious behavior

At risk population

- Individuals with history of enteral nutrition
- Older adults

- Premature infants

Associated conditions

- Acquired anatomic defects
- Brain injuries
- Cerebral palsy
- Conditions with significant muscle hypotonia
- Congenital heart disease
- Cranial nerve involvement
- Developmental disabilities
- Esophageal achalasia
- Gastroesophageal reflux disease
- Laryngeal diseases
- Mechanical obstruction
- Nasal defect

- Nasopharyngeal cavity defect
- Neurological problems
- Neuromuscular diseases
- Oropharynx abnormality
- Pharmaceutical preparations
- Prolonged intubation
- Respiratory condition
- Tracheal defect
- Trauma
- Upper airway anomaly
- Vocal cord dysfunction

2. Nutrition

Domain 2 • Class 4 • Diagnosis Code 00179

Risk for unstable blood glucose level

Focus of the diagnosis: blood glucose level
Approved 2006 • Revised 2013, 2017, 2020 • Level of Evidence 3.2

Definition
Susceptible to variation in serum levels of glucose from the normal range, which may compromise health.

Risk factors
- Excessive stress
- Excessive weight gain
- Excessive weight loss
- Inadequate adherence to treatment regimen
- Inadequate blood glucose self-monitoring
- Inadequate diabetes self-management
- Inadequate dietary intake
- Inadequate knowledge of disease management
- Inadequate knowledge of modifiable factors
- Ineffective medication self-management
- Sedentary lifestyle

At risk population
- Individuals experiencing rapid growth period
- Individuals in intensive care units
- Individuals of African descent
- Individuals with altered mental status
- Individuals with compromised physical health status
- Individuals with delayed cognitive development
- Individuals with family history of diabetes mellitus
- Individuals with history of autoimmune disorders
- Individuals with history of gestational diabetes
- Individuals with history of hypoglycemia
- Individuals with history of pre-pregnancy overweight
- Low birth weight infants
- Native American individuals
- Pregnant women > 22 years of age
- Premature infants
- Women with hormonal shifts indicative of normal life stage changes

Associated conditions

- Cardiogenic shock
- Diabetes mellitus
- Infections
- Pancreatic diseases
- Pharmaceutical preparations
- Polycystic ovary syndrome
- Pre-eclampsia
- Pregnancy-induced hypertension
- Surgical procedures

2. Nutrition

Original literature support available at www.thieme.com/nanda-i.

Domain 2 • Class 4 • Diagnosis Code 00194

Neonatal hyperbilirubinemia

Focus of the diagnosis: hyperbilirubinemia
Approved 2008 • Revised 2010, 2017 • Level of Evidence 2.1

Definition
The accumulation of unconjugated bilirubin in the circulation (less than 15 ml/dl) that occurs after 24 hours of life.

Defining characteristics
- Abnormal liver function test results
- Bruised skin
- Yellow mucous membranes
- Yellow sclera
- Yellow-orange skin color

Related factors
- Delay in meconium passage
- Inadequate paternal feeding behavior
- Malnourished infants

At risk population
- East Asian neonates
- Low birth weight neonates
- Native American neonates
- Neonates aged ≤ 7 days
- Neonates who are breastfed
- Neonates whose blood groups are incompatible with mothers'
- Neonates whose mothers had gestational diabetes
- Neonates whose sibling had history of jaundice
- Neonates with significant bruising during birth
- Populations living at high altitudes
- Premature neonates

Associated conditions
- Bacterial infections
- Enzyme deficiency
- Impaired metabolism
- Internal bleeding
- Liver malfunction
- Prenatal infection
- Sepsis
- Viral infection

Original literature support available at www.thieme.com/nanda-i.

Domain 2 • Class 4 • Diagnosis Code 00230

Risk for neonatal hyperbilirubinemia

Focus of the diagnosis: hyperbilirubinemia
Approved 2010 • Revised 2013, 2017 • Level of Evidence 2.1

2. Nutrition

Definition
Susceptible to the accumulation of unconjugated bilirubin in the circulation (less than 15 ml/dl) that occurs after 24 hours of life which may compromise health.

Risk factors
- Delay in meconium passage
- Inadequate paternal feeding behavior
- Malnourished infants

At risk population
- East Asian neonates
- Low birth weight neonates
- Native American neonates
- Neonates aged ≤ 7 days
- Neonates who are breastfed
- Neonates whose blood groups are incompatible with mothers'
- Neonates whose mothers had gestational diabetes
- Neonates whose sibling had history of jaundice
- Neonates with significant bruising during birth
- Populations living at high altitudes
- Premature neonates

Associated conditions
- Bacterial infections
- Enzyme deficiency
- Impaired metabolism
- Internal bleeding
- Liver malfunction
- Prenatal infection
- Sepsis
- Viral infection

Original literature support available at www.thieme.com/nanda-i.

Domain 2 • Class 4 • Diagnosis Code 00178

Risk for impaired liver function

Focus of the diagnosis: liver function
Approved 2006 • Revised 2008, 2013, 2017 • Level of Evidence 2.1

Definition
Susceptible to a decrease in liver function, which may compromise health.

Risk factors
– Substance misuse

Associated conditions
– Human immunodeficiency virus (HIV) coinfection
– Pharmaceutical preparations
– Viral infection

This diagnosis will retire from the NANDA-I Taxonomy in the 2024–2026 edition if no additional risk factors are developed.

Original literature support available at www.thieme.com/nanda-i.

Domain 2 · Class 4 · Diagnosis Code 00296

Risk for metabolic syndrome

Focus of the diagnosis: metabolic syndrome
Approved 2020 · Level of Evidence 2.1

Definition
Susceptible to developing a cluster of symptoms that increase risk of cardio-vascular disease and type 2 diabetes mellitus, which may compromise health.

Risk factors

- Absence of interest in improving health behaviors
- Average daily physical activity is less than recommended for age and gender
- Body mass index above normal range for age and gender
- Excessive accumulation of fat for age and gender
- Excessive alcohol intake
- Excessive stress
- Inadequate dietary habits
- Inadequate knowledge of modifiable factors
- Inattentive to second-hand smoke
- Smoking

At risk population

- Individuals aged > 30 years
- Individuals with family history of diabetes mellitus
- Individuals with family history of dyslipidemia
- Individuals with family history of hypertension
- Individuals with family history of metabolic syndrome
- Individuals with family history of obesity
- Individuals with family history of unstable blood pressure

Associated conditions

- Hyperuricemia
- Insulin resistance
- Polycystic ovary syndrome

Original literature support available at www.thieme.com/nanda-i.

Domain 2 · Class 5 · Diagnosis Code 00195

Risk for electrolyte imbalance

Focus of the diagnosis: electrolyte balance
Approved 2008 · Revised 2013, 2017 · Level of Evidence 2.1

Definition
Susceptible to changes in serum electrolyte levels, which may compromise health.

Risk factors
- Diarrhea
- Excessive fluid volume
- Inadequate knowledge of modifiable factors
- Insufficient fluid volume
- Vomiting

Associated conditions
- Compromised regulatory mechanism
- Endocrine regulatory dysfunction
- Renal dysfunction
- Treatment regimen

Original literature support available at www.thieme.com/nanda-i.

Domain 2 • Class 5 • Diagnosis Code 00025

Risk for imbalanced fluid volume

Focus of the diagnosis: balanced fluid volume
Approved 1998 • Revised 2008, 2013, 2017, 2020 • Level of Evidence 2.1

Definition
Susceptible to a decrease, increase, or rapid shift from one to the other of intravascular, interstitial and/or intracellular fluid, which may compromise health.

Risk factors
- Altered fluid intake
- Difficulty accessing water
- Excessive sodium intake
- Inadequate knowledge about fluid needs
- Ineffective medication self-management
- Insufficient muscle mass
- Malnutrition

At risk population
- Individuals at extremes of weight
- Individuals with external conditions affecting fluid needs
- Individuals with internal conditions affecting fluid needs
- Women

Associated conditions
- Active fluid volume loss
- Deviations affecting fluid absorption
- Deviations affecting fluid elimination
- Deviations affecting fluid intake
- Deviations affecting vascular permeability
- Excessive fluid loss through normal route
- Fluid loss through abnormal route
- Pharmaceutical preparations
- Treatment regimen

Original literature support available at www.thieme.com/nanda-i.

2. Nutrition

2. Nutrition

Domain 2 • Class 5 • Diagnosis Code 00027

Deficient fluid volume

Focus of the diagnosis: fluid volume
Approved 1978 • Revised 1996, 2017, 2020 • Level of Evidence 2.1

Definition
Decreased intravascular, interstitial, and/or intracellular fluid. This refers to dehydration, water loss alone without change in sodium.

Defining characteristics

- Altered mental status
- Altered skin turgor
- Decreased blood pressure
- Decreased pulse pressure
- Decreased pulse volume
- Decreased tongue turgor
- Decreased urine output
- Decreased venous filling
- Dry mucous membranes
- Dry skin
- Increased body temperature
- Increased heart rate
- Increased serum hematocrit levels
- Increased urine concentration
- Sudden weight loss
- Sunken eyes
- Thirst
- Weakness

Related factors

- Difficulty meeting increased fluid volume requirement
- Inadequate access to fluid
- Inadequate knowledge about fluid needs
- Ineffective medication self-management
- Insufficient fluid intake
- Insufficient muscle mass
- Malnutrition

At risk population

- Individuals at extremes of weight
- Individuals with external conditions affecting fluid needs
- Individuals with internal conditions affecting fluid needs
- Women

Associated conditions

- Active fluid volume loss
- Deviations affecting fluid absorption
- Deviations affecting fluid elimination
- Deviations affecting fluid intake
- Excessive fluid loss through normal route
- Fluid loss through abnormal route
- Pharmaceutical preparations
- Treatment regimen

Domain 2 • Class 5 • Diagnosis Code 00028

Risk for deficient fluid volume

Focus of the diagnosis: fluid volume
Approved 1978 • Revised 2010, 2013, 2017, 2020 • Level of Evidence 2.1

Definition
Susceptible to experiencing decreased intravascular, interstitial, and/or intracellular fluid volumes, which may compromise health.

Risk factors
- Difficulty meeting increased fluid volume requirement
- Inadequate access to fluid
- Inadequate knowledge about fluid needs
- Ineffective medication self-management
- Insufficient fluid intake
- Insufficient muscle mass
- Malnutrition

At risk population
- Individuals at extremes of weight
- Individuals with external conditions affecting fluid needs
- Individuals with internal conditions affecting fluid needs
- Women

Associated conditions
- Active fluid volume loss
- Deviations affecting fluid absorption
- Deviations affecting fluid elimination
- Deviations affecting fluid intake
- Excessive fluid loss through normal route
- Fluid loss through abnormal route
- Pharmaceutical preparations
- Treatment regimen

2. Nutrition

Domain 2 • Class 5 • Diagnosis Code 00026

Excess fluid volume

Focus of the diagnosis: fluid volume
Approved 1982 • Revised 1996, 2013, 2017, 2020 • Level of Evidence 2.1

Definition
Surplus retention of fluid.

Defining characteristics

- Adventitious breath sounds
- Altered blood pressure
- Altered mental status
- Altered pulmonary artery pressure
- Altered respiratory pattern
- Altered urine specific gravity
- Anxiety
- Azotemia
- Decreased serum hematocrit levels
- Decreased serum hemoglobin level
- Edema
- Hepatomegaly
- Increased central venous pressure
- Intake exceeds output
- Jugular vein distension
- Oliguria
- Pleural effusion
- Positive hepatojugular reflex
- Presence of S3 heart sound
- Psychomotor agitation
- Pulmonary congestion
- Weight gain over short period of time

Related factors

- Excessive fluid intake
- Excessive sodium intake
- Ineffective medication self-management

Associated conditions

- Deviations affecting fluid elimination
- Pharmaceutical preparations

Original literature support available at www.thieme.com/nanda-i.

Domain 3.
Elimination and exchange

Secretion and excretion of waste products from the body

Class 1. Urinary function
The process of secretion, reabsorption, and excretion of urine

Class 2. Gastrointestinal function
The process of absorption and excretion of the end products of digestion

Class 3. Integumentary function
The process of secretion and excretion through the skin

Code	Diagnosis	Page
	This class does not currently contain any diagnoses	

Class 4. Respiratory function
The process of exchange of gases and removal of the end products of metabolism

Code	Diagnosis	Page
00030	Impaired gas exchange	270

NANDA International, Inc. Nursing Diagnoses: Definitions and Classification 2021–2023, 12th Edition. Edited by T. Heather Herdman, Shigemi Kamitsuru, and Camila Takáo Lopes. © 2021 NANDA International, Inc. Published 2021 by Thieme Medical Publishers, Inc., New York. Companion website: www.thieme.com/nanda-i.

Domain 3 • Class 1 • Diagnosis Code 00297

Disability-associated urinary incontinence

Focus of the diagnosis: disability-associated incontinence
Approved 2020 • Level of Evidence 2.3

> **Definition**
> Involuntary loss of urine not associated with any pathology or problem related to the urinary system.

Defining characteristics

- Adaptive behaviors to avoid others' recognition of urinary incontinence
- Mapping routes to public bathrooms prior to leaving home
- Time required to reach toilet is too long after sensation of urge
- Use of techniques to prevent urination
- Voiding prior to reaching toilet

Related factors

- Avoidance of non-hygienic toilet use
- Caregiver inappropriately implements bladder training techniques
- Cognitive dysfunction
- Difficulty finding the bathroom
- Difficulty obtaining timely assistance to bathroom
- Embarrassment regarding toilet use in social situations
- Environmental constraints that interfere with continence
- Habitually suppresses urge to urinate
- Impaired physical mobility
- Impaired postural balance
- Inadequate motivation to maintain continence
- Increased fluid intake
- Neurobehavioral manifestations
- Pelvic floor disorders

At risk population

- Children
- Older adults

Associated conditions

- Heart diseases
- Impaired coordination
- Impaired hand dexterity
- Intellectual disability
- Neuromuscular diseases
- Osteoarticular diseases
- Pharmaceutical preparations
- Psychological disorder
- Vision disorders

Original literature support available at www.thieme.com/nanda-i.

Domain 3 • Class 1 • Diagnosis Code 00016

Impaired urinary elimination

Focus of the diagnosis: elimination
Approved 1973 • Revised 2006, 2017, 2020 • Level of Evidence 3.1

Definition
Dysfunction in urine elimination.

Defining characteristics
- Dysuria
- Frequent voiding
- Nocturia
- Urinary hesitancy
- Urinary incontinence
- Urinary retention
- Urinary urgency

Related factors
- Alcohol consumption
- Altered environmental factor
- Caffeine consumption
- Environmental constraints
- Fecal impaction
- Improper toileting posture
- Ineffective toileting habits
- Insufficient privacy
- Involuntary sphincter relaxation
- Obesity
- Pelvic organ prolapse
- Smoking
- Use of aspartame
- Weakened bladder muscle
- Weakened supportive pelvic structure

At risk population
- Older adults
- Women

Associated conditions
- Anatomic obstruction
- Diabetes mellitus
- Sensory motor impairment
- Urinary tract infection

Original literature support available at www.thieme.com/nanda-i.

Domain 3 • Class 1 • Diagnosis Code 00310

Mixed urinary incontinence

Focus of the diagnosis: incontinence
Approved 2020 • Level of Evidence 2.3

> **Definition**
> Involuntary loss of urine in combination with or following a strong sensation or urgency to void, and also with activities that increase intra-abdominal pressure.

Defining characteristics
- Expresses incomplete bladder emptying
- Involuntary loss of urine upon coughing
- Involuntary loss of urine upon effort
- Involuntary loss of urine upon laughing
- Involuntary loss of urine upon physical exertion
- Involuntary loss of urine upon sneezing
- Nocturia
- Urinary urgency

Related factors
- Incompetence of the bladder neck
- Incompetence of the urethral sphincter
- Overweight
- Pelvic organ prolapse
- Skeletal muscular atrophy
- Smoking
- Weak anterior wall of the vagina

At risk population
- Individuals with chronic cough
- Individuals with one type of urinary incontinence
- Multiparous women
- Older adults
- Women experiencing menopause
- Women giving birth vaginally

Associated conditions
- Diabetes mellitus
- Estrogen deficiency
- Motor disorders
- Pelvic floor disorders
- Prolonged urinary incontinence
- Surgery for stress urinary incontinence
- Urethral sphincter injury

Original literature support available at www.thieme.com/nanda-i.

Domain 3 • Class 1 • Diagnosis Code 00017

Stress urinary incontinence

Focus of the diagnosis: incontinence
Approved 1986 • Revised 2006, 2017, 2020 • Level of Evidence 2.3

> **Definition**
> Involuntary loss of urine with activities that increase intra-abdominal pressure, which is not associated with urgency to void.

Defining characteristics

- Involuntary loss of urine in the absence of detrusor contraction
- Involuntary loss of urine in the absence of overdistended bladder
- Involuntary loss of urine upon coughing
- Involuntary loss of urine upon effort
- Involuntary loss of urine upon laughing
- Involuntary loss of urine upon physical exertion
- Involuntary loss of urine upon sneezing

Related factors

- Overweight
- Pelvic floor disorders
- Pelvic organ prolapse

At risk population

- Individuals who perform high-intensity physical exercise
- Multiparous women
- Pregnant women
- Women experiencing menopause
- Women giving birth vaginally

Associated conditions

- Damaged pelvic floor muscles
- Degenerative changes in pelvic floor muscles
- Intrinsic urethral sphincter deficiency
- Nervous system diseases
- Prostatectomy
- Urethral sphincter injury

Original literature support available at www.thieme.com/nanda-i.

Domain 3 • Class 1 • Diagnosis Code 00019

Urge urinary incontinence

Focus of the diagnosis: incontinence
Approved 1986 • Revised 2006, 2017, 2020 • Level of Evidence 2.3

Definition
Involuntary loss of urine in combination with or following a strong sensation or urgency to void.

Defining characteristics
- Decreased bladder capacity
- Feeling of urgency with triggered stimulus
- Increased urinary frequency
- Involuntary loss of urine before reaching toilet
- Involuntary loss of urine with bladder contractions
- Involuntary loss of urine with bladder spasms
- Involuntary loss of varying volumes of urine between voids, with urgency
- Nocturia

Related factors
- Alcohol consumption
- Anxiety
- Caffeine consumption
- Carbonated beverage consumption
- Fecal impaction
- Ineffective toileting habits
- Involuntary sphincter relaxation
- Overweight
- Pelvic floor disorders
- Pelvic organ prolapse

At risk population
- Individuals exposed to abuse
- Individuals with history of urinary urgency during childhood
- Older adults
- Women
- Women experiencing menopause

Associated conditions
- Atrophic vaginitis
- Bladder outlet obstruction
- Depression
- Diabetes mellitus
- Nervous system diseases
- Nervous system trauma
- Overactive pelvic floor
- Pharmaceutical preparations
- Treatment regimen
- Urologic diseases

Original literature support available at www.thieme.com/nanda-i.

Domain 3 • Class 1 • Diagnosis Code 00022

Risk for urge urinary incontinence

Focus of the diagnosis: incontinence
Approved 1998 • Revised 2008, 2013, 2017, 2020 • Level of Evidence 2.2

Definition
Susceptible to involuntary passage of urine occurring soon after a strong sensation or urgency to void, which may compromise health.

Risk factors
- Alcohol consumption
- Anxiety
- Caffeine consumption
- Carbonated beverage consumption
- Fecal impaction
- Ineffective toileting habits
- Involuntary sphincter relaxation
- Overweight
- Pelvic floor disorders
- Pelvic organ prolapse

At risk population
- Individuals exposed to abuse
- Individuals with history of urinary urgency during childhood
- Older adults
- Women
- Women experiencing menopause

Associated conditions
- Atrophic vaginitis
- Bladder outlet obstruction
- Depression
- Diabetes mellitus
- Nervous system diseases
- Nervous system trauma
- Overactive pelvic floor
- Pharmaceutical preparations
- Treatment regimen
- Urologic diseases

Original literature support available at www.thieme.com/nanda-i.

Domain 3 • Class 1 • Diagnosis Code 00023

Urinary retention

Focus of the diagnosis: retention
Approved 1986 • Revised 2017, 2020 • Level of Evidence 3.1

Definition
Incomplete emptying of the bladder.

Defining characteristics
- Absence of urinary output
- Bladder distention
- Dysuria
- Increased daytime urinary frequency
- Minimal void volume
- Overflow incontinence
- Reports sensation of bladder fullness
- Reports sensation of residual urine
- Weak urine stream

Related factors
- Environmental constraints
- Fecal impaction
- Improper toileting posture
- Inadequate relaxation of pelvic floor muscles
- Insufficient privacy
- Pelvic organ prolapse
- Weakened bladder muscle

At risk population
- Puerperal women

Associated conditions
- Benign prostatic hyperplasia
- Diabetes mellitus
- Nervous system diseases
- Pharmaceutical preparations
- Urinary tract obstruction

Domain 3 • Class 1 • Diagnosis Code 00322

Risk for urinary retention

Focus of the diagnosis: retention
Approved 2020 • Level of Evidence 3.1

Definition
Susceptible to incomplete emptying of the bladder.

Risk factors
- Environmental constraints
- Fecal impaction
- Improper toileting posture
- Inadequate relaxation of pelvic floor muscles
- Insufficient privacy
- Pelvic organ prolapse
- Weakened bladder muscle

At risk population
- Puerperal women

Associated conditions
- Benign prostatic hyperplasia
- Diabetes mellitus
- Nervous system diseases
- Pharmaceutical preparations
- Urinary tract obstruction

Original literature support available at www.thieme.com/nanda-i.

Domain 3 • Class 2 • Diagnosis Code 00011

Constipation

Focus of the diagnosis: constipation
Approved 1975 • Revised 1998, 2017, 2020 • Level of Evidence 3.1

Definition
Infrequent or difficult evacuation of feces.

Defining characteristics
- Evidence of symptoms in standardized diagnostic criteria
- Hard stools
- Lumpy stools
- Need for manual maneuvers to facilitate defecation
- Passing fewer than three stools a week
- Sensation of anorectal obstruction
- Sensation of incomplete evacuation
- Straining with defecation

Related factors
- Altered regular routine
- Average daily physical activity is less than recommended for age and gender
- Cognitive dysfunction
- Communication barriers
- Habitually suppresses urge to defecate
- Impaired physical mobility
- Impaired postural balance
- Inadequate knowledge of modifiable factors
- Inadequate toileting habits
- Insufficient fiber intake
- Insufficient fluid intake
- Insufficient privacy
- Stressors
- Substance misuse

At risk population
- Individuals admitted to hospital
- Individuals experiencing prolonged hospitalization
- Individuals in aged care settings
- Individuals in the early postoperative period
- Older adults
- Pregnant women
- Women

Associated conditions
- Blockage in the colon
- Blockage in the rectum
- Depression
- Developmental disabilities
- Digestive system diseases
- Endocrine system diseases
- Heart diseases
- Mental disorders

- Muscular diseases
- Nervous system diseases
- Neurocognitive disorders
- Pelvic floor disorders
- Pharmaceutical preparations
- Radiotherapy
- Urogynecological disorders

Domain 3 • Class 2 • Diagnosis Code 00015

Risk for constipation

Focus of the diagnosis: constipation
Approved 1998 • Revised 2013, 2017, 2020 • Level of Evidence 3.2

Definition
Susceptible to infrequent or difficult evacuation of feces, which may compromise health.

Risk factors
- Altered regular routine
- Average daily physical activity is less than recommended for age and gender
- Cognitive dysfunction
- Communication barriers
- Habitually suppresses urge to defecate
- Impaired physical mobility
- Impaired postural balance
- Inadequate knowledge of modifiable factors
- Inadequate toileting habits
- Insufficient fiber intake
- Insufficient fluid intake
- Insufficient privacy
- Stressors
- Substance misuse

At risk population
- Individuals admitted to hospital
- Individuals experiencing prolonged hospitalization
- Individuals in aged care settings
- Individuals in the early postoperative period
- Older adults
- Pregnant women
- Women

Associated conditions
- Blockage in the colon
- Blockage in the rectum
- Depression
- Developmental disabilities
- Digestive system diseases
- Endocrine system diseases
- Heart diseases
- Mental disorders
- Muscular diseases
- Nervous system diseases
- Neurocognitive disorders
- Pelvic floor disorders
- Pharmaceutical preparations
- Radiotherapy
- Urogynecological disorders

Domain 3 • Class 2 • Diagnosis Code 00012

Perceived constipation

Focus of the diagnosis: constipation
Approved 1988 • Revised 2020 • Level of Evidence 2.1

Definition
Self-diagnosis of infrequent or difficult evacuation of feces combined with abuse of methods to ensure a daily bowel movement.

Defining characteristics
- Enema misuse
- Expects bowel movement at same time daily
- Laxative misuse
- Suppository misuse

Related factors
- Cultural health beliefs
- Deficient knowledge about normal evacuation patterns
- Disturbed thought processes
- Family health beliefs

Domain 3 • Class 2 • Diagnosis Code 00235

Chronic functional constipation

Focus of the diagnosis: functional constipation
Approved 2013 • Revised 2017 • Level of Evidence 2.2

> **Definition**
> Infrequent or difficult evacuation of feces, which has been present for at least 3 of the prior 12 months.

Defining characteristics

General

- Distended abdomen
- Fecal impaction
- Leakage of stool with digital stimulation
- Pain with defecation
- Palpable abdominal mass
- Positive fecal occult blood test
- Prolonged straining
- Type 1 or 2 on Bristol Stool Chart

Adult: Presence of ≥ 2 of the following symptoms on Rome III classification system:

- Lumpy or hard stools in ≥ 25% defecations
- Manual maneuvers to facilitate ≥ 25% of defecations (digital manipulation, pelvic floor support)
- Sensation of anorectal obstruction/blockage for ≥ 25% of defecations
- Sensation of incomplete evacuation for ≥ 25% of defecations
- Straining during ≥ 25% of defecations
- ≤ 3 evacuations per week

Child > 4 years: Presence of ≥ 2 criteria on Rome III Pediatric classification system for ≥ 2 months:

- Large diameter stools that may obstruct the toilet
- Painful or hard bowel movements
- Presence of large fecal mass in the rectum
- Stool retentive posturing
- ≤ 2 defecations per week
- ≥ 1 episode of fecal incontinence per week

Child ≤ 4 years: Presence of ≥ 2 criteria on Rome III Pediatric classification system for ≥ 1 month:

- Large diameter stools that may obstruct the toilet
- Painful or hard bowel movements

- Presence of large fecal mass in the rectum
- Stool retentive posturing

- ≤ 2 defecations per week
- ≥ 1 episode of fecal incontinence per week

Related factors

- Decreased food intake
- Dehydration
- Diet disproportionally high in fat
- Diet disproportionally high in protein
- Frail elderly syndrome
- Habitually suppresses urge to defecate
- Impaired physical mobility

- Inadequate dietary intake
- Inadequate knowledge of modifiable factors
- Insufficient fiber intake
- Insufficient fluid intake
- Low caloric intake
- Sedentary lifestyle

At risk population

- Older adults

- Pregnant women

Associated conditions

- Amyloidosis
- Anal fissure
- Anal stricture
- Autonomic neuropathy
- Chronic intestinal pseudo-obstruction
- Chronic renal insufficiency
- Colorectal cancer
- Depression
- Dermatomyositis
- Diabetes mellitus
- Extra intestinal mass
- Hemorrhoids
- Hirschprung's disease
- Hypercalcemia
- Hypothyroidism
- Inflammatory bowel disease
- Ischemic stenosis
- Multiple sclerosis

- Myotonic dystrophy
- Neurocognitive disorders
- Panhypopituitarism
- Paraplegia
- Parkinson's disease
- Pelvic floor disorders
- Perineal damage
- Pharmaceutical preparations
- Polypharmacy
- Porphyria
- Postinflammatory stenosis
- Proctitis
- Scleroderma
- Slow colon transit time
- Spinal cord injuries
- Stroke
- Surgical stenosis

Original literature support available at www.thieme.com/nanda-i.

Domain 3 • Class 2 • Diagnosis Code 00236

Risk for chronic functional constipation

Focus of the diagnosis: functional constipation
Approved 2013 • Revised 2017 • Level of Evidence 2.2

3. Elimination and exchange

> **Definition**
> Susceptible to infrequent or difficult evacuation of feces, which has been present nearly 3 of the prior 12 months, which may compromise health.

Risk factors

- Decreased food intake
- Dehydration
- Diet disproportionally high in fat
- Diet disproportionally high in protein
- Frail elderly syndrome
- Habitually suppresses urge to defecate
- Impaired physical mobility
- Inadequate dietary intake
- Inadequate knowledge of modifiable factors
- Insufficient fiber intake
- Insufficient fluid intake
- Low caloric intake
- Sedentary lifestyle

At risk population

- Older adults
- Pregnant women

Associated conditions

- Amyloidosis
- Anal fissure
- Anal stricture
- Autonomic neuropathy
- Chronic intestinal pseudo-obstruction
- Chronic renal insufficiency
- Colorectal cancer
- Depression
- Dermatomyositis
- Diabetes mellitus
- Extra intestinal mass
- Hemorrhoids
- Hirschsprung's disease
- Hypercalcemia
- Hypothyroidism
- Inflammatory bowel disease
- Ischemic stenosis
- Multiple sclerosis
- Myotonic dystrophy
- Neurocognitive disorders
- Panhypopituitarism
- Paraplegia
- Parkinson's disease
- Pelvic floor disorders
- Perineal damage
- Pharmaceutical preparations
- Polypharmacy
- Porphyria
- Postinflammatory stenosis

- Proctitis
- Scleroderma
- Slow colon transit time
- Spinal cord injuries
- Stroke
- Surgical stenosis

Original literature support available at www.thieme.com/nanda-i.

Domain 3 • Class 2 • Diagnosis Code 00319

Impaired bowel continence

Focus of the diagnosis: continence
Approved 2020 • Level of Evidence 3.1

> **Definition**
> Inability to hold stool, to sense the presence of stool in the rectum, to relax and store stool when having a bowel movement is not convenient.

Defining characteristics
- Abdominal discomfort
- Bowel urgency
- Fecal staining
- Impaired ability to expel formed stool despite recognition of rectal fullness
- Inability to delay defecation
- Inability to hold flatus
- Inability to reach toilet in time
- Inattentive to urge to defecate
- Silent leakage of stool during activities

Related factors
- Avoidance of non-hygienic toilet use
- Constipation
- Dependency for toileting
- Diarrhea
- Difficulty finding the bathroom
- Difficulty obtaining timely assistance to bathroom
- Embarrassment regarding toilet use in social situations
- Environmental constraints that interfere with continence
- Generalized decline in muscle tone
- Impaired physical mobility
- Impaired postural balance
- Inadequate dietary habits
- Inadequate motivation to maintain continence
- Incomplete emptying of bowel
- Laxative misuse
- Stressors

At risk population
- Older adults
- Women giving birth vaginally
- Women giving birth with obstetrical extraction

Associated conditions
- Anal trauma
- Congenital abnormalities of the digestive system
- Diabetes mellitus
- Neurocognitive disorders
- Neurological diseases
- Physical inactivity
- Prostatic diseases

- Rectum trauma
- Spinal cord injuries

- Stroke

Original literature support available at www.thieme.com/nanda-i.

Domain 3 • Class 2 • Diagnosis Code 00013

Diarrhea

Focus of the diagnosis: diarrhea
Approved 1975 • Revised 1998, 2017, 2020 • Level of Evidence 3.1

Definition
Passage of three or more loose or liquid stools per day.

Defining characteristics
- Abdominal cramping
- Abdominal pain
- Bowel urgency
- Dehydration
- Hyperactive bowel sounds

Related factors
- Anxiety
- Early formula feeding
- Inadequate access to safe drinking water
- Inadequate access to safe food
- Inadequate knowledge about rotavirus vaccine
- Inadequate knowledge about sanitary food preparation
- Inadequate knowledge about sanitary food storage
- Inadequate personal hygiene practices
- Increased stress level
- Laxative misuse
- Malnutrition
- Substance misuse

At risk population
- Frequent travelers
- Individuals at extremes of age
- Individuals exposed to toxins

Associated conditions
- Critical illness
- Endocrine system diseases
- Enteral nutrition
- Gastrointestinal diseases
- Immunosuppression
- Infections
- Pharmaceutical preparations
- Treatment regimen

Domain 3 • Class 2 • Diagnosis Code 00196

Dysfunctional gastrointestinal motility

Focus of the diagnosis: gastrointestinal motility
Approved 2008 • Revised 2017 • Level of Evidence 2.1

Definition
Increased, decreased, ineffective, or lack of peristaltic activity within the gastro-intestinal tract.

Defining characteristics
- Abdominal cramping
- Abdominal pain
- Absence of flatus
- Acceleration of gastric emptying
- Altered bowel sounds
- Bile-colored gastric residual
- Diarrhea
- Difficulty with defecation
- Distended abdomen
- Hard, formed stool
- Increased gastric residual
- Nausea
- Regurgitation
- Vomiting

Related factors
- Altered water source
- Anxiety
- Eating habit change
- Impaired physical mobility
- Malnutrition
- Sedentary lifestyle
- Stressors
- Unsanitary food preparation

At risk population
- Individuals who ingested contaminated material
- Older adults
- Premature infants

Associated conditions
- Decreased gastrointestinal circulation
- Diabetes mellitus
- Enteral nutrition
- Food intolerance
- Gastroesophageal reflux disease
- Infections
- Pharmaceutical preparations
- Treatment regimen

Original literature support available at www.thieme.com/nanda-i.

Domain 3 • Class 2 • Diagnosis Code 00197

Risk for dysfunctional gastrointestinal motility

Focus of the diagnosis: gastrointestinal motility
Approved 2008 • Revised 2013, 2017 • Level of Evidence 2.1

Definition
Susceptible to increased, decreased, ineffective, or lack of peristaltic activity within the gastrointestinal tract, which may compromise health.

Risk factors
- Altered water source
- Anxiety
- Eating habit change
- Impaired physical mobility
- Malnutrition
- Sedentary lifestyle
- Stressors
- Unsanitary food preparation

At risk population
- Individuals who ingested contaminated material
- Older adults
- Premature infants

Associated conditions
- Decreased gastrointestinal circulation
- Diabetes mellitus
- Enteral nutrition
- Food intolerance
- Gastroesophageal reflux disease
- Infections
- Pharmaceutical preparations
- Treatment regimen

Original literature support available at www.thieme.com/nanda-i.

3. Elimination and exchange

Domain 3 • Class 4 • Diagnosis Code 00030

Impaired gas exchange

Focus of the diagnosis: gas exchange
Approved 1980 • Revised 1996, 1998, 2017, 2020 • Level of Evidence 3.3

Definition
Excess or deficit in oxygenation and/or carbon dioxide elimination.

Defining characteristics

- Abnormal arterial pH
- Abnormal skin color
- Altered respiratory depth
- Altered respiratory rhythm
- Bradypnea
- Confusion
- Decreased carbon dioxide level
- Diaphoresis
- Headache upon awakening
- Hypercapnia
- Hypoxemia
- Hypoxia
- Irritable mood
- Nasal flaring
- Psychomotor agitation
- Somnolence
- Tachycardia
- Tachypnea
- Visual disturbance

Related factors

- Ineffective airway clearance
- Ineffective breathing pattern
- Pain

At risk population

- Premature infants

Associated conditions

- Alveolar-capillary membrane changes
- Asthma
- General anesthesia
- Heart diseases
- Ventilation-perfusion imbalance

Domain 4.
Activity/rest

The production, conservation, expenditure, or balance of energy resources

Class 3. Energy balance
A dynamic state of harmony between intake and expenditure of resources

Code	Diagnosis	Page
00273	Imbalanced energy field	291
00093	Fatigue	292
00154	Wandering	294

Class 4. Cardiovascular/pulmonary responses
Cardiopulmonary mechanisms that support activity/rest

Code	Diagnosis	Page
00032	Ineffective breathing pattern	295
00029	Decreased cardiac output	297
00240	Risk for decreased cardiac output	299
00311	Risk for impaired cardiovascular function	300
00278	Ineffective lymphedema self-management	301
00281	Risk for ineffective lymphedema self-management	303
00033	Impaired spontaneous ventilation	305
00267	Risk for unstable blood pressure	306
00291	Risk for thrombosis	307
00200	Risk for decreased cardiac tissue perfusion	308
00201	Risk for ineffective cerebral tissue perfusion	309
00204	Ineffective peripheral tissue perfusion	310
00228	Risk for ineffective peripheral tissue perfusion	311
00034	Dysfunctional ventilatory weaning response	312
00318	Dysfunctional adult ventilatory weaning response	314

Class 5. Self-care
Ability to perform activities to care for one's body and bodily functions

Code	Diagnosis	Page
00108	Bathing self-care deficit	316
00109	Dressing self-care deficit	317
00102	Feeding self-care deficit	318

NANDA International, Inc. Nursing Diagnoses: Definitions and Classification 2021–2023, 12th Edition.
Edited by T. Heather Herdman, Shigemi Kamitsuru, and Camila Takáo Lopes.
© 2021 NANDA International, Inc. Published 2021 by Thieme Medical Publishers, Inc., New York.
Companion website: www.thieme.com/nanda-i.

Domain 4 • Class 1 • Diagnosis Code 00095

Insomnia

Focus of the diagnosis: insomnia
Approved 2006 • Revised 2017, 2020 • Level of Evidence 3.3

Definition
Inability to initiate or maintain sleep, which impairs functioning.

Defining characteristics

- Altered affect
- Altered attention
- Altered mood
- Early awakening
- Expresses dissatisfaction with quality of life
- Expresses dissatisfaction with sleep
- Expresses forgetfulness
- Expresses need for frequent naps during the day
- Impaired health status
- Increased absenteeism
- Increased accidents
- Insufficient physical endurance
- Nonrestorative sleep-wake cycle

Related factors

- Anxiety
- Average daily physical activity is less than recommended for age and gender
- Caffeine consumption
- Caregiver role strain
- Consumption of sugar-sweetened beverages
- Depressive symptoms
- Discomfort
- Dysfunctional sleep beliefs
- Environmental disturbances
- Fear
- Frequent naps during the day
- Inadequate sleep hygiene
- Lifestyle incongruent with normal circadian rhythms
- Low psychological resilience
- Obesity
- Stressors
- Substance misuse
- Use of interactive electronic devices

At risk population

- Adolescents
- Economically disadvantaged individuals
- Grieving individuals
- Individuals undergoing changes in marital status
- Night shift workers
- Older adults
- Pregnant women in third trimester
- Rotating shift workers
- Women

Associated conditions
- Chronic disease
- Hormonal change
- Pharmaceutical preparations

Original literature support available at www.thieme.com/nanda-i.

Domain 4 • Class 1 • Diagnosis Code 00096

Sleep deprivation

Focus of the diagnosis: sleep
Approved 1998 • Revised 2017

Definition
Prolonged periods of time without sustained natural, periodic suspension of relative consciousness that provides rest.

Defining characteristics
- Altered attention
- Anxiety
- Apathy
- Combativeness
- Confusion
- Decreased functional ability
- Drowsiness
- Expresses distress
- Fatigue
- Fleeting nystagmus
- Hallucinations
- Heightened sensitivity to pain
- Irritable mood
- Lethargy
- Prolonged reaction time
- Psychomotor agitation
- Transient paranoia
- Tremors

Related factors
- Age-related sleep stage shifts
- Average daily physical activity is less than recommended for age and gender
- Discomfort
- Environmental disturbances
- Environmental overstimulation
- Late day confusion
- Nonrestorative sleep-wake cycle
- Sleep terror
- Sleep walking
- Sustained circadian asynchrony
- Sustained inadequate sleep hygiene

At risk population
- Individuals with familial sleep paralysis

Associated conditions
- Conditions with periodic limb movement
- Idiopathic central nervous system hypersomnolence
- Narcolepsy
- Neurocognitive disorders
- Nightmares

- Sleep apnea
- Sleep-related enuresis
- Sleep-related painful erections

- Treatment regimen

This diagnosis will retire from the NANDA-I Taxonomy in the 2024–2026 edition unless additional work is completed to bring it up to a level of evidence 2.1 or higher.

Domain 4 • Class 1 • Diagnosis Code 00165

Readiness for enhanced sleep

Focus of the diagnosis: sleep
Approved 2002 • Revised 2013 • Level of Evidence 2.1

> **Definition**
> A pattern of natural, periodic suspension of relative consciousness to provide rest and sustain a desired lifestyle, which can be strengthened.

Defining characteristics
- Expresses desire to enhance sleep-wake cycle

Domain 4 • Class 1 • Diagnosis Code 00198

Disturbed sleep pattern

Focus of the diagnosis: sleep pattern
Approved 1980 • Revised 1998, 2006 • Level of Evidence 2.1

Definition
Time-limited awakenings due to external factors.

Defining characteristics
- Difficulty in daily functioning
- Difficulty initiating sleep
- Difficulty maintaining sleep state
- Expresses dissatisfaction with sleep
- Expresses tiredness
- Nonrestorative sleep-wake cycle
- Unintentional awakening

Related factors
- Disruption caused by sleep partner
- Environmental disturbances
- Insufficient privacy

Associated conditions
- Immobilization

Domain 4 • Class 2 • Diagnosis Code 00298

Decreased activity tolerance

Focus of the diagnosis: activity tolerance
Approved 2020 • Level of Evidence 3.2

> **Definition**
> Insufficient endurance to complete required or desired daily activities.

Defining characteristics

- Abnormal blood pressure response to activity
- Abnormal heart rate response to activity
- Anxious when activity is required
- Electrocardiogram change

- Exertional discomfort
- Exertional dyspnea
- Expresses fatigue
- Generalized weakness

Related factors

- Decreased muscle strength
- Depressive symptoms
- Fear of pain
- Imbalance between oxygen supply/demand
- Impaired physical mobility
- Inexperience with an activity

- Insufficient muscle mass
- Malnutrition
- Pain
- Physical deconditioning
- Sedentary lifestyle

At risk population

- Individuals with history of decreased activity tolerance

- Older adults

Associated conditions

- Neoplasms
- Neurodegenerative diseases
- Respiration disorders

- Traumatic brain injuries
- Vitamin D deficiency

Original literature support available at www.thieme.com/nanda-i.

Domain 4 • Class 2 • Diagnosis Code 00299

Risk for decreased activity tolerance

Focus of the diagnosis: activity tolerance
Approved 2020 • Level of Evidence 3.2

> **Definition**
> Susceptible to experiencing insufficient endurance to complete required or desired daily activities.

Risk factors

- Decreased muscle strength
- Depressive symptoms
- Fear of pain
- Imbalance between oxygen supply/demand
- Impaired physical mobility
- Inexperience with an activity
- Insufficient muscle mass
- Malnutrition
- Pain
- Physical deconditioning
- Sedentary lifestyle

At risk population

- Individuals with history of decreased activity tolerance
- Older adults

Associated conditions

- Neoplasms
- Neurodegenerative diseases
- Respiration disorders
- Traumatic brain injuries
- Vitamin D deficiency

Original literature support available at www.thieme.com/nanda-i.

Domain 4 • Class 2 • Diagnosis Code 00040

Risk for disuse syndrome

Focus of the diagnosis: disuse syndrome
Approved 1988 • Revised 2013, 2017

Definition
Susceptible to deterioration of body systems as the result of prescribed or unavoidable musculoskeletal inactivity, which may compromise health.

Risk factors
– Pain

Associated conditions
– Decreased level of consciousness
– Immobilization
– Paralysis
– Prescribed movement restrictions

This diagnosis will retire from the NANDA-I Taxonomy in the 2024–2026 edition unless additional work is completed to bring it up to a level of evidence 2.1 or higher.

Domain 4 • Class 2 • Diagnosis Code 00091

Impaired bed mobility

Focus of the diagnosis: mobility
Approved 1998 • Revised 2006, 2017, 2020 • Level of Evidence 2.1

Definition
Limitation in independent movement from one bed position to another.

Defining characteristics
- Difficulty moving between long sitting and supine positions
- Difficulty moving between prone and supine positions
- Difficulty moving between sitting and supine positions
- Difficulty reaching objects on the bed
- Difficulty repositioning self in bed
- Difficulty returning to the bed
- Difficulty rolling on the bed
- Difficulty sitting on edge of bed
- Difficulty turning from side to side

Related factors
- Cognitive dysfunction
- Decreased flexibility
- Environmental constraints
- Impaired postural balance
- Inadequate angle of headboard
- Inadequate knowledge of mobility strategies
- Insufficient muscle strength
- Obesity
- Pain
- Physical deconditioning

At risk population
- Children
- Individuals experiencing prolonged bed rest
- Individuals in the early postoperative period
- Older adults

Associated conditions
- Artificial respiration
- Critical illness
- Dementia
- Drain tubes
- Musculoskeletal impairment
- Neurodegenerative disorders
- Neuromuscular diseases
- Parkinson's disease
- Pharmaceutical preparations
- Sedation

Original literature support available at www.thieme.com/nanda-i.

Domain 4 • Class 2 • Diagnosis Code 00085

Impaired physical mobility

Focus of the diagnosis: mobility
Approved 1973 • Revised 1998, 2013, 2017 • Level of Evidence 2.1

Definition
Limitation in independent, purposeful movement of the body or of one or more extremities.

Defining characteristics

- Altered gait
- Decreased fine motor skills
- Decreased gross motor skills
- Decreased range of motion
- Difficulty turning
- Engages in substitutions for movement
- Expresses discomfort
- Movement-induced tremor
- Postural instability
- Prolonged reaction time
- Slowed movement
- Spastic movement
- Uncoordinated movement

Related factors

- Anxiety
- Body mass index > 75th percentile appropriate for age and gender
- Cognitive dysfunction
- Cultural belief regarding acceptable activity
- Decreased activity tolerance
- Decreased muscle control
- Decreased muscle strength
- Disuse
- Inadequate environmental support
- Inadequate knowledge of value of physical activity
- Insufficient muscle mass
- Insufficient physical endurance
- Joint stiffness
- Malnutrition
- Neurobehavioral manifestations
- Pain
- Physical deconditioning
- Reluctance to initiate movement
- Sedentary lifestyle

Associated conditions

- Altered bone structure integrity
- Contractures
- Depression
- Developmental disabilities
- Impaired metabolism
- Musculoskeletal impairment
- Neuromuscular diseases
- Pharmaceutical preparations
- Prescribed movement restrictions
- Sensory-perceptual impairment

Original literature support available at www.thieme.com/nanda-i.

Domain 4 • Class 2 • Diagnosis Code 00089

Impaired wheelchair mobility

Focus of the diagnosis: mobility
Approved 1998 • Revised 2006, 2017, 2020 • Level of Evidence 3.4

Definition
Limitation in independent operation of wheelchair within environment.

Defining characteristics

- Difficulty bending forward to pick up object from the floor
- Difficulty folding or unfolding wheelchair
- Difficulty leaning forward to reach for something above head
- Difficulty locking brakes on manual wheelchair
- Difficulty maneuvering wheelchair sideways
- Difficulty moving wheelchair out of an elevator
- Difficulty navigating through hinged door
- Difficulty operating battery charger of power wheelchair
- Difficulty operating power wheelchair on a decline
- Difficulty operating power wheelchair on an incline
- Difficulty operating power wheelchair on curbs
- Difficulty operating power wheelchair on even surface
- Difficulty operating power wheelchair on uneven surface
- Difficulty operating wheelchair backwards
- Difficulty operating wheelchair forward
- Difficulty operating wheelchair in corners
- Difficulty operating wheelchair motors
- Difficulty operating wheelchair on a decline
- Difficulty operating wheelchair on an incline
- Difficulty operating wheelchair on curbs
- Difficulty operating wheelchair on even surface
- Difficulty operating wheelchair on stairs
- Difficulty operating wheelchair on uneven surface
- Difficulty operating wheelchair while carrying an object
- Difficulty performing pressure relief
- Difficulty performing stationary wheelie position
- Difficulty putting feet on the footplates of the wheelchair
- Difficulty rolling across side-slope while in wheelchair
- Difficulty selecting drive mode on power wheelchair
- Difficulty selecting speed on power wheelchair
- Difficulty shifting weight
- Difficulty sitting on wheelchair without losing balance
- Difficulty stopping wheelchair before bumping something
- Difficulty transferring from wheelchair

- Difficulty transferring to wheelchair
- Difficulty turning in place while on wheelie position

Related factors

- Altered mood
- Cognitive dysfunction
- Environmental constraints
- Inadequate adjustment to wheelchair size
- Inadequate knowledge of wheelchair use
- Insufficient muscle strength
- Insufficient physical endurance
- Neurobehavioral manifestations
- Obesity
- Pain
- Physical deconditioning
- Substance misuse
- Unaddressed inadequate vision

At risk population

- Individuals using wheelchair for short time
- Individuals with history of fall from wheelchair
- Older adults

Associated conditions

- Musculoskeletal impairment
- Neuromuscular diseases
- Vision disorders

Original literature support available at www.thieme.com/nanda-i.

Domain 4 • Class 2 • Diagnosis Code 00237

Impaired sitting

Focus of the diagnosis: sitting
Approved 2013 • Revised 2017 • Level of Evidence 2.1

Definition

Limitation of ability to independently and purposefully attain and/or maintain a rest position that is supported by the buttocks and thighs, in which the torso is upright.

Defining characteristics

- Difficulty adjusting position of one or both lower limbs on uneven surface
- Difficulty attaining postural balance
- Difficulty flexing or moving both hips
- Difficulty flexing or moving both knees
- Difficulty maintaining postural balance
- Difficulty stressing torso with body weight

Related factors

- Cognitive dysfunction
- Insufficient energy
- Insufficient muscle strength
- Malnutrition
- Neurobehavioral manifestations
- Pain
- Self-imposed relief posture

Associated conditions

- Impaired metabolism
- Mental disorders
- Neurological disorder
- Orthopedic surgery
- Prescribed posture
- Sarcopenia

Original literature support available at www.thieme.com/nanda-i.

4. Activity/rest

Domain 4 • Class 2 • Diagnosis Code 00238

Impaired standing

Focus of the diagnosis: standing
Approved 2013 • Revised 2017 • Level of Evidence 2.1

Definition
Limitation of ability to independently and purposefully attain and/or maintain the body in an upright position from feet to head.

Defining characteristics
- Difficulty adjusting position of one or both lower limbs on uneven surface
- Difficulty attaining postural balance
- Difficulty extending one or both hips
- Difficulty extending one or both knees
- Difficulty flexing one or both hips
- Difficulty flexing one or both knees
- Difficulty maintaining postural balance
- Difficulty moving one or both hips
- Difficulty moving one or both knees
- Difficulty stressing torso with body weight

Related factors
- Excessive emotional disturbance
- Insufficient energy
- Insufficient muscle strength
- Insufficient physical endurance
- Malnutrition
- Obesity
- Pain
- Self-imposed relief posture

Associated conditions
- Circulatory perfusion disorder
- Impaired metabolism
- Injury to lower extremity
- Neurological disorder
- Prescribed posture
- Sarcopenia
- Surgical procedures

Original literature support available at www.thieme.com/nanda-i.

Domain 4 • Class 2 • Diagnosis Code 00090

Impaired transfer ability

Focus of the diagnosis: transfer ability
Approved 1998 • Revised 2006, 2017 • Level of Evidence 2.1

Definition
Limitation of independent movement between two nearby surfaces.

Defining characteristics

- Difficulty transfering between bed and chair
- Difficulty transfering between bed and standing position
- Difficulty transfering between car and chair
- Difficulty transfering between chair and floor
- Difficulty transfering between chair and standing position
- Difficulty transfering between floor and standing position
- Difficulty transfering between uneven levels
- Difficulty transfering in or out of bath tub
- Difficulty transfering in or out of shower stall
- Difficulty transfering on or off a bedside commode
- Difficulty transfering on or off a toilet

Related factors

- Cognitive dysfunction
- Environmental constraints
- Impaired postural balance
- Inadequate knowledge of transfer techniques
- Insufficient muscle strength
- Neurobehavioral manifestations
- Obesity
- Pain
- Physical deconditioning

Associated conditions

- Musculoskeletal impairment
- Neuromuscular diseases
- Vision disorders

Original literature support available at www.thieme.com/nanda-i.

Domain 4 • Class 2 • Diagnosis Code 00088

Impaired walking

Focus of the diagnosis: walking
Approved 1998 • Revised 2006, 2017 • Level of Evidence 2.1

Definition
Limitation of independent movement within the environment on foot.

Defining characteristics
- Difficulty ambulating on decline
- Difficulty ambulating on incline
- Difficulty ambulating on uneven surface
- Difficulty ambulating required distance
- Difficulty climbing stairs
- Difficulty navigating curbs

Related factors
- Altered mood
- Cognitive dysfunction
- Environmental constraints
- Fear of falling
- Inadequate knowledge of mobility strategies
- Insufficient muscle strength
- Insufficient physical endurance
- Neurobehavioral manifestations
- Obesity
- Pain
- Physical deconditioning

Associated conditions
- Cerebrovascular Disorders
- Impaired postural balance
- Musculoskeletal impairment
- Neuromuscular diseases
- Vision disorders

Original literature support available at www.thieme.com/nanda-i.

Domain 4 • Class 3 • Diagnosis Code 00273

Imbalanced energy field

Focus of the diagnosis: balanced energy field
Approved 2016 • Level of Evidence 2.1

Definition
A disruption in the vital flow of human energy that is normally a continuous whole and is unique, dynamic, creative and nonlinear.

Defining characteristics
- Arrhythmic energy field patterns
- Blockage of the energy flow
- Congested energy field patterns
- Congestion of the energy flow
- Dissonant rhythms of the energy field patterns
- Energy deficit of the energy flow
- Expression of the need to regain the experience of the whole
- Hyperactivity of the energy flow
- Irregular energy field patterns
- Magnetic pull to an area of the energy field
- Pulsating to pounding frequency of the energy field patterns
- Pulsations sensed in the energy flow
- Random energy field patterns
- Rapid energy field patterns
- Slow energy field patterns
- Strong energy field patterns
- Temperature differentials of cold in the energy flow
- Temperature differentials of heat in the energy flow
- Tingling sensed in the energy flow
- Tumultuous energy field patterns
- Unsynchronized rhythms sensed in the energy flow
- Weak energy field patterns

Related factors
- Anxiety
- Discomfort
- Excessive stress
- Interventions that disrupt the energetic pattern or flow
- Pain

At risk population
- Individuals experiencing life transition
- Individuals experiencing personal crisis

Associated conditions
- Impaired health status
- Injury

Original literature support available at www.thieme.com/nanda-i.

Domain 4 • Class 3 • Diagnosis Code 00093

Fatigue

Focus of the diagnosis: fatigue
Approved 1988 • Revised 1998, 2017, 2020 • Level of Evidence 3.2

Definition
An overwhelming sustained sense of exhaustion and decreased capacity for physical and mental work at the usual level.

Defining characteristics
- Altered attention
- Apathy
- Decreased aerobic capacity
- Decreased gait velocity
- Difficulty maintaining usual physical activity
- Difficulty maintaining usual routines
- Disinterested in surroundings
- Drowsiness
- Expresses altered libido
- Expresses demoralization
- Expresses frustration
- Expresses lack of energy
- Expresses nonrelief through usual energy-recovery strategies
- Expresses tiredness
- Expresses weakness
- Inadequate role performance
- Increased physical symptoms
- Increased rest requirement
- Insufficient physical endurance
- Introspection
- Lethargy
- Tiredness

Related factors
- Altered sleep-wake cycle
- Anxiety
- Depressive symptoms
- Environmental constraints
- Increased mental exertion
- Increased physical exertion
- Malnutrition
- Nonstimulating lifestyle
- Pain
- Physical deconditioning
- Stressors

At risk population
- Individuals exposed to negative life event
- Individuals with demanding occupation
- Pregnant women
- Women experiencing labor

Associated conditions
- Anemia
- Chemotherapy
- Chronic disease
- Chronic inflammation

- Dementia
- Fibromyalgia
- Hypothalamus-pituitary-adrenal axis dysregulation
- Myasthenia gravis

- Neoplasms
- Radiotherapy
- Stroke

4. Activity/rest

Domain 4 • Class 3 • Diagnosis Code 00154

Wandering

Focus of the diagnosis: wandering
Approved 2000 • Revised 2017

Definition
Meandering, aimless, or repetitive locomotion that exposes the individual to harm; frequently incongruent with boundaries, limits, or obstacles.

Defining characteristics

- Eloping behavior
- Frequent movement from place to place
- Fretful locomotion
- Haphazard locomotion
- Hyperactivity
- Locomotion interspersed with nonlocomotion
- Locomotion into unauthorized spaces
- Locomotion resulting in getting lost
- Locomotion that cannot be easily dissuaded
- Long periods of locomotion without an apparent destination
- Pacing
- Periods of locomotion interspersed with periods of nonlocomotion
- Persistent locomotion in search of something
- Scanning behavior
- Searching behavior
- Shadowing a caregiver's locomotion
- Trespassing

Related factors

- Altered sleep-wake cycle
- Cognitive dysfunction
- Desire to go home
- Environmental overstimulation
- Neurobehavioral manifestations
- Physiological state
- Separation from familiar environment

At risk population

- Individuals with premorbid behavior

Associated conditions

- Cortical atrophy
- Psychological disorder
- Sedation

This diagnosis will retire from the NANDA-I Taxonomy in the 2024–2026 edition unless additional work is completed to bring it up to a level of evidence 2.1 or higher.

Domain 4 · Class 4 · Diagnosis Code 00032

Ineffective breathing pattern

Focus of the diagnosis: breathing pattern
Approved 1980 · Revised 1996, 1998, 2010, 2017, 2020 · Level of Evidence 3.3

Definition
Inspiration and/or expiration that does not provide adequate ventilation.

Defining characteristics

- Abdominal paradoxical respiratory pattern
- Altered chest excursion
- Altered tidal volume
- Bradypnea
- Cyanosis
- Decreased expiratory pressure
- Decreased inspiratory pressure
- Decreased minute ventilation
- Decreased vital capacity
- Hypercapnia
- Hyperventilation
- Hypoventilation
- Hypoxemia
- Hypoxia
- Increased anterior-posterior chest diameter
- Nasal flaring
- Orthopnea
- Prolonged expiration phase
- Pursed-lip breathing
- Subcostal retraction
- Tachypnea
- Uses accessory muscles to breathe
- Uses three-point position

Related factors

- Anxiety
- Body position that inhibits lung expansion
- Fatigue
- Increased physical exertion
- Obesity
- Pain

At risk population

- Young women

Associated conditions

- Bony deformity
- Chest wall deformity
- Chronic obstructive pulmonary disease
- Critical illness
- Heart diseases
- Hyperventilation syndrome
- Hypoventilation syndrome
- Increased airway resistance
- Increased serum hydrogen concentration
- Musculoskeletal impairment

4. Activity/rest

- Neurological immaturity
- Neurological impairment
- Neuromuscular diseases
- Reduced pulmonary complacency
- Sleep-apnea syndromes
- Spinal cord injuries

Original literature support available at www.thieme.com/nanda-i.

Domain 4 • Class 4 • Diagnosis Code 00029

Decreased cardiac output

Focus of the diagnosis: cardiac output
Approved 1975 • Revised 1996, 2000, 2017

Definition
Inadequate volume of blood pumped by the heart to meet the metabolic demands of the body.

Defining characteristics
Altered Heart Rate/Rhythm

- Bradycardia
- Electrocardiogram change

- Heart palpitations
- Tachycardia

Altered Preload

- Decreased central venous pressure
- Decreased pulmonary artery wedge pressure
- Edema
- Fatigue
- Heart murmur

- Increased central venous pressure
- Increased pulmonary artery wedge pressure
- Jugular vein distension
- Weight gain

Altered Afterload

- Abnormal skin color
- Altered blood pressure
- Clammy skin
- Decreased peripheral pulses
- Decreased pulmonary vascular resistance
- Decreased systemic vascular resistance

- Dyspnea
- Increased pulmonary vascular resistance
- Increased systemic vascular resistance
- Oliguria
- Prolonged capillary refill

Altered Contractility

- Adventitious breath sounds
- Coughing
- Decreased cardiac index
- Decreased ejection fraction
- Decreased left ventricular stroke work index

- Decreased stroke volume index
- Orthopnea
- Paroxysmal nocturnal dyspnea
- Presence of S3 heart sound
- Presence of S4 heart sound

Behavioral/Emotional

– Anxiety   – Psychomotor agitation

Related factors

– To be developed

Associated conditions

– Altered afterload   – Altered heart rhythm
– Altered contractility   – Altered preload
– Altered heart rate   – Altered stroke volume

This diagnosis will retire from the NANDA-I Taxonomy in the 2024–2026 edition unless additional work is completed to bring it up to a level of evidence 2.1 or higher.

Domain 4 • Class 4 • Diagnosis Code 00240

Risk for decreased cardiac output

Focus of the diagnosis: cardiac output
Approved 2013 • Revised 2017 • Level of Evidence 2.1

Definition
Susceptible to inadequate volume of blood pumped by the heart to meet metabolic demands of the body, which may compromise health.

Risk factors
- To be developed

Associated conditions
- Altered afterload
- Altered contractility
- Altered heart rate
- Altered heart rhythm
- Altered preload
- Altered stroke volume

This diagnosis will retire from the NANDA-I Taxonomy in the 2024–2026 edition if no modifiable risk factors are developed.

Original literature support available at www.thieme.com/nanda-i.

Domain 4 • Class 4 • Diagnosis Code 00311

Risk for impaired cardiovascular function

Focus of the diagnosis: cardiovascular function
Approved 2020 • Level of Evidence 3.4

Definition
Susceptible to disturbance in substance transport, body homeostasis, tissue metabolic residue removal, and organ function, which may compromise health.

Risk factors

- Anxiety
- Average daily physical activity is less than recommended for age and gender
- Body mass index above normal range for age and gender
- Excessive accumulation of fat for age and gender
- Excessive alcohol intake
- Excessive stress
- Inadequate dietary habits
- Inadequate knowledge of modifiable factors
- Inattentive to second-hand smoke
- Ineffective blood glucose level management
- Ineffective blood pressure management
- Ineffective lipid balance management
- Smoking
- Substance misuse

At risk population

- Economically disadvantaged individuals
- Individuals with family history of diabetes mellitus
- Individuals with family history of dyslipidemia
- Individuals with family history of hypertension
- Individuals with family history of metabolic syndrome
- Individuals with family history of obesity
- Individuals with history of cardio-vascular event
- Men
- Older adults
- Postmenopausal women

Associated conditions

- Depression
- Diabetes mellitus
- Dyslipidemia
- Hypertension
- Insulin resistance
- Pharmaceutical preparations

Original literature support available at www.thieme.com/nanda-i.

Domain 4 • Class 4 • Diagnosis Code 00278

Ineffective lymphedema self-management

Focus of the diagnosis: lymphedema self-management
Approved 2020 • Level of Evidence 2.1

Definition
Unsatisfactory management of symptoms, treatment regimen, physical, psychosocial, and spiritual consequences and lifestyle changes inherent in living with edema related to obstruction or disorders of lymph vessels or nodes.

Defining characteristics

Lymphedema Signs

- Fibrosis in affected limb
- Recurring infections
- Swelling in affected limb

Lymphedema Symptoms

- Expresses dissatisfaction with quality of life
- Reports feeling of discomfort in affected limb
- Reports feeling of heaviness in affected limb
- Reports feeling of tightness in affected limb

Behaviors

- Average daily physical activity is less than recommended for age and gender
- Inadequate manual lymph drainage
- Inadequate protection of affected area
- Inappropriate application of night-time bandaging
- Inappropriate diet
- Inappropriate skin care
- Inappropriate use of compression garments
- Inattentive to carrying heavy objects
- Inattentive to extreme temperatures
- Inattentive to lymphedema signs
- Inattentive to lymphedema symptoms
- Inattentive to sunlight exposure
- Reduced range of motion of affected limb
- Refuses to apply night-time bandages
- Refuses to use compression garments

Related factors

- Cognitive dysfunction
- Competing demands
- Competing lifestyle preferences
- Conflict between health behaviors and social norms
- Decreased perceived quality of life

- Difficulty accessing community resources
- Difficulty managing complex treatment regimen
- Difficulty navigating complex health care systems
- Difficulty with decision-making
- Inadequate commitment to a plan of action
- Inadequate health literacy
- Inadequate knowledge of treatment regimen
- Inadequate number of cues to action
- Inadequate role models
- Inadequate social support

- Limited ability to perform aspects of treatment regimen
- Low self efficacy
- Negative feelings toward treatment regimen
- Neurobehavioral manifestations
- Nonacceptance of condition
- Perceived barrier to treatment regimen
- Perceived social stigma associated with condition
- Unrealistic perception of seriousness of condition
- Unrealistic perception of susceptibility to sequelae
- Unrealistic perception of treatment benefit

At risk population

- Adolescents
- Children
- Economically disadvantaged individuals
- Individuals with history of ineffective health self-management

- Individuals with limited decision-making experience
- Individuals with low educational level
- Older adults

Associated conditions

- Chemotherapy
- Chronic venous insufficiency
- Developmental disabilities
- Infections
- Invasive procedure
- Major surgery

- Neoplasms
- Obesity
- Radiotherapy
- Removal of lymph nodes
- Trauma

Original literature support available at www.thieme.com/nanda-i.

Domain 4 • Class 4 • Diagnosis Code 00281

Risk for ineffective lymphedema self-management

Focus of the diagnosis: lymphedema self-management
Approved 2020 • Level of Evidence 2.1

Definition
Susceptible to unsatisfactory management of symptoms, treatment regimen, physical, psychosocial and spiritual consequences and lifestyle changes inherent in living with edema related to obstruction or disorders of lymph vessels or nodes, which may compromise health.

Risk factors

- Cognitive dysfunction
- Competing demands
- Competing lifestyle preferences
- Conflict between health behaviors and social norms
- Decreased perceived quality of life
- Difficulty accessing community resources
- Difficulty managing complex treatment regimen
- Difficulty navigating complex health care systems
- Difficulty with decision-making
- Inadequate commitment to a plan of action
- Inadequate health literacy
- Inadequate knowledge of treatment regimen
- Inadequate number of cues to action
- Inadequate role models
- Inadequate social support
- Limited ability to perform aspects of treatment regimen
- Low self efficacy
- Negative feelings toward treatment regimen
- Neurobehavioral manifestations
- Nonacceptance of condition
- Perceived barrier to treatment regimen
- Perceived social stigma associated with condition
- Unrealistic perception of seriousness of condition
- Unrealistic perception of susceptibility to sequelae
- Unrealistic perception of treatment benefit

At risk population

- Adolescents
- Children
- Economically disadvantaged individuals
- Individuals with history of ineffective health self-management
- Individuals with limited decision-making experience
- Individuals with low educational level
- Older adults

Associated conditions

- Chemotherapy
- Chronic venous insufficiency
- Developmental disabilities
- Infections
- Invasive procedure
- Major surgery
- Neoplasms
- Obesity
- Radiotherapy
- Removal of lymph nodes
- Trauma

Original literature support available at www.thieme.com/nanda-i.

Domain 4 • Class 4 • Diagnosis Code 00033

Impaired spontaneous ventilation

Focus of the diagnosis: spontaneous ventilation
Approved 1992 • Revised 2017

Definition
Inability to initiate and/or maintain independent breathing that is adequate to support life.

Defining characteristics
- Apprehensiveness
- Decreased arterial oxygen saturation
- Decreased cooperation
- Decreased partial pressure of oxygen
- Decreased tidal volume
- Increased accessory muscle use
- Increased heart rate
- Increased metabolic rate
- Increased partial pressure of carbon dioxide (PCO_2)
- Psychomotor agitation

Related factors
- Respiratory muscle fatigue

Associated conditions
- Impaired metabolism

This diagnosis will retire from the NANDA-I Taxonomy in the 2024–2026 edition unless additional work is completed to bring it up to a level of evidence 2.1 or higher.

Domain 4 • Class 4 • Diagnosis Code 00267

Risk for unstable blood pressure

Focus of the diagnosis: stable blood pressure
Approved 2016 • Level of Evidence 2.1

Definition
Susceptible to fluctuating forces of blood flowing through arterial vessels, which may compromise health.

Risk factors
- Inconsistency with medication regimen
- Orthostasis

Associated conditions
- Adverse effect of pharmaceutical preparations
- Adverse effects of cocaine
- Cardiac dysrhythmia
- Cushing Syndrome
- Fluid retention
- Fluid shifts
- Hormonal change
- Hyperparathyroidism
- Hyperthyroidism
- Hypothyroidism
- Increased intracranial pressure
- Pharmaceutical preparations
- Rapid absorption and distribution of pharmaceutical preparations
- Sympathetic responses

Original literature support available at www.thieme.com/nanda-i.

Domain 4 • Class 4 • Diagnosis Code 00291

Risk for thrombosis

Focus of the diagnosis: thrombosis
Approved 2020 • Level of Evidence 2.1

Definition
Susceptible to obstruction of a blood vessel by a thrombus that can break off and lodge in another vessel, which may compromise health.

Risk factors
- Atherogenic diet
- Dehydration
- Excessive stress
- Impaired physical mobility
- Inadequate knowledge of modifiable factors
- Ineffective management of preventive measures
- Ineffective medication self-management
- Obesity
- Sedentary lifestyle
- Smoking

At risk population
- Economically disadvantaged individuals
- Individuals aged ≥ 60 years
- Individuals with family history of thrombotic disease
- Individuals with history of thrombotic disease
- Pregnant women
- Women < 6 weeks postpartum

Associated conditions
- Atherosclerosis
- Autoimmune diseases
- Blood coagulation disorders
- Chronic inflammation
- Critical illness
- Diabetes mellitus
- Dyslipidemias
- Endovascular procedures
- Heart diseases
- Hematologic diseases
- High acuity illness
- Hormonal therapy
- Hyperhomocysteinemia
- Infections
- Kidney diseases
- Medical devices
- Metabolic syndrome
- Neoplasms
- Surgical procedures
- Trauma
- Vascular diseases

Original literature support available at www.thieme.com/nanda-i.

Domain 4 • Class 4 • Diagnosis Code 00200

Risk for decreased cardiac tissue perfusion

Focus of the diagnosis: tissue perfusion
Approved 2008 • Revised 2013, 2017 • Level of Evidence 2.1

Definition
Susceptible to a decrease in cardiac (coronary) circulation, which may compromise health.

Risk factors
– Inadequate knowledge of modifiable factors
– Substance misuse

At risk population
– Individuals with family history of cardiovascular disease

Associated conditions
– Cardiac tamponade
– Cardiovascular surgery
– Coronary artery spasm
– Diabetes mellitus
– Elevated C-reactive protein
– Hyperlipidemia
– Hypertension
– Hypovolemia
– Hypoxemia
– Hypoxia
– Pharmaceutical preparations

Original literature support available at www.thieme.com/nanda-i.

Domain 4 • Class 4 • Diagnosis Code 00201

Risk for ineffective cerebral tissue perfusion

Focus of the diagnosis: tissue perfusion
Approved 2008 • Revised 2013, 2017 • Level of Evidence 2.1

Definition
Susceptible to a decrease in cerebral tissue circulation, which may compromise health.

Risk factors
– Substance misuse

At risk population
– Individuals with history of recent myocardial infarction

Associated conditions
– Abnormal serum partial thromboplastin time
– Abnormal serum prothrombin time
– Akinetic left ventricular wall segment
– Arterial dissection
– Atherosclerosis
– Atrial fibrillation
– Atrial myxoma
– Brain injuries
– Brain neoplasm
– Carotid stenosis
– Cerebral aneurysm
– Coagulopathy
– Dilated cardiomyopathy
– Disseminated intravascular coagulopathy
– Embolism
– Hypercholesterolemia
– Hypertension
– Infective endocarditis
– Mechanical prosthetic valve
– Mitral stenosis
– Pharmaceutical preparations
– Sick sinus syndrome
– Treatment regimen

4. Activity/rest

This diagnosis will retire from the NANDA-I Taxonomy in the 2024–2026 edition if no additional risk factors are developed.

Original literature support available at www.thieme.com/nanda-i.

Domain 4 • Class 4 • Diagnosis Code 00204

Ineffective peripheral tissue perfusion

Focus of the diagnosis: tissue perfusion
Approved 2008 • Revised 2010, 2017 • Level of Evidence 2.1

> **Definition**
> Decrease in blood circulation to the periphery, which may compromise health.

Defining characteristics

- Absence of peripheral pulses
- Altered motor function
- Altered skin characteristic
- Ankle-brachial index < 0.90
- Capillary refill time > 3 seconds
- Color does not return to lowered limb after 1 minute leg elevation
- Decreased blood pressure in extremities
- Decreased pain-free distances during a 6-minute walk test
- Decreased peripheral pulses
- Delayed peripheral wound healing
- Distance in the 6-minute walk test below normal range
- Edema
- Extremity pain
- Femoral bruit
- Intermittent claudication
- Paresthesia
- Skin color pales with limb elevation

Related factors

- Excessive sodium intake
- Inadequate knowledge of disease process
- Inadequate knowledge of modifiable factors
- Sedentary lifestyle
- Smoking

Associated conditions

- Diabetes mellitus
- Endovascular procedures
- Hypertension
- Trauma

Original literature support available at www.thieme.com/nanda-i.

Domain 4 • Class 4 • Diagnosis Code 00228

Risk for ineffective peripheral tissue perfusion

Focus of the diagnosis: tissue perfusion
Approved 2010 • Revised 2013, 2017 • Level of Evidence 2.1

Definition
Susceptible to a decrease in blood circulation to the periphery, which may compromise health.

Risk factors
- Excessive sodium intake
- Inadequate knowledge of disease process
- Inadequate knowledge of modifiable factors
- Sedentary lifestyle
- Smoking

Associated conditions
- Diabetes mellitus
- Endovascular procedures
- Hypertension
- Trauma

Original literature support available at www.thieme.com/nanda-i.

4. Activity/rest

Domain 4 • Class 4 • Diagnosis Code 00034

Dysfunctional ventilatory weaning response

Focus of the diagnosis: ventilatory weaning response
Approved 1992 • Revised 2017

Definition
Inability to adjust to lowered levels of mechanical ventilator support that interrupts and prolongs the weaning process.

Defining characteristics

Mild

- Breathing discomfort
- Expresses feeling warm
- Fatigue
- Fear of machine malfunction
- Increased focus on breathing
- Mildly increased respiratory rate over baseline
- Perceived need for increased oxygen
- Psychomotor agitation

Moderate

- Abnormal skin color
- Apprehensiveness
- Blood pressure increased from baseline (< 20 mmHg)
- Decreased air entry on auscultation
- Diaphoresis
- Difficulty cooperating
- Difficulty responding to coaching
- Facial expression of fear
- Heart rate increased from baseline (< 20 beats/min)
- Hyperfocused on activities
- Minimal use of respiratory accessory muscles
- Moderately increased respiratory rate over baseline

Severe

- Adventitious breath sounds
- Asynchronized breathing with the ventilator
- Blood pressure increased from baseline (≥ to 20 mmHg)
- Deterioration in arterial blood gases from baseline
- Gasping breaths
- Heart rate increased from baseline (≥ 20 beats/min)
- Paradoxical abdominal breathing
- Profuse diaphoresis
- Shallow breathing
- Significantly increased respiratory rate above baseline
- Uses significant respiratory accessory muscles

Related factors

Physiological Factors

- Altered sleep-wake cycle
- Ineffective airway clearance
- Malnutrition
- Pain

Psychological

- Anxiety
- Decreased motivation
- Fear
- Hopelessness
- Inadequate knowledge of weaning process
- Inadequate trust in health care professional
- Low self-esteem
- Powerlessness
- Uncertainty about ability to wean

Situational

- Environmental disturbances
- Inappropriate pace of weaning process
- Uncontrolled episodic energy demands

At risk population

- Individuals with history of unsuccessful weaning attempt
- Individuals with history of ventilator dependence > 4 days

Associated conditions

- Decreased level of consciousness

This diagnosis was originally developed for neonates. This diagnosis will retire from the NANDA-I Taxonomy in the 2024–2026 edition unless additional work on neonates and/or children is completed to bring it up to a level of evidence 2.1 or higher.

Domain 4 • Class 4 • Diagnosis Code 00318

Dysfunctional adult ventilatory weaning response

Focus of the diagnosis: ventilatory weaning response
Approved 2020 • Level of Evidence 3.2

Definition
Inability of individuals > 18 years of age, who have required mechanical ventilation at least 24 hours, to successfully transition to spontaneous ventilation.

Defining characteristics

Early Response (< 30 minutes)

- Adventitious breath sounds
- Audible airway secretions
- Decreased blood pressure (< 90 mmHg or > 20% reduction from baseline)
- Decreased heart rate (> 20% reduction from baseline)
- Decreased oxygen saturation (< 90% when fraction of inspired oxygen ratio > 40%)
- Expresses apprehensiveness
- Expresses distress
- Expresses fear of machine malfunction
- Expresses feeling warm
- Hyperfocused on activities

- Increased blood pressure (systolic pressure > 180 mmHg or > 20% from baseline)
- Increased in heart rate (> 140 bpm or > 20% from baseline)
- Increased respiratory rate (> 35 rpm or > 50% over baseline)
- Nasal flaring
- Panting
- Paradoxical abdominal breathing
- Perceived need for increased oxygen
- Psychomotor agitation
- Shallow breathing
- Uses significant respiratory accessory muscles
- Wide-eyed appearance

Intermediate Response (30-90 minutes)

- Decreased pH (< 7.32 or > 0.07 reduction from baseline)
- Diaphoresis
- Difficulty cooperating with instructions

- Hypercapnia (> 50 mmHg increase in partial pressure of carbon dioxide or > 8 mmHg increase from baseline)
- Hypoxemia (Partial pressure of oxygen 50% or oxygen > 6 L/min)

Late Response (> 90 minutes)

- Cardiorespiratory arrest
- Cyanosis

- Fatigue
- Recent onset arrhythmias

Related factors

- Altered sleep-wake cycle
- Excessive airway secretions
- Ineffective cough
- Malnutrition

At risk population

- Individuals with history of failed weaning attempt
- Individuals with history of lung diseases
- Individuals with history of prolonged dependence on ventilator
- Individuals with history of unplanned extubation
- Individuals with unfavorable pre-extubation indexes
- Older adults

Associated conditions

- Acid-base imbalance
- Anemia
- Cardiogenic shock
- Decreased level of consciousness
- Diaphragm dysfunction acquired in the intensive care unit
- Endocrine system diseases
- Heart diseases
- High acuity illness
- Hyperthermia
- Hypoxemia
- Infections
- Neuromuscular diseases
- Pharmaceutical preparations
- Water-electrolyte imbalance

4. Activity/rest

Original literature support available at www.thieme.com/nanda-i.

Domain 4 • Class 5 • Diagnosis Code 00108

Bathing self-care deficit

Focus of the diagnosis: bathing self-care
Approved 1980 • Revised 1998, 2008, 2017 • Level of Evidence 2.1

Definition
Inability to independently complete cleansing activities.

Defining characteristics
- Difficulty accessing bathroom
- Difficulty accessing water
- Difficulty drying body
- Difficulty gathering bathing supplies
- Difficulty regulating bath water
- Difficulty washing body

Related factors
- Anxiety
- Cognitive dysfunction
- Decreased motivation
- Environmental constraints
- Impaired physical mobility
- Neurobehavioral manifestations
- Pain
- Weakness

At risk population
- Older adults

Associated conditions
- Impaired ability to perceive body part
- Impaired ability to perceive spatial relationships
- Musculoskeletal diseases
- Neuromuscular diseases

Domain 4 • Class 5 • Diagnosis Code 00109

Dressing self-care deficit

Focus of the diagnosis: dressing self-care
Approved 1980 • Revised 1998, 2008, 2017 • Level of Evidence 2.1

Definition
Inability to independently put on or remove clothing.

Defining characteristics

- Difficulty choosing clothing
- Difficulty fastening clothing
- Difficulty gathering clothing
- Difficulty maintaining appearance
- Difficulty picking up clothing
- Difficulty putting clothing on lower body
- Difficulty putting clothing on upper body
- Difficulty putting on various items of clothing
- Difficulty removing clothing item
- Difficulty using assistive device
- Difficulty using zipper

Related factors

- Anxiety
- Cognitive dysfunction
- Decreased motivation
- Discomfort
- Environmental constraints
- Fatigue
- Neurobehavioral manifestations
- Pain
- Weakness

Associated conditions

- Musculoskeletal impairment
- Neuromuscular diseases

Domain 4 • Class 5 • Diagnosis Code 00102

Feeding self-care deficit

Focus of the diagnosis: feeding self-care
Approved 1980 • Revised 1998, 2008, 2017 • Level of Evidence 2.1

Definition
Inability to eat independently.

Defining characteristics

- Difficulty bringing food to mouth
- Difficulty chewing food
- Difficulty getting food onto utensil
- Difficulty handling utensils
- Difficulty manipulating food in mouth
- Difficulty opening containers
- Difficulty picking up cup
- Difficulty preparing food
- Difficulty self-feeding a complete meal
- Difficulty self-feeding in an acceptable manner
- Difficulty swallowing food
- Difficulty swallowing sufficient amount of food
- Difficulty using assistive device

Related factors

- Anxiety
- Cognitive dysfunction
- Decreased motivation
- Discomfort
- Environmental constraints
- Fatigue
- Neurobehavioral manifestations
- Pain
- Weakness

Associated conditions

- Musculoskeletal impairment
- Neuromuscular diseases

Domain 4 • Class 5 • Diagnosis Code 00110

Toileting self-care deficit

Focus of the diagnosis: toileting self-care
Approved 1980 • Revised 1998, 2008, 2017 • Level of Evidence 2.1

Definition
Inability to independently perform tasks associated with bowel and bladder elimination.

Defining characteristics
- Difficulty completing toilet hygiene
- Difficulty flushing toilet
- Difficulty manipulating clothing for toileting
- Difficulty reaching toilet
- Difficulty rising from toilet
- Difficulty sitting on toilet

Related factors
- Anxiety
- Cognitive dysfunction
- Decreased motivation
- Environmental constraints
- Fatigue
- Impaired physical mobility
- Impaired transfer ability
- Neurobehavioral manifestations
- Pain
- Weakness

Associated conditions
- Musculoskeletal impairment
- Neuromuscular diseases

4. Activity/rest

Domain 4 • Class 5 • Diagnosis Code 00182

Readiness for enhanced self-care

Focus of the diagnosis: self-care
Approved 2006 • Revised 2013 • Level of Evidence 2.1

Definition
A pattern of performing activities for oneself to meet health-related goals, which can be strengthened.

Defining characteristics
- Expresses desire to enhance independence with health
- Expresses desire to enhance independence with life
- Expresses desire to enhance independence with personal development
- Expresses desire to enhance independence with well-being
- Expresses desire to enhance knowledge of self-care strategies
- Expresses desire to enhance self-care

Original literature support available at www.thieme.com/nanda-i.

Domain 4 • Class 5 • Diagnosis Code 00193

Self-neglect

Focus of the diagnosis: self-neglect
Approved 2008 • Revised 2017 • Level of Evidence 2.1

Definition
A constellation of culturally framed behaviors involving one or more self-care activities in which there is a failure to maintain a socially accepted standard of health and well-being (Gibbons, Lauder & Ludwick, 2006).

Defining characteristics
- Inadequate environmental hygiene
- Inadequate personal hygiene
- Nonadherence to health activity

Related factors
- Cognitive dysfunction
- Fear of institutionalization
- Impaired executive function
- Inability to maintain control
- Lifestyle choice
- Neurobehavioral manifestations
- Stressors
- Substance misuse

Associated conditions
- Capgras syndrome
- Frontal lobe dysfunction
- Functional impairment
- Learning disability
- Malingering
- Mental disorders
- Psychotic disorders

Original literature support available at www.thieme.com/nanda-i.

Domain 5.
Perception/cognition

The human processing system including attention, orientation, sensation, perception, cognition, and communication

Class 1. Attention
Mental readiness to notice or observe

Code	Diagnosis	Page
00123	Unilateral neglect	325

Class 2. Orientation
Awareness of time, place, and person

Code	Diagnosis	Page
	This class does not currently contain any diagnoses	

Class 3. Sensation/perception
Receiving information through the senses of touch, taste, smell, vision, hearing, and kinesthesia, and the comprehension of sensory data resulting in naming, associating, and/or pattern recognition

Code	Diagnosis	Page
	This class does not currently contain any diagnoses	

Class 4. Cognition
Use of memory, learning, thinking, problem-solving, abstraction, judgment, insight, intellectual capacity, calculation, and language

Code	Diagnosis	Page
00128	Acute confusion	326
00173	Risk for acute confusion	327
00129	Chronic confusion	328

Class 5. Communication
Sending and receiving verbal and nonverbal information

NANDA International, Inc. Nursing Diagnoses: Definitions and Classification 2021–2023, 12th Edition.
Edited by T. Heather Herdman, Shigemi Kamitsuru, and Camila Takáo Lopes.
© 2021 NANDA International, Inc. Published 2021 by Thieme Medical Publishers, Inc., New York.
Companion website: www.thieme.com/nanda-i.

Domain 5 • Class 1 • Diagnosis Code 00123

Unilateral neglect

Focus of the diagnosis: unilateral neglect
Approved 1986 • Revised 2006, 2017 • Level of Evidence 2.1

Definition
Impairment in sensory and motor response, mental representation, and spatial attention of the body, and the corresponding environment, characterized by inattention to one side and overattention to the opposite side. Left-side neglect is more severe and persistent than right-side neglect.

Defining characteristics
- Altered safety behavior on neglected side
- Disturbed sound lateralization
- Failure to dress neglected side
- Failure to eat food from portion of plate on neglected side
- Failure to groom neglected side
- Failure to move eyes in the neglected hemisphere
- Failure to move head in the neglected hemisphere
- Failure to move limbs in the neglected hemisphere
- Failure to move trunk in the neglected hemisphere
- Failure to notice people approaching from the neglected side
- Hemianopsia
- Impaired performance on line bisection tests
- Impaired performance on line cancellation tests
- Impaired performance on target cancellation tests
- Left hemiplegia from cerebrovascular accident
- Marked deviation of the eyes to stimuli on the non-neglected side
- Marked deviation of the trunk to stimuli on the non-neglected side
- Omission of drawing on the neglected side
- Perseveration
- Representational neglect
- Substitution of letters to form alternative words when reading
- Transfer of pain sensation to the non-neglected side
- Unaware of positioning of neglected limb
- Unilateral visuospatial neglect
- Uses vertical half of page only when writing

Related factors
- To be developed

Associated conditions
- Brain injuries

This diagnosis will retire from the NANDA-I Taxonomy in the 2024–2026 edition if no related factors are developed. Original literature support available at www.thieme.com/nanda-i.

5. Perception/cognition

Domain 5 • Class 4 • Diagnosis Code 00128

Acute confusion

Focus of the diagnosis: confusion
Approved 1994 • Revised 2006, 2017 • Level of Evidence 2.1

Definition
Reversible disturbances of consciousness, attention, cognition and perception that develop over a short period of time, and which last less than 3 months.

Defining characteristics
- Altered psychomotor performance
- Cognitive dysfunction
- Difficulty initiating goal-directed behavior
- Difficulty initiating purposeful behavior
- Hallucinations
- Inadequate follow-through with goal-directed behavior
- Inadequate follow-through with purposeful behavior
- Misperception
- Neurobehavioral manifestations
- Psychomotor agitation

Related factors
- Altered sleep-wake cycle
- Dehydration
- Impaired physical mobility
- Inappropriate use of physical restraint
- Malnutrition
- Pain
- Sensory deprivation
- Substance misuse
- Urinary retention

At risk population
- Individuals aged ≥ 60 years
- Individuals with history of cerebral vascular accident
- Men

Associated conditions
- Decreased level of consciousness
- Impaired metabolism
- Infections
- Neurocognitive disorders
- Pharmaceutical preparations

Original literature support available at www.thieme.com/nanda-i.

Domain 5 • Class 4 • Diagnosis Code 00173

Risk for acute confusion

Focus of the diagnosis: confusion
Approved 2006 • Revised 2013, 2017 • Level of Evidence 2.2

Definition
Susceptible to reversible disturbances of consciousness, attention, cognition and perception that develop over a short period of time, which may compromise health.

Risk factors
- Altered sleep-wake cycle
- Dehydration
- Impaired physical mobility
- Inappropriate use of physical restraint
- Malnutrition
- Pain
- Sensory deprivation
- Substance misuse
- Urinary retention

At risk population
- Individuals aged ≥ 60 years
- Individuals with history of cerebral vascular accident
- Men

Associated conditions
- Decreased level of consciousness
- Impaired metabolism
- Infections
- Neurocognitive disorders
- Pharmaceutical preparations

Original literature support available at www.thieme.com/nanda-i.

Domain 5 • Class 4 • Diagnosis Code 00129

Chronic confusion

Focus of the diagnosis: confusion
Approved 1994 • Revised 2017, 2020 • Level of Evidence 3.1

Definition
Irreversible, progressive, insidious disturbances of consciousness, attention, cognition, and perception, which last more than 3 months.

Defining characteristics
- Altered personality
- Difficulty retrieving information when speaking
- Difficulty with decision-making
- Impaired executive functioning skills
- Impaired psychosocial functioning
- Inability to perform at least one daily activity
- Incoherent speech
- Long-term memory loss
- Marked change in behavior
- Short-term memory loss

Related factors
- Chonic sorrow
- Sedentary lifestyle
- Substance misuse

At risk population
- Individuals aged ≥ 60 years

Associated conditions
- Central nervous system diseases
- Human immunodeficiency virus infections
- Mental disorders
- Neurocognitive disorders
- Stroke

Original literature support available at www.thieme.com/nanda-i.

Domain 5 • Class 4 • Diagnosis Code 00251

Labile emotional control

Focus of the diagnosis: emotional control
Approved 2013 • Revised 2017 • Level of Evidence 2.1

Definition
Uncontrollable outbursts of exaggerated and involuntary emotional expression.

Defining characteristics

- Absence of eye contact
- Crying
- Excessive crying without feeling sadness
- Excessive laughing without feeling happiness
- Expresses embarrassment regarding emotional expression
- Expression of emotion incongruent with triggering factor
- Impaired nonverbal communication
- Involuntary crying
- Involuntary laughing
- Social alienation
- Uncontrollable crying
- Uncontrollable laughing
- Withdrawal from occupational situation

Related factors

- Altered self-esteem
- Excessive emotional disturbance
- Fatigue
- Inadequate knowledge about symptom control
- Inadequate knowledge of disease
- Insufficient muscle strength
- Social distress
- Stressors
- Substance misuse

Associated conditions

- Brain injuries
- Functional impairment
- Mental disorders
- Mood disorders
- Musculoskeletal impairment
- Pharmaceutical preparations
- Physical disability

Original literature support available at www.thieme.com/nanda-i.

Domain 5 • Class 4 • Diagnosis Code 00222

Ineffective impulse control

Focus of the diagnosis: impulse control
Approved 2010 • Revised 2017 • Level of Evidence 2.1

Definition

A pattern of performing rapid, unplanned reactions to internal or external stimuli without regard for the negative consequences of these reactions to the impulsive individual or to others.

Defining characteristics

- Acting without thinking
- Asking personal questions despite discomfort of others
- Dangerous behavior
- Gambling addiction
- Impaired ability to regulate finances
- Inappropriate sharing of personal details
- Irritable mood
- Overly familiar with strangers
- Sensation seeking
- Sexual promiscuity
- Temper outbursts

Related factors

- Cognitive dysfunction
- Hopelessness
- Mood disorders
- Neurobehavioral manifestations
- Smoking
- Substance misuse

Associated conditions

- Altered development
- Developmental disabilities
- Neurocognitive disorders
- Personality disorders

Original literature support available at www.thieme.com/nanda-i.

Domain 5 • Class 4 • Diagnosis Code 00126

Deficient knowledge

Focus of the diagnosis: knowledge
Approved 1980 • Revised 2017, 2020 • Level of Evidence 2.3

Definition
Absence of cognitive information related to a specific topic, or its acquisition.

Defining characteristics
- Inaccurate follow-through of instruction
- Inaccurate performance on a test
- Inaccurate statements about a topic
- Inappropriate behavior

Related factors
- Anxiety
- Cognitive dysfunction
- Depressive symptoms
- Inadequate access to resources
- Inadequate awareness of resources
- Inadequate commitment to learning
- Inadequate information
- Inadequate interest in learning
- Inadequate knowledge of resources
- Inadequate participation in care planning
- Inadequate trust in health care professional
- Low self efficacy
- Misinformation
- Neurobehavioral manifestations

At risk population
- Economically disadvantaged individuals
- Illiterate individuals
- Individuals with low educational level

Associated conditions
- Depression
- Developmental disabilities
- Neurocognitive disorders

Domain 5 • Class 4 • Diagnosis Code 00161

Readiness for enhanced knowledge

Focus of the diagnosis: knowledge
Approved 2002 • Level of Evidence 2.1

Definition
A pattern of cognitive information related to a specific topic, or its acquisition, which can be strengthened.

Defining characteristics
- Expresses desire to enhance learning

Domain 5 • Class 4 • Diagnosis Code 00131

Impaired memory

Focus of the diagnosis: memory
Approved 1994 • Revised 2017, 2020 • Level of Evidence 3.1

Definition
Persistent inability to remember or recall bits of information or skills, while maintaining the capacity to independently perform activities of daily living.

Defining characteristics

- Consistently forgets to perform a behavior at the scheduled time
- Difficulty acquiring a new skill
- Difficulty acquiring new information
- Difficulty recalling events
- Difficulty recalling factual information
- Difficulty recalling familiar names
- Difficulty recalling familiar objects
- Difficulty recalling familiar words
- Difficulty recalling if a behavior was performed
- Difficulty retaining a new skill
- Difficulty retaining new information

Related factors

- Depressive symptoms
- Inadequate intellectual stimulation
- Inadequate motivation
- Inadequate social support
- Social isolation
- Water-electrolyte imbalance

At risk population

- Economically disadvantaged individuals
- Individuals aged ≥ 60 years
- Individuals with low educational level

Associated conditions

- Anemia
- Brain hypoxia
- Cognition disorders

Original literature support available at www.thieme.com/nanda-i.

Domain 5 • Class 4 • Diagnosis Code 00279

Disturbed thought process

Focus of the diagnosis: thought process
Approved 2020 • Level of Evidence 2.3

Definition
Disruption in cognitive functioning that affects the mental processes involved in developing concepts and categories, reasoning, and problem solving .

Defining characteristics
- Difficulty communicating verbally
- Difficulty performing instrumental activities of daily living
- Disorganized thought sequence
- Expresses unreal thoughts
- Impaired interpretation of events
- Impaired judgment
- Inadequate emotional response to situations
- Limited ability to find solutions to everyday situations
- Limited ability to make decisions
- Limited ability to perform expected social roles
- Limited ability to plan activities
- Limited impulse control ability
- Obsessions
- Phobic disorders
- Suspicions

Related factors
- Acute confusion
- Anxiety
- Disorientation
- Fear
- Grieving
- Non-psychotic depressive symptoms
- Pain
- Stressors
- Substance misuse
- Unaddressed trauma

At risk population
- Economically disadvantaged individuals
- Individuals in the early postoperative period
- Older adults
- Pregnant women

Associated conditions
- Brain injuries
- Critical illness
- Hallucinations
- Mental disorders
- Neurodegenerative disorders
- Pharmaceutical preparations

Original literature support available at www.thieme.com/nanda-i.

Domain 5 • Class 5 • Diagnosis Code 00157

Readiness for enhanced communication

Focus of the diagnosis: communication
Approved 2002 • Revised 2013 • Level of Evidence 2.1

> **Definition**
> A pattern of exchanging information and ideas with others, which can be strengthened.

Defining characteristics
- Expresses desire to enhance communication

Domain 5 • Class 5 • Diagnosis Code 00051

Impaired verbal communication

Focus of the diagnosis: verbal communication
Approved 1983 • Revised 1996, 1998, 2017, 2020 • Level of Evidence 3.2

> **Definition**
> Decreased, delayed, or absent ability to receive, process, transmit, and/or use a system of symbols.

Defining characteristics

- Absence of eye contact
- Agraphia
- Alternative communication
- Anarthria
- Aphasia
- Augmentative communication
- Decline of speech productivity
- Decline of speech rate
- Decreased willingness to partici-pate in social interaction
- Difficulty comprehending communication
- Difficulty establishing social interaction
- Difficulty maintaining communication
- Difficulty using body expressions
- Difficulty using facial expressions
- Difficulty with selective attention
- Displays negative emotions
- Dysarthria
- Dysgraphia
- Dyslalia
- Dysphonia
- Fatigued by conversation
- Impaired ability to speak
- Impaired ability to use body expressions
- Impaired ability to use facial expressions
- Inability to speak language of caregiver
- Inappropriate verbalization
- Obstinate refusal to speak
- Slurred speech

Related factors

- Altered self-concept
- Cognitive dysfunction
- Dyspnea
- Emotional lability
- Environmental constraints
- Inadequate stimulation
- Low self-esteem
- Perceived vulnerability
- Psychological barriers
- Values incongruent with cultural norms

At risk population

- Individuals facing physical barriers
- Individuals in the early postopera-tive period
- Individuals unable to verbalize
- Individuals with communication barriers
- Individuals without a significant other

Associated conditions

- Altered perception
- Central nervous system diseases
- Developmental disabilities
- Flaccid facial paralysis
- Hemifacial spasm
- Motor neuron disease
- Neoplasms
- Neurocognitive disorders
- Oropharyngeal defect
- Peripheral nervous system diseases
- Psychotic disorders
- Respiratory muscle weakness
- Sialorrhea
- Speech disorders
- Tongue diseases
- Tracheostomy
- Treatment regimen
- Velopharyngeal insufficiency
- Vocal cord dysfunction

Domain 6.
Self-perception

Awareness about the self

Class 1. Self-concept
The perception(s) about the total self

Code	Diagnosis	Page
00124	Hopelessness	341
00185	Readiness for enhanced hope	343
00174	Risk for compromised human dignity	344
00121	Disturbed personal identity	345
00225	Risk for disturbed personal identity	346
00167	Readiness for enhanced self-concept	347

Class 2. Self-esteem
Assessment of one's own worth, capability, significance, and success

Code	Diagnosis	Page
00119	Chronic low self-esteem	348
00224	Risk for chronic low self-esteem	350
00120	Situational low self-esteem	351
00153	Risk for situational low self-esteem	353

Class 3. Body image
A mental image of one's own body

Code	Diagnosis	Page
00118	Disturbed body image	355

NANDA International, Inc. Nursing Diagnoses: Definitions and Classification 2021–2023, 12th Edition.
Edited by T. Heather Herdman, Shigemi Kamitsuru, and Camila Takáo Lopes.

Domain 6 • Class 1 • Diagnosis Code 00124

Hopelessness

Focus of the diagnosis: hope
Approved 1986 • Revised 2017, 2020 • Level of Evidence 2.1

Definition
The feeling that one will not experience positive emotions, or an improvement in one's condition.

Defining characteristics

- Anorexia
- Avoidance behaviors
- Decreased affective display
- Decreased initiative
- Decreased response to stimuli
- Decreased verbalization
- Depressive symptoms
- Expresses despondency
- Expresses diminished hope
- Expresses feeling of uncertain future
- Expresses inadequate motivation for the future
- Expresses negative expectations about self
- Expresses negative expectations about the future
- Expresses sense of incompetency in meeting goals
- Inadequate involvement with self-care
- Overestimates the likelihood of unfortunate events
- Passivity
- Reports altered sleep-wake cycle
- Suicidal behaviors
- Unable to imagine life in the future
- Underestimates the occurrence of positive events

Related factors

- Chronic stress
- Fear
- Inadequate social support
- Loss of belief in spiritual power
- Loss of belief in transcendent values
- Low self efficacy
- Prolonged immobility
- Social isolation
- Unaddressed violence
- Uncontrolled severe disease symptoms

At risk population

- Adolescents
- Displaced individuals
- Economically disadvantaged individuals
- Individuals experiencing infertility
- Individuals experiencing significant loss
- Individuals with history of attempted suicide
- Individuals with history of being abandoned

6. Self-perception

- Older adults
- Unemployed individuals

Associated conditions
- Critical illness
- Depression
- Deterioration in physiological condition
- Feeding and eating disorders
- Mental disorders
- Neoplasms
- Terminal illness

Domain 6 • Class 1 • Diagnosis Code 00185

Readiness for enhanced hope

Focus of the diagnosis: hope
Approved 2006 • Revised 2013, 2020 • Level of Evidence 3.2

Definition
A pattern of expectations and desires for mobilizing energy to achieve positive outcomes, or avoid a potentially threatening or negative situation, which can be strengthened.

Defining characteristics
- Expresses desire to enhance ability to set achievable goals
- Expresses desire to enhance belief in possibilities
- Expresses desire to enhance congruency of expectation with goal
- Expresses desire to enhance deep inner strength
- Expresses desire to enhance giving and receiving of care
- Expresses desire to enhance giving and receiving of love
- Expresses desire to enhance initiative
- Expresses desire to enhance involvement with self-care
- Expresses desire to enhance positive outlook on life
- Expresses desire to enhance problem-solving to meet goal
- Expresses desire to enhance sense of meaning in life
- Expresses desire to enhance spirituality

6. Self-perception

Original literature support available at www.thieme.com/nanda-i.

Domain 6 • Class 1 • Diagnosis Code 00174

Risk for compromised human dignity

Focus of the diagnosis: human dignity
Approved 2006 • Revised 2013 • Level of Evidence 2.1

Definition
Susceptible for perceived loss of respect and honor, which may compromise health.

Risk factors

- Dehumanization
- Disclosure of confidential information
- Exposure of the body
- Humiliation
- Inadequate understanding of health information
- Insufficient privacy
- Intrusion by clinician
- Loss of control over body function
- Perceived social stigma
- Values incongruent with cultural norms

At risk population

- Individuals with limited decision-making experience

Original literature support available at www.thieme.com/nanda-i.

Domain 6 · Class 1 · Diagnosis Code 00121

Disturbed personal identity

Focus of the diagnosis: personal identity
Approved 1978 · Revised 2008, 2017 · Level of Evidence 2.1

Definition
Inability to maintain an integrated and complete perception of self.

Defining characteristics
- Altered body image
- Confusion about cultural values
- Confusion about goals
- Confusion about ideological values
- Delusional description of self
- Expresses feeling of emptiness
- Expresses feeling of strangeness
- Fluctuating feelings about self
- Impaired ability to distinguish between internal and external stimuli
- Inadequate interpersonal relations
- Inadequate role performance
- Inconsistent behavior
- Ineffective coping strategies
- Reports social discrimination

Related factors
- Altered social role
- Cult indoctrination
- Dysfunctional family processes
- Gender conflict
- Low self-esteem
- Perceived social discrimination
- Values incongruent with cultural norms

At risk population
- Individuals experiencing developmental transition
- Individuals experiencing situational crisis
- Individuals exposed to toxic chemicals

Associated conditions
- Dissociative identity disorder
- Mental disorders
- Neurocognitive disorders
- Pharmaceutical preparations

6. Self-perception

Original literature support available at www.thieme.com/nanda-i.

Domain 6 • Class 1 • Diagnosis Code 00225

Risk for disturbed personal identity

Focus of the diagnosis: personal identity
Approved 2010 • Revised 2013, 2017 • Level of Evidence 2.1

Definition
Susceptible to the inability to maintain an integrated and complete perception of self, which may compromise health.

Risk factors
- Altered social role
- Cult indoctrination
- Dysfunctional family processes
- Gender conflict
- Low self-esteem
- Perceived social discrimination
- Values incongruent with cultural norms

At risk population
- Individuals experiencing developmental transition
- Individuals experiencing situational crisis
- Individuals exposed to toxic chemicals

Associated conditions
- Dissociative identity disorder
- Mental disorders
- Neurocognitive disorders
- Pharmaceutical preparations

Original literature support available at www.thieme.com/nanda-i.

6. Self-perception

Domain 6 • Class 1 • Diagnosis Code 00167

Readiness for enhanced self-concept

Focus of the diagnosis: self-concept
Approved 2002 • Revised 2013 • Level of Evidence 2.1

> **Definition**
> A pattern of perceptions or ideas about the self, which can be strengthened.

Defining characteristics

- Expresses desire to enhance acceptance of limitations
- Expresses desire to enhance acceptance of strengths
- Expresses desire to enhance body image satisfaction
- Expresses desire to enhance confidence in abilities
- Expresses desire to enhance congruence between actions and words
- Expresses desire to enhance role performance
- Expresses desire to enhance satisfaction with personal identity
- Expresses desire to enhance satisfaction with sense of worth
- Expresses desire to enhance self-esteem

6. Self-perception

Domain 6 • Class 2 • Diagnosis Code 00119

Chronic low self-esteem

Focus of the diagnosis: self-esteem
Approved 1988 • Revised 1996, 2008, 2017, 2020 • Level of Evidence 3.2

Definition
Long-standing negative perception of self-worth, self-acceptance, self-respect, competence, and attitude toward self.

Defining characteristics
- Dependent on others' opinions
- Depressive symptoms
- Excessive guilt
- Excessive seeking of reassurance
- Expresses loneliness
- Hopelessness
- Insomnia
- Loneliness
- Nonassertive behavior
- Overly conforming behaviors
- Reduced eye contact
- Rejects positive feedback
- Reports repeated failures
- Rumination
- Self-negating verbalizations
- Shame
- Suicidal ideation
- Underestimates ability to deal with situation

Related factors
- Decreased mindful acceptance
- Difficulty managing finances
- Disturbed body image
- Fatigue
- Fear of rejection
- Impaired religiosity
- Inadequate affection received
- Inadequate attachment behavior
- Inadequate family cohesiveness
- Inadequate group membership
- Inadequate respect from others
- Inadequate sense of belonging
- Inadequate social support
- Ineffective communication skills
- Insufficient approval from others
- Low self efficacy
- Maladaptive grieving
- Negative resignation
- Repeated negative reinforcement
- Spiritual incongruence
- Stigmatization
- Stressors
- Values incongruent with cultural norms

At risk population
- Economically disadvantaged individuals
- Individuals experiencing repeated failure
- Individuals exposed to traumatic situation
- Individuals with difficult developmental transition

- Individuals with history of being abandoned
- Individuals with history of being abused
- Individuals with history of being neglected
- Individuals with history of loss

Associated conditions

- Depression
- Functional impairment
- Mental disorders
- Physical illness

Original literature support available at www.thieme.com/nanda-i.

Domain 6 • Class 2 • Diagnosis Code 00224

Risk for chronic low self-esteem

Focus of the diagnosis: self-esteem
Approved 2010 • Revised 2013, 2017, 2020 • Level of Evidence 3.2

Definition
Susceptible to long-standing negative perception of self-worth, self-acceptance, self-respect, competence, and attitude toward self, which may compromise health.

Risk factors
- Decreased mindful acceptance
- Difficulty managing finances
- Disturbed body image
- Fatigue
- Fear of rejection
- Impaired religiosity
- Inadequate affection received
- Inadequate attachment behavior
- Inadequate family cohesiveness
- Inadequate group membership
- Inadequate respect from others
- Inadequate sense of belonging
- Inadequate social support
- Ineffective communication skills
- Insufficient approval from others
- Low self efficacy
- Maladaptive grieving
- Negative resignation
- Repeated negative reinforcement
- Spiritual incongruence
- Stigmatization
- Stressors
- Values incongruent with cultural norms

At risk population
- Economically disadvantaged individuals
- Individuals experiencing repeated failure
- Individuals exposed to traumatic situation
- Individuals with difficult developmental transition
- Individuals with history of being abandoned
- Individuals with history of being abused
- Individuals with history of being neglected
- Individuals with history of loss

Associated conditions
- Depression
- Functional impairment
- Mental disorders
- Physical illness

Original literature support available at www.thieme.com/nanda-i.

Domain 6 · Class 2 · Diagnosis Code 00120

Situational low self-esteem

Focus of the diagnosis: self-esteem
Approved 1988 · Revised 1996, 2000, 2017, 2020 · Level of Evidence 3.2

Definition
Change from positive to negative perception of self-worth, self-acceptance, self-respect, competence, and attitude toward self in response to a current situation.

Defining characteristics
- Depressive symptoms
- Expresses loneliness
- Helplessness
- Indecisive behavior
- Insomnia
- Loneliness
- Nonassertive behavior
- Purposelessness
- Rumination
- Self-negating verbalizations
- Underestimates ability to deal with situation

Related factors
- Behavior incongruent with values
- Decrease in environmental control
- Decreased mindful acceptance
- Difficulty accepting alteration in social role
- Difficulty managing finances
- Disturbed body image
- Fatigue
- Fear of rejection
- Impaired religiosity
- Inadequate attachment behavior
- Inadequate family cohesiveness
- Inadequate respect from others
- Inadequate social support
- Ineffective communication skills
- Low self efficacy
- Maladaptive perfectionism
- Negative resignation
- Powerlessness
- Stigmatization
- Stressors
- Unrealistic self-expectations
- Values incongruent with cultural norms

At risk population
- Individuals experiencing a change in living environment
- Individuals experiencing alteration in body image
- Individuals experiencing alteration in economic status
- Individuals experiencing alteration in role function
- Individuals experiencing death of a significant other
- Individuals experiencing divorce
- Individuals experiencing new additions to the family
- Individuals experiencing repeated failure

6. Self-perception

- Individuals experiencing unplanned pregnancy
- Individuals with difficult developmental transition
- Individuals with history of being abandoned
- Individuals with history of being abused
- Individuals with history of being neglected
- Individuals with history of loss
- Individuals with history of rejection

Associated conditions

- Depression
- Functional impairment
- Mental disorders
- Physical illness

Domain 6 • Class 2 • Diagnosis Code 00153

Risk for situational low self-esteem

Focus of the diagnosis: self-esteem
Approved 2000 • Revised 2013, 2017, 2020 • Level of Evidence 3.2

> **Definition**
> Susceptible to change from positive to negative perception of self-worth, self-acceptance, self-respect, competence, and attitude toward self in response to a current situation, which may compromise health.

Risk factors

- Behavior incongruent with values
- Decrease in environmental control
- Decreased mindful acceptance
- Difficulty accepting alteration in social role
- Difficulty managing finances
- Disturbed body image
- Fatigue
- Fear of rejection
- Impaired religiosity
- Inadequate attachment behavior
- Inadequate family cohesiveness
- Inadequate respect from others
- Inadequate social support
- Individuals experiencing repeated failure
- Ineffective communication skills
- Low self efficacy
- Maladaptive perfectionism
- Negative resignation
- Powerlessness
- Stigmatization
- Stressors
- Unrealistic self-expectations
- Values incongruent with cultural norms

At risk population

- Individuals experiencing a change in living environment
- Individuals experiencing alteration in body image
- Individuals experiencing alteration in economic status
- Individuals experiencing alteration in role function
- Individuals experiencing death of a significant other
- Individuals experiencing divorce
- Individuals experiencing new additions to the family
- Individuals experiencing unplanned pregnancy
- Individuals with difficult developmental transition
- Individuals with history of being abandoned
- Individuals with history of being abused
- Individuals with history of being neglected
- Individuals with history of loss
- Individuals with history of rejection

Associated conditions

- Depression
- Functional impairment
- Mental disorders
- Physical illness

Domain 6 • Class 3 • Diagnosis Code 00118

Disturbed body image

Focus of the diagnosis: body image
Approved 1973 • Revised 1998, 2017, 2020 • Level of Evidence 3.2

Definition
Negative mental picture of one's physical self.

Defining characteristics

- Altered proprioception
- Altered social involvement
- Avoids looking at one's body
- Avoids touching one's body
- Consistently compares oneself with others
- Depressive symptoms
- Expresses concerns about sexuality
- Expresses fear of reaction by others
- Expresses preoccupation with change
- Expresses preoccupation with missing body part
- Focused on past appearance
- Focused on past function
- Focused on past strength
- Frequently weighs self
- Hides body part
- Monitors changes in one's body
- Names body part
- Names missing body part
- Neglects nonfunctioning body part
- Nonverbal response to body changes
- Nonverbal response to perceived body changes
- Overexposes body part
- Perceptions that reflect an altered view of appearance
- Refuses to acknowledge change
- Reports feeling one has failed in life
- Social anxiety
- Uses impersonal pronouns to describe body part
- Uses impersonal pronouns to describe missing body part

Related factors

- Body consciousness
- Cognitive dysfunction
- Conflict between spiritual beliefs and treatment regimen
- Conflict between values and cultural norms
- Distrust of body function
- Fear of disease recurrence
- Low self efficacy
- Low self-esteem
- Obesity
- Residual limb pain
- Unrealistic perception of treatment outcome
- Unrealistic self-expectations

At risk population

- Cancer survivors
- Individuals experiencing altered body weight
- Individuals experiencing developmental transition
- Individuals experiencing puberty
- Individuals with altered body function
- Individuals with scars
- Individuals with stomas
- Women

Associated conditions

- Binge-eating disorder
- Chronic pain
- Fibromyalgia
- Human immunodeficiency virus infections
- Impaired psychosocial functioning
- Mental disorders
- Surgical procedures
- Treatment regimen
- Wounds and injuries

Domain 7.
Role relationship

The positive and negative connections or associations between people or groups of people and the means by which those connections are demonstrated

Class 1. Caregiving roles
Socially expected behavior patterns by people providing care who are not health care professionals

Code	Diagnosis	Page
00056	Impaired parenting	359
00057	Risk for impaired parenting	361
00164	Readiness for enhanced parenting	363
00061	Caregiver role strain	364
00062	Risk for caregiver role strain	367

Class 2. Family relationships
Associations of people who are biologically related or related by choice

Code	Diagnosis	Page
00058	Risk for impaired attachment	369
00283	Disturbed family identity syndrome	370
00284	Risk for disturbed family identity syndrome	372
00063	Dysfunctional family processes	373
00060	Interrupted family processes	376
00159	Readiness for enhanced family processes	377

Class 3. Role performance
Quality of functioning in socially expected behavior patterns

NANDA International, Inc. Nursing Diagnoses: Definitions and Classification 2021–2023, 12th Edition.
Edited by T. Heather Herdman, Shigemi Kamitsuru, and Camila Takáo Lopes.
© 2021 NANDA International, Inc. Published 2021 by Thieme Medical Publishers, Inc., New York.
Companion website: www.thieme.com/nanda-i.

Domain 7 · Class 1 · Diagnosis Code 00056

Impaired parenting

Focus of the diagnosis: parenting
Approved 1978 · Revised 1998, 2017, 2020 · Level of Evidence 3.1

> **Definition**
> Limitation of primary caregiver to nurture, protect, and promote optimal growth and development of the child, through a consistent, empathic exercise of authority and appropriate behavior in response to the child's needs.

Defining characteristics

Parental Externalizing Symptoms

- Hostile parenting behaviors
- Impulsive behaviors
- Intrusive behaviors
- Negative communication

Parental Internalizing Symptoms

- Decreased engagement in parent-child relations
- Decreased positive temperament
- Decreased subjective attention quality
- Extreme mood swings
- Failure to provide safe home environment
- Inadequate response to infant behavioral cues
- Inappropriate child-care arrangements
- Rejects child
- Social alienation

Infant or Child

- Anxiety
- Conduct problems
- Delayed cognitive development
- Depressive symptoms
- Difficulty establishing healthy intimate interpersonal relations
- Difficulty functioning socially
- Difficulty regulating emotion
- Extreme mood alterations
- Low academic performance
- Obesity
- Role reversal
- Somatic complaints
- Substance misuse

Related factors

- Altered parental role
- Decreased emotion recognition abilities
- Depressive symptoms
- Difficulty managing complex treatment regimen
- Dysfunctional family processes
- Emotional vacillation

- High use of internet-connected devices
- Inadequate knowledge about child development
- Inadequate knowledge about child health maintenance
- Inadequate parental role model
- Inadequate problem-solving skills
- Inadequate social support
- Inadequate transportation
- Inattentive to child's needs

- Increased anxiety symptoms
- Low self efficacy
- Marital conflict
- Nonrestorative sleep-wake cycle
- Perceived economic strain
- Social isolation
- Substance misuse
- Unaddressed intimate partner violence

At risk population
Parent

- Adolescents
- Economically disadvantaged individuals
- Homeless individuals
- Individuals experiencing family substance misuse
- Individuals experiencing situational crisis
- Individuals with family history of post-traumatic shock
- Individuals with history of being abused

- Individuals with history of being abusive
- Individuals with history of being neglected
- Individuals with history of exposure to violence
- Individuals with history of inadequate prenatal care
- Individuals with history of prenatal stress
- Individuals with low educational level
- Sole parents

Infant or Child

- Children experiencing prolonged separation from parent
- Children with difficult temperament

- Children with gender other than that desired by parent
- Children with history of hospitalization in neonatal intensive care
- Premature infants

Associated conditions
Parent

- Depression

- Mental disorders

Infant or Child

- Behavioral disorder
- Complex treatment regimen

- Emotional disorder
- Neurodevelopmental disabilities

Domain 7 • Class 1 • Diagnosis Code 00057

Risk for impaired parenting

Focus of the diagnosis: parenting
Approved 1978 • Revised 1998, 2013, 2017, 2020 • Level of Evidence 3.1

Definition
Primary caregiver susceptible to a limitation to nurture, protect, and promote optimal growth and development of the child, through a consistent, empathic exercise of authority and appropriate behavior in response to the child's needs.

Risk factors

- Altered parental role
- Decreased emotion recognition abilities
- Depressive symptoms
- Difficulty managing complex treatment regimen
- Dysfunctional family processes
- Emotional vacillation
- High use of internet-connected devices
- Inadequate knowledge about child development
- Inadequate knowledge about child health maintenance
- Inadequate parental role model
- Inadequate problem-solving skills
- Inadequate social support
- Inadequate transportation
- Inattentive to child's needs
- Increased anxiety symptoms
- Low self efficacy
- Marital conflict
- Nonrestorative sleep-wake cycle
- Perceived economic strain
- Social isolation
- Substance misuse
- Unaddressed intimate partner violence

At risk population

Parent

- Adolescents
- Economically disadvantaged individuals
- Homeless individuals
- Individuals experiencing family substance misuse
- Individuals experiencing situational crisis
- Individuals with family history of post-traumatic shock
- Individuals with history of being abused
- Individuals with history of being abusive
- Individuals with history of being neglected
- Individuals with history of exposure to violence
- Individuals with history of inadequate prenatal care
- Individuals with history of prenatal stress
- Individuals with low educational level
- Sole parents

Infant or Child

- Children experiencing prolonged separation from parent
- Children with difficult temperament

- Children with gender other than that desired by parent
- Children with history of hospitalization in neonatal intensive care
- Premature infants

Associated conditions

Parent

- Depression

- Mental disorders

Infant or Child

- Behavioral disorder
- Complex treatment regimen

- Emotional disorder
- Neurodevelopmental disabilities

Domain 7 • Class 1 • Diagnosis Code 00164

Readiness for enhanced parenting

Focus of the diagnosis: parenting
Approved 2002 • Revised 2013, 2020 • Level of Evidence 2.1

Definition
A pattern of primary caregiver to nurture, protect, and promote optimal growth and development of the child, through a consistent, empathic exercise of authority and appropriate behavior in response to the child's needs, which can be strengthened.

Defining characteristics

- Expresses desire to enhance acceptance of child
- Expresses desire to enhance attention quality
- Expresses desire to enhance child health maintenance
- Expresses desire to enhance child-care arrangements
- Expresses desire to enhance engagement with child
- Expresses desire to enhance home environmental safety
- Expresses desire to enhance mood stability
- Expresses desire to enhance parent-child relations
- Expresses desire to enhance patience
- Expresses desire to enhance positive communication
- Expresses desire to enhance positive parenting behaviors
- Expresses desire to enhance positive temperament
- Expresses desire to enhance response to infant behavioral cues

Domain 7 • Class 1 • Diagnosis Code 00061

Caregiver role strain

Focus of the diagnosis: role strain
Approved 1992 • Revised 1998, 2000, 2017 • Level of Evidence 2.1

> **Definition**
> Difficulty in fulfilling care responsibilities, expectations and/or behaviors for family or significant others.

Defining characteristics

Caregiving Activities

- Apprehensive about future ability to provide care
- Apprehensive about future health of care receiver
- Apprehensive about potential institutionalization of care receiver
- Apprehensive about well-being of care receiver if unable to provide care

- Difficulty completing required tasks
- Difficulty performing required tasks
- Dysfunctional change in caregiving activities
- Preoccupation with care routine

Caregiver Health Status: Physiological

- Fatigue
- Gastrointestinal distress
- Headache
- Hypertension

- Rash
- Reports altered sleep-wake cycle
- Weight change

Caregiver Health Status: Emotional

- Depressive symptoms
- Emotional lability
- Expresses anger
- Expresses frustration
- Impatience

- Insufficient time to meet personal needs
- Nervousness
- Somatization

Caregiver Health Status: Socioeconomic

- Altered leisure activities
- Isolation

- Low work productivity
- Refuses career advancement

Caregiver-Care Receiver Relationship

- Difficulty watching care receiver with illness
- Sadness about altered interpersonal relations with care receiver

- Uncertainty about alteration in interpersonal relations with care receiver

Family Processes

- Family conflict

- Reports concern about family member(s)

Related factors
Caregiver Factors

- Competing role commitments
- Depressive symptoms
- Inadequate fulfillment of others' expectations
- Inadequate fulfillment of self-expectations
- Inadequate knowledge about community resources
- Inadequate psychological resilience
- Inadequate recreation
- Ineffective coping strategies

- Inexperience with caregiving
- Insufficient physical endurance
- Insufficient privacy
- Not developmentally ready for caregiver role
- Physical conditions
- Social isolation
- Stressors
- Substance misuse
- Unrealistic self-expectations

Care Receiver Factors

- Discharged home with significant needs
- Increased care needs
- Loss of independence
- Problematic behavior

- Substance misuse
- Unpredictability of illness trajectory
- Unstable health status

Caregiver-Care Receiver Relationship

- Abusive interpersonal relations
- Codependency
- Inadequate interpersonal relations
- Unaddressed abuse

- Unrealistic care receiver expectations
- Violent interpersonal relations

Caregiving Activities

- Altered nature of care activities
- Around-the-clock care responsibilities
- Complexity of care activities
- Excessive caregiving activities

- Extended duration of caregiving required
- Inadequate assistance
- Inadequate equipment for providing care

7. Role relationship

- Inadequate physical environment for providing care
- Inadequate respite for caregiver

- Insufficient time
- Unpredictability of care situation

Family Processes

- Family isolation
- Ineffective family adaptation
- Pattern of family dysfunction

- Pattern of family dysfunction prior to the caregiving situation
- Pattern of ineffective family coping

Socioeconomic

- Difficulty accessing assistance
- Difficulty accessing community resources
- Difficulty accessing support
- Inadequate community resources

- Inadequate social support
- Inadequate transportation
- Social alienation

At risk population

- Care receiver with developmental disabilities
- Caregiver delivering care to partner
- Caregiver with developmental disabilities

- Female caregiver
- Individuals delivering care to infants born prematurely
- Individuals experiencing financial crisis

Associated conditions

Caregiver Factors

- Impaired health status

- Psychological disorder

Care Receiver Factors

- Chronic disease
- Cognitive dysfunction
- Congenital disorders

- Illness severity
- Mental disorders

7. Role relationship

Domain 7 • Class 1 • Diagnosis Code 00062

Risk for caregiver role strain

Focus of the diagnosis: role strain
Approved 1992 • Revised 2010, 2013, 2017 • Level of Evidence 2.1

Definition
Susceptible to difficulty in fulfilling care responsibilities, expectations, and/or behaviors for family or significant others, which may compromise health.

Risk factors

Caregiver Factors

- Competing role commitments
- Depressive symptoms
- Inadequate fulfillment of others' expectations
- Inadequate fulfillment of self-expectations
- Inadequate knowledge about community resources
- Inadequate psychological resilience
- Inadequate recreation
- Ineffective coping strategies
- Inexperience with caregiving
- Insufficient physical endurance
- Insufficient privacy
- Not developmentally ready for caregiver role
- Physical conditions
- Stressors
- Substance misuse
- Unrealistic self-expectations
- Unstable health status

Care Receiver Factors

- Discharged home with significant needs
- Increased care needs
- Loss of independence
- Problematic behavior
- Substance misuse
- Unpredictability of illness trajectory
- Unstable health condition

Caregiver-Care Receiver Relationship

- Abusive interpersonal relations
- Codependency
- Inadequate interpersonal relations
- Unaddressed abuse
- Unrealistic care receiver expectations
- Violent interpersonal relations

Caregiving Activities

- Altered nature of care activities
- Around-the-clock care responsibilities

7. Role relationship

- Complexity of care activities
- Excessive caregiving activities
- Extended duration of caregiving required
- Inadequate assistance
- Inadequate equipment for providing care

- Inadequate physical environment for providing care
- Inadequate respite for caregiver
- Insufficient time
- Unpredictability of care situation

Family Processes

- Family isolation
- Ineffective family adaptation
- Pattern of family dysfunction

- Pattern of family dysfunction prior to the caregiving situation
- Pattern of ineffective family coping

Socioeconomic

- Difficulty accessing assistance
- Difficulty accessing community resources
- Difficulty accessing support
- Inadequate community resources

- Inadequate social support
- Inadequate transportation
- Social alienation
- Social isolation

At risk population

- Care receiver with developmental disabilities
- Care receiver's condition inhibits conversation
- Caregiver delivering care to partner

- Caregiver with developmental disabilities
- Female caregiver
- Individuals delivering care to infants born prematurely
- Individuals experiencing financial crisis

Associated conditions

Caregiver Factors

- Impaired health status

- Psychological disorder

Care Receiver Factors

- Chronic disease
- Cognitive dysfunction
- Congenital disorders

- Illness severity
- Mental disorders

Domain 7 · Class 2 · Diagnosis Code 00058

Risk for impaired attachment

Focus of the diagnosis: attachment
Approved 1994 · Revised 2008, 2013, 2017 · Level of Evidence 2.1

Definition
Susceptible to disruption of the interactive process between parent or significant other and child that fosters the development of a protective and nurturing reciprocal relationship.

Risk factors
- Anxiety
- Child's illness prevents effective initiation of parental contact
- Disorganized infant behavior
- Inability of parent to meet personal needs
- Insufficient privacy
- Parent's illness prevents effective initiation of infant contact
- Parent-child separation
- Parental conflict resulting from disorganized infant behavior
- Physical barrier
- Substance misuse

At risk population
- Premature infants

Domain 7 • Class 2 • Diagnosis Code 00283

Disturbed family identity syndrome

Focus of the diagnosis: disturbed family identity syndrome
Approved 2020 • Level of Evidence 2.1

> **Definition**
> Inability to maintain an ongoing interactive, communicative process of creating and maintaining a shared collective sense of the meaning of the family.

Defining characteristics

- Decisional conflict (00083)
- Disabled family coping (00073)
- Disturbed personal identity (00121)
- Dysfunctional family processes (00063)
- Impaired resilience (00210)
- Ineffective childbearing process (00221)
- Ineffective relationship (00223)
- Ineffective sexuality pattern (00065)
- Interrupted family processes (00060)

Related factors

- Ambivalent family relations
- Different coping styles among family members
- Disrupted family rituals
- Disrupted family roles
- Excessive stress
- Inadequate social support
- Inconsistent management of therapeutic regimen among family members
- Ineffective coping strategies
- Ineffective family communication
- Perceived danger to value system
- Perceived social discrimination
- Sexual dysfunction
- Unaddressed domestic violence
- Unrealistic expectations
- Values incongruent with cultural norms

At risk population

- Blended families
- Economically disadvantaged families
- Families experiencing infertility
- Families with history of domestic violence
- Families with incarcerated member
- Families with member experiencing alteration in health status
- Families with member experiencing developmental crisis
- Families with member experiencing situational crisis
- Families with member living far from relatives
- Families with member with history of adoption
- Families with member with intimacy dysfunction
- Families with unemployed members

Associated conditions
- Infertility treatment regimen

Original literature support available at www.thieme.com/nanda-i.

Domain 7 • Class 2 • Diagnosis Code 00284

Risk for disturbed family identity syndrome

Focus of the diagnosis: disturbed family identity syndrome
Approved 2020 • Level of Evidence 2.1

Definition

Susceptible to an inability to maintain an ongoing interactive, communicative process of creating and maintaining a shared collective sense of the meaning of the family, which may compromise family members' health .

Risk factors

- Ambivalent family relations
- Different coping styles among family members
- Disrupted family rituals
- Disrupted family roles
- Excessive stress
- Inadequate social support
- Inconsistent management of therapeutic regimen among family members
- Ineffective coping strategies
- Ineffective family communication
- Perceived danger to value system
- Perceived social discrimination
- Sexual dysfunction
- Unaddressed domestic violence
- Unrealistic expectations
- Values incongruent with cultural norms

At risk population

- Blended families
- Economically disadvantaged families
- Families experiencing infertility
- Families with history of domestic violence
- Families with incarcerated member
- Families with member experiencing alteration in health status
- Families with member experiencing developmental crisis
- Families with member experiencing situational crisis
- Families with member living far from relatives
- Families with member with history of adoption
- Families with member with intimacy dysfunction
- Families with unemployed members

Associated conditions

- Infertility treatment regimen

Original literature support available at www.thieme.com/nanda-i.

Domain 7 • Class 2 • Diagnosis Code 00063

Dysfunctional family processes

Focus of the diagnosis: family processes
Approved 1994 • Revised 2008, 2017 • Level of Evidence 2.1

Definition
Family functioning which fails to support the well-being of its members.

Defining characteristics
Behavioral Factors

- Altered academic performance
- Altered attention
- Conflict avoidance
- Contradictory communication pattern
- Controlling communication pattern
- Criticizing others
- Decreased physical contact
- Denies problems
- Difficulty accepting a wide range of feelings
- Difficulty accepting help
- Difficulty adapting to change
- Difficulty dealing constructively with traumatic experiences
- Difficulty expressing a wide range of feelings
- Difficulty having fun
- Difficulty meeting the emotional needs of members
- Difficulty meeting the security needs of members
- Difficulty meeting the spiritual needs of its members
- Difficulty receiving help appropriately
- Difficulty with intimate interpersonal relations
- Difficulty with life-cycle transition
- Enabling substance misuse pattern
- Escalating conflict
- Harsh self-judgment
- Immaturity
- Inadequate communication skills
- Inadequate knowledge about substance misuse
- Inappropriate anger expression
- Loss of independence
- Lying
- Maladaptive grieving
- Manipulation
- Nicotine addiction
- Orientation favors tension relief rather than goal attainment
- Paradoxical communication pattern
- Pattern of broken promises
- Power struggles
- Psychomotor agitation
- Rationalization
- Refuses to accept personal responsibility
- Refuses to get help
- Seeks affirmation
- Seeks approval
- Self-blame
- Social isolation
- Special occasions centered on substance misuse
- Stress-related physical illness
- Substance misuse
- Unreliable behavior

7. Role relationship

- Verbal abuse of children
- Verbal abuse of parent

- Verbal abuse of partner

Feelings

- Anxiety
- Confuses love and pity
- Confusion
- Depressive symptoms
- Dissatisfaction
- Emotionally controlled by others
- Expresses anger
- Expresses distress
- Expresses embarrassment
- Expresses fear
- Expresses feeling abandoned
- Expresses feeling of failure
- Expresses feeling unloved
- Expresses frustration
- Expresses insecurity
- Expresses lingering resentment
- Expresses loneliness
- Expresses shame
- Expresses tension
- Hopelessness

- Hostility
- Loss
- Loss of identity
- Low self-esteem
- Mistrust of others
- Moodiness
- Powerlessness
- Rejection
- Reports feeling different from others
- Reports feeling emotionally isolated
- Reports feeling guilty
- Reports feeling misunderstood
- Repressed emotions
- Taking responsibility for substance misuser's behavior
- Unhappiness
- Worthlessness

Roles and Relationships

- Altered family relations
- Altered role function
- Chronic family problems
- Closed communication system
- Conflict between partners
- Deterioration in family relations
- Diminished ability of family members to relate to each other for mutual growth and maturation
- Disrupted family rituals
- Disrupted family roles
- Family denial
- Family disorganization
- Inadequate family cohesiveness

- Inadequate family respect for autonomy of its members
- Inadequate family respect for individuality of its members
- Inadequate interpersonal relations skills
- Inconsistent parenting
- Ineffective communication with partner
- Neglects obligation to family member
- Pattern of rejection
- Perceived inadequate parental support
- Triangulating family relations

Related factors

- Addictive personality
- Inadequate problem-solving skills

- Ineffective coping strategies
- Perceived vulnerability

At risk population

- Economically disadvantaged families
- Families with history of resistance to treatment regimen
- Families with member with history of substance misuse
- Families with members with genetic predisposition to substance misuse

Associated conditions

- Depression
- Developmental disabilities
- Intimacy dysfunction
- Surgical procedures

Domain 7 • Class 2 • Diagnosis Code 00060

Interrupted family processes

Focus of the diagnosis: family processes
Approved 1982 • Revised 1998, 2017

Definition
Break in the continuity of family functioning which fails to support the well-being of its members.

Defining characteristics
- Altered affective responsiveness
- Altered communication pattern
- Altered family conflict resolution
- Altered family satisfaction
- Altered interpersonal relations
- Altered intimacy
- Altered participation in decision-making
- Altered participation in problem-solving
- Altered somatization
- Altered stress-reduction behavior
- Assigned tasks change
- Decreased emotional support availability
- Decreased mutual support
- Ineffective task completion
- Power alliance change
- Reports conflict with community resources
- Reports isolation from community resources
- Ritual change

Related factors
- Altered community interaction
- Altered family role
- Difficulty dealing with power shift among family members

At risk population
- Families with altered finances
- Families with altered social status
- Families with member experiencing developmental crisis
- Families with member experiencing developmental transition
- Families with member experiencing situational crisis
- Families with member experiencing situational transition

Associated conditions
- Altered health status

This diagnosis will retire from the NANDA-I Taxonomy in the 2024–2026 edition unless additional work is completed to bring it up to a level of evidence 2.1 or higher.

Domain 7 • Class 2 • Diagnosis Code 00159

Readiness for enhanced family processes

Focus of the diagnosis: family processes
Approved 2002 • Revised 2013 • Level of Evidence 2.1

Definition
A pattern of family functioning to support the well-being of its members, which can be strengthened.

Defining characteristics
- Expresses desire to enhance balance between personal autonomy and family cohesiveness
- Expresses desire to enhance communication pattern
- Expresses desire to enhance energy level of family to support activities of daily living
- Expresses desire to enhance family adaptation to change
- Expresses desire to enhance family dynamics
- Expresses desire to enhance family psychological resilience
- Expresses desire to enhance growth of family members
- Expresses desire to enhance interdependence with community
- Expresses desire to enhance maintenance of boundaries between family members
- Expresses desire to enhance respect for family members
- Expresses desire to enhance safety of family members

Domain 7 • Class 3 • Diagnosis Code 00223

Ineffective relationship

Focus of the diagnosis: relationship
Approved 2010 • Revised 2017 • Level of Evidence 2.1

Definition
A pattern of mutual partnership that is insufficient to provide for each other's needs.

Defining characteristics

- Delayed attainment of developmental goals appropriate for family life-cycle stage
- Expresses dissatisfaction with complementary interpersonal relations between partners
- Expresses dissatisfaction with emotional need fulfillment between partners
- Expresses dissatisfaction with idea sharing between partners
- Expresses dissatisfaction with information sharing between partners
- Expresses dissatisfaction with physical need fulfillment between partners
- Imbalance in autonomy between partners
- Imbalance in collaboration between partners
- Inadequate mutual respect between partners
- Inadequate mutual support in daily activities between partners
- Inadequate understanding of partner's compromised functioning
- Partner not identified as support person
- Reports unsatisfactory communication with partner

Related factors

- Inadequate communication skills
- Stressors
- Substance misuse
- Unrealistic expectations

At risk population

- Individuals experiencing developmental crisis
- Individuals with history of domestic violence
- Individuals with incarcerated intimate partner

Associated conditions

- Cognitive dysfunction in one partner

Original literature support available at www.thieme.com/nanda-i.

7. Role relationship

Domain 7 • Class 3 • Diagnosis Code 00229

Risk for ineffective relationship

Focus of the diagnosis: relationship
Approved 2010 • Revised 2013, 2017 • Level of Evidence 2.1

Definition
Susceptible to developing a pattern that is insufficient for providing a mutual partnership to provide for each other's needs.

Risk factors
– Inadequate communication skills
– Stressors
– Substance misuse
– Unrealistic expectations

At risk population
– Individuals experiencing developmental crisis
– Individuals with history of domestic violence
– Individuals with incarcerated intimate partner

Associated conditions
– Cognitive dysfunction in one partner

Original literature support available at www.thieme.com/nanda-i.

7. Role relationship

Domain 7 · Class 3 · Diagnosis Code 00207

Readiness for enhanced relationship

Focus of the diagnosis: relationship
Approved 2006 · Revised 2013 · Level of Evidence 2.1

Definition
A pattern of mutual partnership to provide for each other's needs, which can be strengthened.

Defining characteristics

- Expresses desire to enhance autonomy between partners
- Expresses desire to enhance collaboration between partners
- Expresses desire to enhance communication between partners
- Expresses desire to enhance emotional need fulfillment for each partner
- Expresses desire to enhance mutual respect between partners
- Expresses desire to enhance satisfaction with complementary interpersonal relations between partners
- Expresses desire to enhance satisfaction with emotional need fulfillment for each partner
- Expresses desire to enhance satisfaction with idea sharing between partners
- Expresses desire to enhance satisfaction with information sharing between partners
- Expresses desire to enhance satisfaction with physical need fulfillment for each partner
- Expresses desire to enhance understanding of partner's functional impairment

Original literature support available at www.thieme.com/nanda-i.

7. Role relationship

Domain 7 • Class 3 • Diagnosis Code 00064

Parental role conflict

Focus of the diagnosis: role conflict
Approved 1988 • Revised 2017

Definition
Parental experience of role confusion and conflict in response to crisis.

Defining characteristics
- Anxiety
- Disrupted caregiver routines
- Expresses fear
- Expresses frustration
- Perceived inadequacy to provide for child's needs
- Perceived loss of control over decisions relating to child
- Reluctance to participate in usual caregiver activities
- Reports concern about change in parental role
- Reports concern about family
- Reports feeling guilty

Related factors
- Interruptions in family life due to home treatment regimen
- Intimidated by invasive modalities
- Intimidated by restrictive modalities
- Parent-child separation

At risk population
- Individuals living in nontraditional setting
- Individuals undergoing changes in marital status
- Parents with child requiring home care for special needs

7. Role relationship

Domain 7 • Class 3 • Diagnosis Code 00055

Ineffective role performance

Focus of the diagnosis: role performance
Approved 1978 • Revised 1996, 1998, 2017

Definition
A pattern of behavior and self-expression that does not match the environmental context, norms, and expectations.

Defining characteristics
- Altered pattern of responsibility
- Altered perception of role by others
- Altered role perception
- Altered role resumption
- Anxiety
- Depressive symptoms
- Domestic violence
- Harassment
- Inadequate confidence
- Inadequate external support for role enactment
- Inadequate knowledge of role requirements
- Inadequate motivation
- Inadequate opportunity for role enactment
- Inadequate self-management
- Inadequate skills
- Inappropriate developmental expectations
- Ineffective adaptation to change
- Ineffective coping strategies
- Ineffective role performance
- Perceived social discrimination
- Pessimism
- Powerlessness
- Reports social discrimination
- Role ambivalence
- Role denial
- Role dissatisfaction
- System conflict
- Uncertainty

Related factors
- Altered body image
- Conflict
- Fatigue
- Inadequate health resources
- Inadequate psychosocial support system
- Inadequate rewards
- Inadequate role models
- Inadequate role preparation
- Inadequate role socialization
- Inappropriate linkage with the health care system
- Low self-esteem
- Pain
- Role conflict
- Role confusion
- Role strain
- Stressors
- Substance misuse
- Unaddressed domestic violence
- Unrealistic role expectations

At risk population

- Economically disadvantaged individuals
- Individuals with developmental level inappropriate for role expectation
- Individuals with high demand job role
- Individuals with low educational level

Associated conditions

- Depression
- Neurological defect
- Personality disorders
- Physical illness
- Psychosis

This diagnosis will retire from the NANDA-I Taxonomy in the 2024–2026 edition unless additional work is completed to bring it up to a level of evidence 2.1 or higher.

Domain 7 • Class 3 • Diagnosis Code 00052

Impaired social interaction

Focus of the diagnosis: social interaction
Approved 1986 • Revised 2017, 2020 • Level of Evidence 2.1

Definition
Insufficient or excessive quantity or ineffective quality of social exchange.

Defining characteristics

- Anxiety during social interaction
- Dysfunctional interaction with others
- Expresses difficulty establishing satisfactory reciprocal interpersonal relations
- Expresses difficulty functioning socially
- Expresses difficulty performing social roles
- Expresses discomfort in social situations
- Expresses dissatisfaction with social connection
- Family reports altered interaction
- Inadequate psychosocial support system
- Inadequate use of social status toward others
- Low levels of social activities
- Minimal interaction with others
- Reports unsatisfactory social engagement
- Unhealthy competitive focus
- Unwillingness to cooperate with others

Related factors

- Altered self-concept
- Cognitive dysfunction
- Depressive symptoms
- Disturbed thought processes
- Environmental constraints
- Impaired physical mobility
- Inadequate communication skills
- Inadequate knowledge about how to enhance mutuality
- Inadequate personal hygiene
- Inadequate social skills
- Inadequate social support
- Maladaptive grieving
- Neurobehavioral manifestations
- Sociocultural dissonance

At risk population

- Individuals without a significant other

Associated conditions

- Halitosis
- Mental diseases
- Neurodevelopmental disorders
- Therapeutic isolation

Domain 8.
Sexuality

Sexual identity, sexual function, and reproduction

Class 1.   Sexual identity
The state of being a specific person in regard to sexuality and/or gender

Code	Diagnosis	Page
	This class does not currently contain any diagnoses	

Class 2.   Sexual function
The capacity or ability to participate in sexual activities

Code	Diagnosis	Page
00059	Sexual dysfunction	386
00065	Ineffective sexuality pattern	387

Class 3.   Reproduction
Any process by which human beings are produced

Code	Diagnosis	Page
00221	Ineffective childbearing process	388
00227	Risk for ineffective childbearing process	390
00208	Readiness for enhanced childbearing process	391
00209	Risk for disturbed maternal-fetal dyad	392

NANDA International, Inc. Nursing Diagnoses: Definitions and Classification 2021–2023, 12th Edition.
Edited by T. Heather Herdman, Shigemi Kamitsuru, and Camila Takáo Lopes.
© 2021 NANDA International, Inc. Published 2021 by Thieme Medical Publishers, Inc., New York.
Companion website: www.thieme.com/nanda-i.

Domain 8 • Class 2 • Diagnosis Code 00059

Sexual dysfunction

Focus of the diagnosis: sexual function
Approved 1980 • Revised 2006, 2017 • Level of Evidence 2.1

Definition
A state in which an individual experiences a change in sexual function during the sexual response phases of desire, arousal, and/or orgasm, which is viewed as unsatisfying, unrewarding, or inadequate.

Defining characteristics
- Altered interest in others
- Altered self-interest
- Altered sexual activity
- Altered sexual excitation
- Altered sexual role
- Altered sexual satisfaction
- Decreased sexual desire
- Perceived sexual limitation
- Seeks confirmation of desirability
- Undesired alteration in sexual function

Related factors
- Inaccurate information about sexual function
- Inadequate knowledge about sexual function
- Inadequate role models
- Insufficient privacy
- Perceived vulnerability
- Unaddressed abuse
- Value conflict

At risk population
- Individuals without a significant other

Associated conditions
- Altered body function
- Altered body structure

Original literature support available at www.thieme.com/nanda-i.

Domain 8 • Class 2 • Diagnosis Code 00065

Ineffective sexuality pattern

Focus of the diagnosis: sexuality pattern
Approved 1986 • Revised 2006, 2017 • Level of Evidence 2.1

Definition
Expressions of concern regarding own sexuality.

Defining characteristics
- Altered sexual activity
- Altered sexual behavior
- Altered sexual partner relations
- Altered sexual role
- Difficulty with sexual activity
- Difficulty with sexual behavior
- Value conflict

Related factors
- Conflict about sexual orientation
- Conflict about variant preference
- Fear of pregnancy
- Fear of sexually transmitted infection
- Impaired sexual partner relations
- Inadequate alternative sexual strategies
- Inadequate role models
- Insufficient privacy

At risk population
- Individuals without a significant other

8. Sexuality

Original literature support available at www.thieme.com/nanda-i.

Domain 8 • Class 3 • Diagnosis Code 00221

Ineffective childbearing process

Focus of the diagnosis: childbearing process
Approved 2010 • Revised 2017 • Level of Evidence 2.1

Definition
Inability to prepare for and/or maintain a healthy pregnancy, childbirth process and care of the newborn for ensuring well-being.

Defining characteristics

During Pregnancy

- Failure to utilize social support
- Inadequate attachment behavior
- Inadequate prenatal care
- Inadequate prenatal lifestyle
- Inadequate preparation of newborn care items
- Inadequate preparation of the home environment
- Inadequate respect for unborn baby
- Ineffective management of unpleasant symptoms in pregnancy
- Unrealistic expectations about labor and delivery

During Labor and Delivery

- Decreased proactivity during labor and delivery
- Failure to utilize social support
- Inadequate attachment behavior
- Inadequate lifestyle for stage of labor
- Inappropriate response to onset of labor

After Birth

- Failure to utilize social support
- Inadequate attachment behavior
- Inadequate baby care techniques
- Inadequate infant clothing
- Inappropriate baby feeding techniques
- Inappropriate breast care
- Inappropriate lifestyle
- Unsafe environment for an infant

Related factors

- Domestic violence
- Inadequate knowledge of childbearing process
- Inadequate mental preparation for parenting
- Inadequate parental role model
- Inadequate prenatal care
- Inadequate social support
- Inconsistent prenatal health visits
- Low maternal confidence
- Maternal malnutrition
- Maternal powerlessness

- Maternal psychological distress
- Substance misuse
- Unrealistic birth plan
- Unsafe environment

At risk population

- Individuals experiencing unplanned pregnancy
- Individuals experiencing unwanted pregnancy

Original literature support available at www.thieme.com/nanda-i.

Domain 8 • Class 3 • Diagnosis Code 00227

Risk for ineffective childbearing process

Focus of the diagnosis: childbearing process
Approved 2010 • Revised 2013, 2017 • Level of Evidence 2.1

Definition
Susceptible to an inability to prepare for and/or maintain a healthy pregnancy, childbirth process and care of the newborn for ensuring well-being.

Risk factors
- Inadequate knowledge of childbearing process
- Inadequate mental preparation for parenting
- Inadequate parental role model
- Inadequate prenatal care
- Inadequate social support
- Inconsistent prenatal health visits
- Low maternal confidence
- Maternal malnutrition
- Maternal powerlessness
- Maternal psychological distress
- Substance misuse
- Unaddressed domestic violence
- Unrealistic birth plan
- Unsafe environment

At risk population
- Individuals experiencing unplanned pregnancy
- Individuals experiencing unwanted pregnancy

Domain 8 • Class 3 • Diagnosis Code 00208

Readiness for enhanced childbearing process

Focus of the diagnosis: childbearing process
Approved 2008 • Revised 2013 • Level of Evidence 2.1

Definition
A pattern of preparing for and maintaining a healthy pregnancy, childbirth process and care of the newborn for ensuring well-being which can be strengthened.

Defining characteristics

During Pregnancy

- Expresses desire to enhance knowledge of childbearing process
- Expresses desire to enhance management of unpleasant pregnancy symptoms
- Expresses desire to enhance prenatal lifestyle
- Expresses desire to enhance preparation for newborn

During Labor and Delivery

- Expresses desire to enhance lifestyle appropriate for stage of labor
- Expresses desire to enhance proactivity during labor and delivery

After Birth

- Expresses desire to enhance attachment behavior
- Expresses desire to enhance baby care techniques
- Expresses desire to enhance baby feeding techniques
- Expresses desire to enhance breast care
- Expresses desire to enhance environmental safety for the baby
- Expresses desire to enhance postpartum lifestyle
- Expresses desire to enhance use of support system

Original literature support available at www.thieme.com/nanda-i.

8. Sexuality

Domain 8 • Class 3 • Diagnosis Code 00209

Risk for disturbed maternal-fetal dyad

Focus of the diagnosis: maternal-fetal dyad
Approved 2008 • Revised 2013, 2017 • Level of Evidence 2.1

Definition
Susceptible to a disruption of the symbiotic mother-fetal relationship as a result of comorbid or pregnancy-related conditions, which may compromise health.

Risk factors
- Inadequate prenatal care
- Substance misuse
- Unaddressed abuse

Associated conditions
- Compromised fetal oxygen transport
- Glucose metabolism disorders
- Pregnancy complication
- Treatment regimen

Original literature support available at www.thieme.com/nanda-i.

Domain 9.
Coping/stress tolerance

Contending with life events/life processes

Class 3. Neurobehavioral stress
Behavioral responses reflecting nerve and brain function

NANDA International, Inc. Nursing Diagnoses: Definitions and Classification 2021–2023, 12th Edition.
Edited by T. Heather Herdman, Shigemi Kamitsuru, and Camila Takáo Lopes.
© 2021 NANDA International, Inc. Published 2021 by Thieme Medical Publishers, Inc., New York.
Companion website: www.thieme.com/nanda-i.

Domain 9 • Class 1 • Diagnosis Code 00260

Risk for complicated immigration transition

Focus of the diagnosis: immigration transition
Approved 2016 • Level of Evidence 2.1

Definition
Susceptible to experiencing negative feelings (loneliness, fear, anxiety) in response to unsatisfactory consequences and cultural barriers to one's immigration transition, which may compromise health.

Risk factors
- Abusive landlord
- Available work below educational preparation
- Communication barriers
- Cultural barriers
- Inadequate knowledge about accessing resources
- Inadequate social support
- Non-related persons within household
- Overcrowded housing
- Overt social discrimination
- Parent-child conflicts related to enculturation
- Unsanitary housing

At risk population
- Individuals experiencing forced migration
- Individuals experiencing labor exploitation
- Individuals experiencing precarious economic situation
- Individuals exposed to hazardous work conditions with inadequate training
- Individuals living far from significant others
- Individuals with undocumented immigration status
- Individuals with unfulfilled expectations of immigration

Original literature support available at www.thieme.com/nanda-i.

Domain 9 • Class 1 • Diagnosis Code 00141

Post-trauma syndrome

Focus of the diagnosis: post-trauma syndrome
Approved 1986 • Revised 1998, 2010, 2017 • Level of Evidence 2.1

Definition
Sustained maladaptive response to a traumatic, overwhelming event.

Defining characteristics
- Aggressive behaviors
- Alienation
- Altered attention
- Altered mood
- Anxiety (00146)
- Avoidance behaviors
- Compulsive behavior
- Denial
- Depressive symptoms
- Dissociative amnesia
- Enuresis
- Exaggerated startle response
- Expresses anger
- Expresses numbness
- Expresses shame
- Fear (00148)
- Flashbacks
- Gastrointestinal irritation
- Headache
- Heart palpitations
- Hopelessness (00124)
- Horror
- Hypervigilance
- Intrusive dreams
- Intrusive thoughts
- Irritable mood
- Neurosensory irritability
- Nightmares
- Panic attacks
- Rage
- Reports feeling guilty
- Repression
- Substance misuse

Related factors
- Diminished ego strength
- Environment not conducive to needs
- Exaggerated sense of responsibility
- Inadequate social support
- Perceives event as traumatic
- Self-injurious behavior
- Survivor role

At risk population
- Individuals displaced from home
- Individuals experiencing prolonged duration of traumatic event
- Individuals exposed to disaster
- Individuals exposed to epidemic
- Individuals exposed to event involving multiple deaths
- Individuals exposed to event outside the range of usual human experience

9. Coping/stress tolerance

- Individuals exposed to serious accident
- Individuals exposed to war
- Individuals in human service occupations
- Individuals suffering serious threat
- Individuals who witnessed mutilation
- Individuals who witnessed violent death
- Individuals whose loved ones suffered serious injuries
- Individuals whose loved ones suffered serious threats
- Individuals with destructed home
- Individuals with history of being a prisoner of war
- Individuals with history of being abused
- Individuals with history of criminal victimization
- Individuals with history of detachment
- Individuals with history of torture

Associated conditions

- Depression

This diagnosis will retire from the NANDA-I Taxonomy in the 2024–2026 edition unless additional work is completed to meet definition of a syndrome.

9. Coping/stress tolerance

Domain 9 • Class 1 • Diagnosis Code 00145

Risk for post-trauma syndrome

Focus of the diagnosis: post-trauma syndrome
Approved 1998 • Revised 2013, 2017 • Level of Evidence 2.1

Definition
Susceptible to sustained maladaptive response to a traumatic, overwhelming event, which may compromise health.

Risk factors
- Diminished ego strength
- Environment not conducive to needs
- Exaggerated sense of responsibility
- Inadequate social support
- Perceives event as traumatic
- Self-injurious behavior
- Survivor role

At risk population
- Individuals displaced from home
- Individuals experiencing prolonged duration of traumatic event
- Individuals exposed to disaster
- Individuals exposed to epidemic
- Individuals exposed to event involving multiple deaths
- Individuals exposed to event outside the range of usual human experience
- Individuals exposed to serious accident
- Individuals exposed to war
- Individuals in human service occupations
- Individuals suffering serious threat
- Individuals who witnessed mutilation
- Individuals who witnessed violent death
- Individuals whose loved ones suffered serious injuries
- Individuals whose loved ones suffered serious threats
- Individuals with destructed home
- Individuals with history of being a prisoner of war
- Individuals with history of being abused
- Individuals with history of criminal victimization
- Individuals with history of torture

Associated conditions
- Depression

This diagnosis will retire from the NANDA-I Taxonomy in the 2024–2026 edition unless additional work along with Post-trauma syndrome (00141) is completed .

Domain 9 • Class 1 • Diagnosis Code 00142

Rape-trauma syndrome

Focus of the diagnosis: rape-trauma syndrome
Approved 1980 • Revised 1998, 2017

Definition
Sustained maladaptive response to a forced, violent, sexual penetration against the victim's will and consent.

Defining characteristics
- Aggressive behaviors
- Altered interpersonal relations
- Anger behaviors
- Anxiety (00146)
- Cardiogenic shock
- Confusion
- Denial
- Depressive symptoms
- Difficulty with decision-making
- Disordered thinking
- Expresses anger
- Expresses embarrassment
- Expresses shame
- Fear (00148)
- Humiliation
- Hypervigilance
- Loss of independence
- Low self-esteem
- Mood variability
- Muscle spasm
- Muscle tension
- Nightmares
- Paranoia
- Perceived vulnerability
- Phobic disorders
- Physical trauma
- Powerlessness (00125)
- Psychomotor agitation
- Reports altered sleep-wake cycle
- Reports feeling guilty
- Self-blame
- Sexual dysfunction (00059)
- Substance misuse
- Thoughts of revenge

Related factors
- To be developed

At risk population
- Individuals who experienced rape
- Individuals with history of suicide attempt

Associated conditions
- Depression
- Dissociative identity disorder

This diagnosis will retire from the NANDA-I Taxonomy in the 2023–2024 edition unless additional work is completed to bring it up to a level of evidence 2.1 or higher.

9. Coping/stress tolerance

Domain 9 • Class 1 • Diagnosis Code 00114

Relocation stress syndrome

Focus of the diagnosis: relocation stress syndrome
Approved 1992 • Revised 2000, 2017

> **Definition**
> Physiological and/or psychosocial disturbance following transfer from one environment to another.

Defining characteristics

- Anger behaviors
- Anxiety (00146)
- Decreased self concept
- Depressive symptoms
- Expresses anger
- Expresses frustration
- Fear (00148)
- Increased morbidity
- Increased physical symptoms
- Increased verbalization of needs
- Loss of identity
- Loss of independence
- Low self-esteem
- Pessimism
- Preoccupation
- Reports altered sleep-wake cycle
- Reports concern about relocation
- Reports feeling alone
- Reports feeling insecure
- Reports feeling lonely
- Social alienation
- Unwillingness to move

Related factors

- Communication barriers
- Inadequate control over environment
- Inadequate predeparture counseling
- Inadequate social support
- Ineffective coping strategies
- Powerlessness
- Situational challenge to self-worth
- Social isolation

At risk population

- Individuals facing unpredictability of experience
- Individuals who move from one environment to another
- Individuals with history of loss

Associated conditions

- Depression
- Diminished mental competency
- Impaired health status

- Impaired psychosocial functioning

This diagnosis will retire from the NANDA-I Taxonomy in the 2024–2026 edition unless additional work is completed to bring it to a level of evidence 2.1 or higher.
Original literature support available at www.thieme.com/nanda-i.

Domain 9 • Class 1 • Diagnosis Code 00149

Risk for relocation stress syndrome

Focus of the diagnosis: relocation stress syndrome
Approved 2000 • Revised 2013, 2017

Definition
Susceptible to physiological and/or psychosocial disturbance following transfer from one environment to another, which may compromise health.

Risk factors

- Communication barriers
- Inadequate control over environment
- Inadequate predeparture counseling
- Inadequate social support
- Ineffective coping strategies
- Powerlessness
- Situational challenge to self-worth
- Social isolation

At risk population

- Individuals facing unpredictability of experience
- Individuals who move from one environment to another
- Individuals with history of loss

Associated conditions

- Diminished mental competency
- Impaired health status
- Impaired psychosocial functioning

This diagnosis will retire from the NANDA-I Taxonomy in the 2024–2026 edition unless additional work is completed to bring it to a level of evidence 2.1 or higher.

Domain 9 • Class 2 • Diagnosis Code 00199

Ineffective activity planning

Focus of the diagnosis: activity planning
Approved 2008 • Revised 2017 • Level of Evidence 2.1

Definition
Inability to prepare for a set of actions fixed in time and under certain conditions.

Defining characteristics
- Absence of plan
- Expresses anxiety about a task
- Inadequate health resources
- Inadequate organizational skills
- Pattern of failure
- Reports fear of performing a task
- Unmet goals for chosen activity

Related factors
- Flight behavior when faced with proposed solution
- Hedonism
- Inadequate information processing ability
- Inadequate social support
- Unrealistic perception of event
- Unrealistic perception of personal abilities

At risk population
- Individuals with history of procrastination

9. Coping/stress tolerance

Original literature support available at www.thieme.com/nanda-i.

Domain 9 • Class 2 • Diagnosis Code 00226

Risk for ineffective activity planning

Focus of the diagnosis: activity planning
Approved 2010 • Revised 2013 • Level of Evidence 2.1

Definition
Susceptible to an inability to prepare for a set of actions fixed in time and under certain conditions, which may compromise health.

Risk factors
- Flight behavior when faced with proposed solution
- Hedonism
- Inadequate information processing ability
- Inadequate social support
- Unrealistic perception of event
- Unrealistic perception of personal abilities

At risk population
- Individuals with history of procrastination

Original literature support available at www.thieme.com/nanda-i.

Domain 9 • Class 2 • Diagnosis Code 00146

Anxiety

Focus of the diagnosis: anxiety
Approved 1973 • Revised 1982, 1998, 2017, 2020 • Level of Evidence 3.2

Definition
An emotional response to a diffuse threat in which the individual anticipates nonspecific impending danger, catastrophe, or misfortune.

Defining characteristics
Behavioral/Emotional

- Crying
- Decrease in productivity
- Expresses anguish
- Expresses anxiety about life event changes
- Expresses distress
- Expresses insecurity
- Expresses intense dread
- Helplessness
- Hypervigilance

- Increased wariness
- Insomnia
- Irritable mood
- Nervousness
- Psychomotor agitation
- Reduced eye contact
- Scanning behavior
- Self-focused

Physiological

- Altered respiratory pattern
- Anorexia
- Brisk reflexes
- Chest tightness
- Cold extremities
- Diarrhea
- Dry mouth
- Expresses abdominal pain
- Expresses feeling faint
- Expresses muscle weakness
- Expresses tension
- Facial flushing
- Increased blood pressure

- Increased heart rate
- Increased sweating
- Nausea
- Pupil dilation
- Quivering voice
- Reports altered sleep-wake cycle
- Reports heart palpitations
- Reports tingling in extremities
- Superficial vasoconstriction
- Tremors
- Urinary frequency
- Urinary hesitancy
- Urinary urgency

Cognitive

- Altered attention
- Confusion

- Decreased perceptual field
- Expresses forgetfulness

- Expresses preoccupation
- Reports blocking of thoughts

- Rumination

Related factors
- Conflict about life goals
- Interpersonal transmission
- Pain
- Stressors

- Substance misuse
- Unfamiliar situation
- Unmet needs
- Value conflict

At risk population
- Individuals experiencing developmental crisis
- Individuals experiencing situational crisis
- Individuals exposed to toxins

- Individuals in the perioperative period
- Individuals with family history of anxiety
- Individuals with hereditary predisposition

Associated conditions
- Mental disorders

Domain 9 • Class 2 • Diagnosis Code 00071

Defensive coping

Focus of the diagnosis: coping
Approved 1988 • Revised 2008 • Level of Evidence 2.1

Definition
Repeated projection of falsely positive self-evaluation based on a self-protective pattern that defends against underlying perceived threats to positive self-regard.

Defining characteristics
- Altered reality testing
- Denies problems
- Denies weaknesses
- Difficulty establishing interpersonal relations
- Difficulty maintaining interpersonal relations
- Grandiosity
- Hostile laughter
- Hypersensitivity to a discourtesy
- Hypersensitivity to criticism
- Inadequate follow through with treatment regimen
- Inadequate participation in treatment regimen
- Projection of blame
- Projection of responsibility
- Rationalization of failures
- Reality distortion
- Ridicules others
- Superior attitude toward others

Related factors
- Conflict between self-perception and value system
- Fear of failure
- Fear of humiliation
- Fear of repercussions
- Inadequate confidence in others
- Inadequate psychological resilience
- Inadequate self-confidence
- Inadequate social support
- Uncertainty
- Unrealistic self-expectations

9. Coping/stress tolerance

Original literature support available at www.thieme.com/nanda-i.

Domain 9 • Class 2 • Diagnosis Code 00069

Ineffective coping

Focus of the diagnosis: coping
Approved 1978 • Revised 1998

Definition
A pattern of invalid appraisal of stressors, with cognitive and/or behavioral efforts, that fails to manage demands related to well-being.

Defining characteristics

- Altered affective responsiveness
- Altered attention
- Altered communication pattern
- Destructive behavior toward others
- Destructive behavior toward self
- Difficulty organizing information
- Fatigue
- Frequent illness
- Impaired ability to ask for help
- Impaired ability to attend to information
- Impaired ability to deal with a situation
- Impaired ability to meet basic needs
- Impaired ability to meet role expectation
- Inadequate follow-through with goal-directed behavior
- Inadequate problem resolution
- Inadequate problem-solving skills
- Reports altered sleep-wake cycle
- Reports inadequate sense of control
- Risk-taking behavior
- Substance misuse

Related factors

- High degree of threat
- Inability to conserve adaptive energies
- Inaccurate threat appraisal
- Inadequate confidence in ability to deal with a situation
- Inadequate health resources
- Inadequate preparation for stressor
- Inadequate sense of control
- Inadequate social support
- Ineffective tension release strategies

At risk population

- Individuals experiencing maturational crisis
- Individuals experiencing situational crisis

This diagnosis will retire from the NANDA-I Taxonomy in the 2024–2026 edition unless additional work is completed to bring it up to a level of evidence 2.1 or higher.

Domain 9 • Class 2 • Diagnosis Code 00158

Readiness for enhanced coping

Focus of the diagnosis: coping
Approved 2002 • Revised 2013 • Level of Evidence 2.1

Definition
A pattern of valid appraisal of stressors with cognitive and/or behavioral efforts to manage demands related to well-being, which can be strengthened.

Defining characteristics

- Expresses desire to enhance knowledge of stress management strategies
- Expresses desire to enhance management of stressors
- Expresses desire to enhance social support
- Expresses desire to enhance use of emotion-oriented strategies
- Expresses desire to enhance use of problem-oriented strategies
- Expresses desire to enhance use of spiritual resource

Domain 9 • Class 2 • Diagnosis Code 00077

Ineffective community coping

Focus of the diagnosis: coping
Approved 1994 • Revised 1998, 2017

Definition
A pattern of community activities for adaptation and problem-solving that is unsatisfactory for meeting the demands or needs of the community.

Defining characteristics
- Community does not meet expectations of its members
- Deficient community participation
- Elevated community illness rate
- Excessive community conflict
- Excessive community stress
- High incidence of community problems
- Perceived community powerlessness
- Perceived community vulnerability

Related factors
- Inadequate community problem-solving resources
- Inadequate community resources
- Nonexistent community systems

At risk population
- Community that has experienced a disaster

This diagnosis will retire from the NANDA-I Taxonomy in the 2024–2026 edition unless additional work is completed to bring it up to a level of evidence 2.1 or higher.

Domain 9 • Class 2 • Diagnosis Code 00076

Readiness for enhanced community coping

Focus of the diagnosis: coping
Approved 1994 • Revised 2013

Definition
A pattern of community activities for adaptation and problem-solving for meeting the demands or needs of the community, which can be strengthened.

Defining characteristics
- Expresses desire to enhance availability of community recreation programs
- Expresses desire to enhance availability of community relaxation programs
- Expresses desire to enhance communication among community members
- Expresses desire to enhance communication between groups and larger community
- Expresses desire to enhance community planning for predictable stressors
- Expresses desire to enhance community resources for managing stressors
- Expresses desire to enhance community responsibility for stress management
- Expresses desire to enhance problem-solving for identified issue

9. Coping/stress tolerance

This diagnosis will retire from the NANDA-I Taxonomy in the 2024–2026 edition unless additional work is completed to bring it up to a level of evidence 2.1 or higher.

Domain 9 • Class 2 • Diagnosis Code 00074

Compromised family coping

Focus of the diagnosis: coping
Approved 1980 • Revised 1996, 2017

Definition
An usually supportive primary person (family member, significant other, or close friend) provides insufficient, ineffective, or compromised support, comfort, assistance, or encouragement that may be needed by the client to manage or master adaptive tasks related to his or her health challenge.

Defining characteristics
- Client complaint about support person's response to health problem
- Client reports concern about support person's response to health problem
- Limitation in communication between support person and client
- Protective behavior by support person incongruent with client's abilities
- Protective behavior by support person incongruent with client's need for autonomy
- Support person reports inadequate knowledge
- Support person reports inadequate understanding
- Support person reports preoccupation with own reaction to client's need
- Support person withdraws from client
- Unsatisfactory assistive behaviors of support person

Related factors
- Coexisting situations affecting support person
- Depleted capacity of support person
- Family disorganization
- Inaccurate information presented by others
- Inadequate information available to support person
- Inadequate reciprocal support
- Inadequate support given by client to support person
- Inadequate understanding of information by support person
- Misunderstanding of information by support person
- Preoccupation by support person with concern outside of family

At risk population
- Families with member with altered family role

- Families with support person experiencing depleted capacity due to prolonged disease
- Families with support persons experiencing developmental crisis
- Families with support persons experiencing situational crisis

This diagnosis will retire from the NANDA-I Taxonomy in the 2024–2026 edition if not revised to a LOE 2.1 or higher.

Domain 9 • Class 2 • Diagnosis Code 00073

Disabled family coping

Focus of the diagnosis: coping
Approved 1980 • Revised 1996, 2008 • Level of Evidence 2.1

Definition
Behavior of primary person (family member, significant other, or close friend) that disables his or her capacities and the client's capacities to effectively address tasks essential to either person's adaptation to the health challenge.

Defining characteristics
- Abandons client
- Adopts illness symptoms of client
- Aggressive behaviors
- Depressive symptoms
- Difficulty structuring a meaningful life
- Disregards basic needs of client
- Disregards family relations
- Distorted reality about client's health problem
- Expresses feeling abandoned
- Family behaviors detrimental to well-being
- Hostility
- Impaired individualism
- Inadequate ability to tolerate client
- Loss of client independence
- Neglects treatment regimen
- Performing routines without regard for client's needs
- Prolonged hyperfocus on client
- Psychomotor agitation
- Psychosomatic symptoms

Related factors
- Ambivalent family relations
- Chronically unexpressed feelings by support person
- Differing coping styles between support person and client
- Differing coping styles between support persons

Domain 9 • Class 2 • Diagnosis Code 00075

Readiness for enhanced family coping

Focus of the diagnosis: coping
Approved 1980 • Revised 2013

Definition
A pattern of management of adaptive tasks by primary person (family member, significant other, or close friend) involved with the client's health challenge, which can be strengthened.

Defining characteristics
- Expresses desire to acknowledge growth impact of crisis
- Expresses desire to choose experiences that optimize wellness
- Expresses desire to enhance connection with others who have experienced a similar situation
- Expresses desire to enhance enrichment of lifestyle
- Expresses desire to enhance health promotion

9. Coping/stress tolerance

Domain 9 • Class 2 • Diagnosis Code 00147

Death anxiety

Focus of the diagnosis: death anxiety
Approved 1998 • Revised 2006, 2017, 2020 • Level of Evidence 2.1

Definition
Emotional distress and insecurity, generated by anticipation of death and the process of dying of oneself or significant others, which negatively effects one's quality of life.

Defining characteristics
- Dysphoria
- Expresses concern about caregiver strain
- Expresses concern about the impact of one's death on significant other
- Expresses deep sadness
- Expresses fear of developing terminal illness
- Expresses fear of loneliness
- Expresses fear of loss of mental abilities when dying
- Expresses fear of pain related to dying
- Expresses fear of premature death
- Expresses fear of prolonged dying process
- Expresses fear of separation from loved ones
- Expresses fear of suffering related to dying
- Expresses fear of the dying process
- Expresses fear of the unknown
- Expresses powerlessness
- Reports negative thoughts related to death and dying

Related factors
- Anticipation of adverse consequences of anesthesia
- Anticipation of impact of death on others
- Anticipation of pain
- Anticipation of suffering
- Awareness of imminent death
- Depressive symptoms
- Discussions on the topic of death
- Impaired religiosity
- Loneliness
- Low self-esteem
- Nonacceptance of own mortality
- Spiritual distress
- Uncertainty about encountering a higher power
- Uncertainty about life after death
- Uncertainty about the existence of a higher power
- Uncertainty of prognosis
- Unpleasant physical symptoms

At risk population
- Individuals experiencing terminal care of significant others
- Individuals receiving terminal care

- Individuals with history of adverse experiences with death of significant others
- Individuals with history of near-death experience

- Older adults
- Women
- Young adults

Associated conditions

- Depression
- Stigmatized illnesses with high fear of death

- Terminal illness

Original literature support available at www.thieme.com/nanda-i.

9. Coping/stress tolerance

Domain 9 • Class 2 • Diagnosis Code 00072

Ineffective denial

Focus of the diagnosis: denial
Approved 1988 • Revised 2006 • Level of Evidence 2.1

Definition
Conscious or unconscious attempt to disavow the knowledge or meaning of an event to reduce anxiety and/or fear, leading to the detriment of health.

Defining characteristics
- Delayed search for health care
- Denies fear of death
- Denies fear of disability
- Displaced source of symptoms
- Does not admit impact of disease on life
- Does not perceive relevance of danger
- Does not perceive relevance of symptoms
- Fear displacement regarding impact of condition
- Inappropriate affect
- Minimizes symptoms
- Refuses health care
- Uses dismissive comments when speaking of distressing event
- Uses dismissive gestures when speaking of distressing event
- Uses treatment not advised by health care professional

Related factors
- Anxiety
- Excessive stress
- Fear of death
- Fear of losing personal autonomy
- Fear of separation
- Inadequate emotional support
- Inadequate sense of control
- Ineffective coping strategies
- Perceived inadequacy in dealing with strong emotions
- Threat of unpleasant reality

Original literature support available at www.thieme.com/nanda-i.

Domain 9 • Class 2 • Diagnosis Code 00148

Fear

Focus of the diagnosis: fear
Approved 1980 • Revised 1996, 2000, 2017, 2020 • Level of Evidence 3.2

Definition
Basic, intense emotional response aroused by the detection of imminent threat, involving an immediate alarm reaction (American Psychological Association).

Defining characteristics

Physiological Factors

- Anorexia
- Diaphoresis
- Diarrhea
- Dyspnea
- Increased blood pressure
- Increased heart rate
- Increased respiratory rate
- Increased sweating

- Increased urinary frequency
- Muscle tension
- Nausea
- Pallor
- Pupil dilation
- Vomiting
- Xerostomia

Behavioral/Emotional

- Apprehensiveness
- Concentration on the source of fear
- Decreased self-assurance
- Expresses alarm
- Expresses fear
- Expresses intense dread

- Expresses tension
- Impulsive behaviors
- Increased alertness
- Ineffective impulse control
- Nervousness
- Psychomotor agitation

Related factors

- Communication barriers
- Learned response to threat

- Response to phobic stimulus
- Unfamiliar situation

At risk population

- Children
- Individuals exposed to traumatic situation
- Individuals living in areas with increased violence

- Individuals receiving terminal care
- Individuals separated from social support
- Individuals undergoing surgical procedure

9. Coping/stress tolerance

- Individuals with family history of post-traumatic shock
- Individuals with history of falls
- Older adults
- Pregnant women
- Women
- Women experiencing childbirth

Associated conditions
- Sensation disorders

Domain 9 • Class 2 • Diagnosis Code 00301

Maladaptive grieving

Focus of the diagnosis: grieving
Approved 2020 • Level of Evidence 3.4

Definition
A disorder that occurs after the death of a significant other, in which the experience of distress accompanying bereavement fails to follow sociocultural expectations.

Defining characteristics

- Anxiety
- Decreased life role performance
- Depressive symptoms
- Diminished intimacy levels
- Disbelief
- Excessive stress
- Experiencing symptoms the deceased experienced
- Expresses anger
- Expresses being overwhelmed
- Expresses distress about the deceased person
- Expresses feeling detached from others
- Expresses feeling of emptiness
- Expresses feeling stunned
- Expresses shock
- Fatigue
- Gastrointestinal symptoms
- Grief avoidance
- Increased morbidity
- Longing for the deceased person
- Mistrust of others
- Nonacceptance of a death
- Persistent painful memories
- Preoccupation with thoughts about a deceased person
- Rumination about deceased person
- Searching for a deceased person
- Self-blame

Related factors

- Difficulty dealing with concurrent crises
- Excessive emotional disturbance
- High attachment anxiety
- Inadequate social support
- Low attachment avoidance

At risk population

- Economically disadvantaged individuals
- Individuals experiencing socially unacceptable loss
- Individuals experiencing unexpected sudden death of significant other
- Individuals experiencing violent death of significant other
- Individuals unsatisfied with death notification
- Individuals who witnessed uncontrolled symptoms of the deceased

9. Coping/stress tolerance

- Individuals with history of childhood abuse
- Individuals with history of unresolved grieving
- Individuals with significant predeath dependency on the deceased

- Individuals with strong emotional proximity to the deceased
- Individuals with unresolved conflict with the deceased
- Individuals without paid employment
- Women

Associated conditions

- Anxiety disorders

- Depression

Original literature support available at www.thieme.com/nanda-i.

Domain 9 • Class 2 • Diagnosis Code 00302

Risk for maladaptive grieving

Focus of the diagnosis: grieving
Approved 2020 • Level of Evidence 3.4

Definition
Susceptible to a disorder that occurs after the death of a significant other, in which the experience of distress accompanying bereavement fails to follow sociocultural expectations, which may compromise health.

Risk factors
- Difficulty dealing with concurrent crises
- Excessive emotional disturbance
- High attachment anxiety
- Inadequate social support
- Low attachment avoidance

At risk population
- Economically disadvantaged individuals
- Individuals experiencing socially unacceptable loss
- Individuals experiencing unexpected sudden death of significant other
- Individuals experiencing violent death of significant other
- Individuals unsatisfied with death notification
- Individuals who witnessed uncontrolled symptoms of the deceased
- Individuals with history of childhood abuse
- Individuals with history of unresolved grieving
- Individuals with significant pre-death dependency on the deceased
- Individuals with strong emotional proximity to the deceased
- Individuals with unresolved conflict with the deceased
- Individuals without paid employment
- Women

Associated conditions
- Anxiety disorders
- Depression

Original literature support available at www.thieme.com/nanda-i.

Domain 9 • Class 2 • Diagnosis Code 00285

Readiness for enhanced grieving

Focus of the diagnosis: grieving
Approved 2020 • Level of Evidence 2.1

Definition
A pattern of integration of a new functional reality that arises after an actual, anticipated or perceived significant loss, which can be strengthened.

Defining characteristics

- Expresses desire to carry on legacy of the deceased
- Expresses desire to engage in previous activities
- Expresses desire to enhance coping with pain
- Expresses desire to enhance forgiveness
- Expresses desire to enhance hope
- Expresses desire to enhance personal growth
- Expresses desire to enhance sleep-wake cycle
- Expresses desire to integrate feelings of anger
- Expresses desire to integrate feelings of despair
- Expresses desire to integrate feelings of guilt
- Expresses desire to integrate feelings of remorse
- Expresses desire to integrate positive feelings
- Expresses desire to integrate positive memories of deceased
- Expresses desire to integrate possibilities for a joyful life
- Expresses desire to integrate possibilities for a meaningful life
- Expresses desire to integrate possibilities for a purposeful life
- Expresses desire to integrate possibilities for a satisfactory life
- Expresses desire to integrate the loss
- Expresses desire to invest energy in new interpersonal relations

Domain 9 • Class 2 • Diagnosis Code 00241

Impaired mood regulation

Focus of the diagnosis: mood regulation
Approved 2013 • Revised 2017 • Level of Evidence 2.1

Definition
A mental state characterized by shifts in mood or affect and which is comprised of a constellation of affective, cognitive, somatic, and/or physiologic manifestations varying from mild to severe.

Defining characteristics
- Altered verbal behavior
- Appetite change
- Disinhibition
- Dysphoria
- Excessive guilt
- Excessive self-awareness
- Flight of thoughts
- Hopelessness
- Impaired attention
- Irritable mood
- Psychomotor agitation
- Psychomotor retardation
- Sad affect
- Self-blame
- Social alienation

Related factors
- Altered sleep-wake cycle
- Anxiety
- Difficulty functioning socially
- External factors influencing self concept
- Hypervigilance
- Loneliness
- Pain
- Recurrent thoughts of death
- Recurrent thoughts of suicide
- Social isolation
- Substance misuse
- Weight change

Associated conditions
- Chronic disease
- Functional impairment
- Psychosis

Original literature support available at www.thieme.com/nanda-i.

9. Coping/stress tolerance

Domain 9 • Class 2 • Diagnosis Code 00125

Powerlessness

Focus of the diagnosis: power
Approved 1982 • Revised 2010, 2017, 2020 • Level of Evidence 2.2

Definition
A state of actual or perceived loss of control or influence over factors or events that affect one's well-being, personal life, or the society (adapted from American Psychology Association).

Defining characteristics

- Delayed recovery
- Depressive symptoms
- Expresses doubt about role performance
- Expresses frustration about inability to perform previous activities
- Expresses lack of purpose in life
- Expresses shame
- Fatigue
- Loss of independence
- Reports inadequate sense of control
- Social alienation

Related factors

- Anxiety
- Caregiver role strain
- Dysfunctional institutional environment
- Impaired physical mobility
- Inadequate interest in improving one's situation
- Inadequate interpersonal relations
- Inadequate knowledge to manage a situation
- Inadequate motivation to improve one's situation
- Inadequate participation in treatment regimen
- Inadequate social support
- Ineffective coping strategies
- Low self-esteem
- Pain
- Perceived complexity of treatment regimen
- Perceived social stigma
- Social marginalization

At risk population

- Economically disadvantaged individuals
- Individuals exposed to traumatic events

Associated conditions
- Cerebrovascular Disorders
- Cognition disorders
- Critical illness
- Progressive illness
- Unpredictability of illness trajectory

Original literature support available at www.thieme.com/nanda-i.

Domain 9 • Class 2 • Diagnosis Code 00152

Risk for powerlessness

Focus of the diagnosis: power
Approved 2000 • Revised 2010, 2013, 2017, 2020 • Level of Evidence 2.2

Definition

Susceptible to a state of actual or perceived loss of control or influence over factors or events that affect one's well-being, personal life, or the society, which may compromise health (adapted from American Psychology Association).

Risk factors

- Anxiety
- Caregiver role strain
- Dysfunctional institutional environment
- Impaired physical mobility
- Inadequate interest in improving one's situation
- Inadequate interpersonal relations
- Inadequate knowledge to manage a situation
- Inadequate motivation to improve one's situation
- Inadequate participation in treatment regimen
- Inadequate social support
- Ineffective coping strategies
- Low self-esteem
- Pain
- Perceived complexity of treatment regimen
- Perceived social stigma
- Social marginalization

At risk population

- Economically disadvantaged individuals
- Individuals exposed to traumatic events

Associated conditions

- Cerebrovascular Disorders
- Cognition disorders
- Critical illness
- Progressive illness
- Unpredictability of illness trajectory

Original literature support available at www.thieme.com/nanda-i.

Domain 9 • Class 2 • Diagnosis Code 00187

Readiness for enhanced power

Focus of the diagnosis: power
Approved 2006 • Revised 2013 • Level of Evidence 2.1

Definition
A pattern of participating knowingly in change for well-being, which can be strengthened.

Defining characteristics

- Expresses desire to enhance awareness of possible changes
- Expresses desire to enhance decisions that could lead to changes
- Expresses desire to enhance independence by taking action for change
- Expresses desire to enhance involvement in change
- Expresses desire to enhance knowledge for participation in change
- Expresses desire to enhance participation in choices for daily living
- Expresses desire to enhance participation in choices for health
- Expresses desire to enhance power

9. Coping/stress tolerance

Original literature support available at www.thieme.com/nanda-i.

Domain 9 • Class 2 • Diagnosis Code 00210

Impaired resilience

Focus of the diagnosis: resilience
Approved 2008 • Revised 2017 • Level of Evidence 2.1

Definition
Decreased ability to recover from perceived adverse or changing situations, through a dynamic process of adaptation.

Defining characteristics
- Decreased interest in academic activities
- Decreased interest in vocational activities
- Depressive symptoms
- Expresses shame
- Impaired health status
- Inadequate sense of control
- Ineffective coping strategies
- Ineffective integration
- Low self-esteem
- Renewed elevation of distress
- Reports feeling guilty
- Social isolation

Related factors
- Altered family relations
- Community violence
- Disrupted family rituals
- Disrupted family roles
- Dysfunctional family processes
- Inadequate health resources
- Inadequate social support
- Inconsistent parenting
- Ineffective family adaptation
- Ineffective impulse control
- Multiple coexisting adverse situations
- Perceived vulnerability
- Substance misuse

At risk population
- Economically disadvantaged individuals
- Individuals experiencing a new crisis
- Individuals experiencing chronic crisis
- Individuals exposed to violence
- Individuals who are members of an ethnic minority
- Individuals whose parents have mental disorders
- Individuals with history of exposure to violence
- Individuals with large families
- Mothers with low educational level
- Women

Associated conditions
- Intellectual disability
- Psychological disorder

Original literature support available at www.thieme.com/nanda-i.

Domain 9 • Class 2 • Diagnosis Code 00211

Risk for impaired resilience

Focus of the diagnosis: resilience
Approved 2008 • Revised 2013, 2017 • Level of Evidence 2.1

Definition
Susceptible to decreased ability to recover from perceived adverse or changing situations, through a dynamic process of adaptation, which may compromise health.

Risk factors
- Altered family relations
- Community violence
- Disrupted family rituals
- Disrupted family roles
- Dysfunctional family processes
- Inadequate health resources
- Inadequate social support

- Inconsistent parenting
- Ineffective family adaptation
- Ineffective impulse control
- Multiple coexisting adverse situations
- Perceived vulnerability
- Substance misuse

At risk population
- Economically disadvantaged individuals
- Individuals experiencing a new crisis
- Individuals experiencing chronic crisis
- Individuals exposed to violence
- Individuals who are members of an ethnic minority

- Individuals whose parents have mental disorders
- Individuals with history of exposure to violence
- Individuals with large families
- Mothers with low educational level
- Women

Associated conditions
- Intellectual disability

- Psychological disorder

Original literature support available at www.thieme.com/nanda-i.

Domain 9 • Class 2 • Diagnosis Code 00212

Readiness for enhanced resilience

Focus of the diagnosis: resilience
Approved 2008 • Revised 2013 • Level of Evidence 2.1

Definition
A pattern of ability to recover from perceived adverse or changing situations, through a dynamic process of adaptation, which can be strengthened.

Defining characteristics

- Expresses desire to enhance available resources
- Expresses desire to enhance communication skills
- Expresses desire to enhance environmental safety
- Expresses desire to enhance goal-setting
- Expresses desire to enhance interpersonal relations
- Expresses desire to enhance involvement in activities
- Expresses desire to enhance own responsibility for action
- Expresses desire to enhance positive outlook
- Expresses desire to enhance progress toward goal
- Expresses desire to enhance psychological resilience
- Expresses desire to enhance self-esteem
- Expresses desire to enhance sense of control
- Expresses desire to enhance support system
- Expresses desire to enhance use of conflict management strategies
- Expresses desire to enhance use of coping skills
- Expresses desire to enhance use of resources

Original literature support available at www.thieme.com/nanda-i.

Domain 9 • Class 2 • Diagnosis Code 00137

Chronic sorrow

Focus of the diagnosis: sorrow
Approved 1998 • Revised 2017

Definition
Cyclical, recurring, and potentially progressive pattern of pervasive sadness experienced (by a parent, caregiver, individual with chronic illness or disability) in response to continual loss, throughout the trajectory of an illness or disability.

Defining characteristics
- Expresses feeling that interferes with well-being
- Overwhelming negative feelings
- Sadness

Related factors
- Disability management crisis
- Illness management crisis
- Missed milestones
- Missed opportunities

At risk population
- Individuals experiencing developmental crisis
- Individuals experiencing loss of significant other
- Individuals working in caregiver role for prolonged period of time

Associated conditions
- Chronic disability
- Chronic disease

This diagnosis will retire from the NANDA-I Taxonomy in the 2024–2026 edition unless additional work is completed to bring it up to a level of evidence 2.1 or higher.

Domain 9 • Class 2 • Diagnosis Code 00177

Stress overload

Focus of the diagnosis: stress
Approved 2006 • Level of Evidence 3.2

Definition
Excessive amounts and types of demands that require action.

Defining characteristics
- Difficulty with decision-making
- Expresses feeling pressured
- Expresses increased anger
- Expresses tension
- Impaired functioning
- Increased impatience
- Negative impact from stress

Related factors
- Inadequate resources
- Repeated stressors
- Stressors

Original literature support available at www.thieme.com/nanda-i.

9. Coping/stress tolerance

Domain 9 • Class 3 • Diagnosis Code 00258

Acute substance withdrawal syndrome

Focus of the diagnosis: acute substance withdrawal syndrome
Approved 2016 • Level of Evidence 2.1

Definition
Serious, multifactorial sequelae following abrupt cessation of an addictive compound.

Defining characteristics
– Acute confusion (00128)
– Anxiety (00146)
– Disturbed sleep pattern (00198)
– Nausea (00134)
– Risk for electrolyte imbalance (00195)
– Risk for injury (00035)

Related factors
– Developed dependence to addictive substance
– Excessive use of an addictive substance over time
– Malnutrition
– Sudden cessation of an addictive substance

At risk population
– Individuals with history of withdrawal symptoms
– Older adults

Associated conditions
– Significant comorbidity

Original literature support available at www.thieme.com/nanda-i.

Domain 9 • Class 3 • Diagnosis Code 00259

Risk for acute substance withdrawal syndrome

Focus of the diagnosis: acute substance withdrawal syndrome
Approved 2016 • Level of Evidence 2.1

Definition
Susceptible to serious, multifactorial sequelae following abrupt cessation of an addictive compound, which may compromise health.

Risk factors
- Developed dependence to addictive substance
- Excessive use of an addictive substance over time
- Malnutrition
- Sudden cessation of an addictive substance

At risk population
- Individuals with history of withdrawal symptoms
- Older adults

Associated conditions
- Significant comorbidity

9. Coping/stress tolerance

Original literature support available at www.thieme.com/nanda-i.

Domain 9 · Class 3 · Diagnosis Code 00009

Autonomic dysreflexia

Focus of the diagnosis: autonomic dysreflexia
Approved 1988 · Revised 2017

Definition

Life-threatening, uninhibited sympathetic response of the nervous system to a noxious stimulus after a spinal cord injury at the 7th thoracic vertebra (T7) or above.

Defining characteristics

- Blurred vision
- Bradycardia
- Chest pain
- Chilling
- Conjunctival congestion
- Diaphoresis above the injury
- Diffuse pain in different areas of the head
- Horner's syndrome
- Metallic taste in mouth
- Nasal congestion
- Pallor below injury
- Paresthesia
- Paroxysmal hypertension
- Pilomotor reflex
- Red blotches on skin above the injury
- Tachycardia

Related factors

Gastrointestinal Stimuli

- Bowel distention
- Constipation
- Difficult passage of feces
- Digital stimulation
- Enemas
- Fecal impaction
- Suppositories

Integumentary Stimuli

- Cutaneous stimulation
- Skin irritation
- Sunburn
- Wound

Musculoskeletal-Neurological Stimuli

- Irritating stimuli below level of injury
- Muscle spasm
- Painful stimuli below level of injury
- Pressure over bony prominence
- Pressure over genitalia
- Range of motion exercises

Regulatory-Situational Stimuli

- Constrictive clothing
- Environmental temperature fluctuations

- Positioning

Reproductive-Urological Stimuli

- Bladder distention
- Bladder spasm

- Instrumentation
- Sexual intercourse

Other Factors

- Inadequate caregiver knowledge of disease process

- Inadequate knowledge of disease process

At risk population

- Individuals exposed to environmental temperature extremes
- Men with spinal cord injury or lesion who are experiencing ejaculation

- Women with spinal cord injury or lesion who are experiencing labor
- Women with spinal cord injury or lesion who are menstruating
- Women with spinal cord injury or lesion who are pregnant

Associated conditions

- Bone fractures
- Detrusor sphincter dyssynergia
- Digestive system diseases
- Epididymitis
- Heterotopic bone
- Ovarian cyst
- Pharmaceutical preparations

- Renal calculi
- Substance withdrawal
- Surgical procedures
- Urinary catheterization
- Urinary tract infection
- Venous thromboembolism

9. Coping/stress tolerance

This diagnosis will retire from the NANDA-I Taxonomy in the 2024–2026 edition unless additional work is completed to bring it up to a level of evidence 2.1 or higher.

Domain 9 • Class 3 • Diagnosis Code 00010

Risk for autonomic dysreflexia

Focus of the diagnosis: autonomic dysreflexia
Approved 1998 • Revised 2000, 2013, 2017

Definition
Susceptible to life-threatening, uninhibited response of the sympathetic nervous system post-spinal shock, in an individual with spinal cord injury or lesion at the 6th thoracic vertebra (T6) or above (has been demonstrated in patients with injuries at the 7th thoracic vertebra [T7] and the 8th thoracic vertebra [T8]), which may compromise health.

Risk factors
Gastrointestinal Stimuli

- Bowel distention
- Constipation
- Difficult passage of feces
- Digital stimulation
- Enemas
- Fecal impaction
- Suppositories

Integumentary Stimuli

- Cutaneous stimulation
- Skin irritation
- Sunburn
- Wound

Musculoskeletal-Neurological Stimuli

- Irritating stimuli below level of injury
- Muscle spasm
- Painful stimuli below level of injury
- Pressure over bony prominence
- Pressure over genitalia
- Range of motion exercises

Regulatory-Situational Stimuli

- Constrictive clothing
- Environmental temperature fluctuations
- Positioning

Reproductive-Urological Stimuli

- Bladder distention
- Bladder spasm
- Instrumentation
- Sexual intercourse

Other Factors
- Inadequate caregiver knowledge of disease process
- Inadequate knowledge of disease process

At risk population
- Individuals with spinal cord injury or lesion exposed to extremes of environmental temperature
- Men with spinal cord injury or lesion who are experiencing ejaculation
- Women with spinal cord injury or lesion who are experiencing labor
- Women with spinal cord injury or lesion who are menstruating
- Women with spinal cord injury or lesion who are pregnant

Associated conditions
- Bone fractures
- Detrusor sphincter dyssynergia
- Digestive system diseases
- Epididymitis
- Heterotopic bone
- Ovarian cyst
- Pharmaceutical preparations
- Renal calculi
- Substance withdrawal
- Surgical procedures
- Urinary catheterization
- Urinary tract infection
- Venous thromboembolism

This diagnosis will retire from the NANDA-I Taxonomy in the 2024–2026 edition unless additional work is completed to bring it up to a level of evidence 2.1 or higher.

Domain 9 • Class 3 • Diagnosis Code 00264

Neonatal abstinence syndrome

Focus of the diagnosis: neonatal abstinence syndrome
Approved 2016 • Level of Evidence 2.1

Definition
A constellation of withdrawal symptoms observed in newborns as a result of in-utero exposure to addicting substances, or as a consequence of postnatal pharmacological pain management.

Defining characteristics
- Diarrhea (00013)
- Disorganized infant behavior (00116)
- Disturbed sleep pattern (00198)
- Impaired comfort (00214)
- Neurobehavioral stress
- Risk for aspiration (00039)
- Risk for impaired attachment (00058)
- Risk for impaired skin integrity (00047)
- Risk for ineffective thermoregulation (00274)
- Risk for injury (00035)

Related factors
- To be developed

At risk population
- Neonates exposed to maternal substance misuse in utero
- Neonates iatrogenically exposed to substance for pain control
- Premature neonates

The Finnegan Neonatal Abstinence Scoring Tool (FNAST) is recommended for assessment of withdrawal symptoms and for making decisions related to the plan of care. An FNAST score of 8 or greater, in combination with a history of in-utero substance exposure, is often used to make the diagnosis of Neonatal Abstinence Syndrome. This instrument was developed and is used predominantly in the U.S. and other western countries, so it may not be appropriate to recommend for the international community. This diagnosis will retire from the NANDA-I Taxonomy in the 2024–2026 edition if no related factors are developed.

Original literature support available at www.thieme.com/nanda-i.

Domain 9 • Class 3 • Diagnosis Code 00116

Disorganized infant behavior

Focus of the diagnosis: organized behavior
Approved 1994 • Revised 1998, 2017

Definition
Disintegration of the physiological and neurobehavioral systems of functioning.

Defining characteristics

Attention-Interaction System

- Impaired response to sensory stimuli

Motor System

- Altered primitive reflexes
- Exaggerated startle response
- Fidgeting
- Finger splaying
- Fisting
- Hands to face behavior
- Hyperextension of extremities
- Impaired motor tone
- Maintains hands to face position
- Tremor
- Twitching
- Uncoordinated movement

Physiological

- Abnormal skin color
- Arrhythmia
- Bradycardia
- Inability to tolerate rate of feedings
- Inability to tolerate volume of feedings
- Oxygen desaturation
- Tachycardia
- Time-out signals

Regulatory Problems

- Impaired ability to inhibit startle reflex
- Irritable mood

State-Organization System

- Active-awake state
- Diffuse alpha electroencephalo-gram (EEG) activity with eyes closed
- Irritable crying
- Quiet-awake state
- State oscillation

9. Coping/stress tolerance

Related factors

- Caregiver misreading infant cues
- Environmental overstimulation
- Feeding intolerance
- Inadequate caregiver knowledge of behavioral cues
- Inadequate containment within environment
- Inadequate physical environment
- Insufficient environmental sensory stimulation
- Malnutrition
- Pain
- Sensory deprivation
- Sensory overstimulation

At risk population

- Infants exposed to teratogen in utero
- Infants with low postmenstrual age
- Premature infants

Associated conditions

- Congenital disorders
- Immature neurological functioning
- Impaired infant motor functioning
- Inborn genetic diseases
- Invasive procedure
- Oral impairment

Domain 9 • Class 3 • Diagnosis Code 00115

Risk for disorganized infant behavior

Focus of the diagnosis: organized behavior
Approved 1994 • Revised 2013, 2017

Definition
Susceptible to disintegration in the pattern of modulation of the physiological and neurobehavioral systems of functioning, which may compromise health.

Risk factors
- Caregiver misreading infant cues
- Environmental overstimulation
- Feeding intolerance
- Inadequate caregiver knowledge of behavioral cues
- Inadequate containment within environment
- Inadequate physical environment
- Insufficient environmental sensory stimulation
- Malnutrition
- Pain
- Sensory deprivation
- Sensory overstimulation

At risk population
- Infants exposed to teratogen in utero
- Infants with low postmenstrual age
- Premature infants

Associated conditions
- Congenital disorders
- Immature neurological functioning
- Impaired infant motor functioning
- Inborn genetic diseases
- Invasive procedure
- Oral impairment

Domain 9 • Class 3 • Diagnosis Code 00117

Readiness for enhanced organized infant behavior

Focus of the diagnosis: organized behavior
Approved 1994 • Revised 2013

Definition
An integrated pattern of modulation of the physiological and neurobehavioral systems of functioning, which can be strengthened.

Defining characteristics

- Primary caregiver expresses desire to enhance cue recognition
- Primary caregiver expresses desire to enhance environmental conditions

- Primary caregiver expresses desire to enhance recognition of infant's self-regulatory behaviors

This diagnosis will retire from the NANDA-I Taxonomy in the 2024–2026 edition unless additional work is completed to bring it up to a level of evidence 2.1 or higher.

Domain 10.
Life principles

Principles underlying conduct, thought, and behavior about acts, customs, or institutions viewed as being true or having intrinsic worth

Class 1. Values
The identification and ranking of preferred modes of conduct or end states

Code	Diagnosis	Page
	This class does not currently contain any diagnoses	

Class 2. Beliefs
Opinions, expectations, or judgments about acts, customs, or institutions viewed as being true or having intrinsic worth

Code	Diagnosis	Page
00068	Readiness for enhanced spiritual well-being	449

Class 3. Value/belief/action congruence
The correspondence or balance achieved among values, beliefs, and actions

Code	Diagnosis	Page
00184	Readiness for enhanced decision-making	451
00083	Decisional conflict	452
00242	Impaired emancipated decision-making	453
00244	Risk for impaired emancipated decision-making	454
00243	Readiness for enhanced emancipated decision-making	455
00175	Moral distress	456
00169	Impaired religiosity	457
00170	Risk for impaired religiosity	458
00171	Readiness for enhanced religiosity	459

NANDA International, Inc. Nursing Diagnoses: Definitions and Classification 2021–2023, 12th Edition.
Edited by T. Heather Herdman, Shigemi Kamitsuru, and Camila Takáo Lopes.
© 2021 NANDA International, Inc. Published 2021 by Thieme Medical Publishers, Inc., New York.
Companion website: www.thieme.com/nanda-i.

Domain 10 • Class 2 • Diagnosis Code 00068

Readiness for enhanced spiritual well-being

Focus of the diagnosis: spiritual well-being
Approved 1994 • Revised 2002, 2013, 2020 • Level of Evidence 2.1

Definition
A pattern of integrating meaning and purpose in life through connections with self, others, the world, and/or a power greater than oneself, which can be strengthened.

Defining characteristics

- Expresses desire to enhance acceptance
- Expresses desire to enhance capacity to self-comfort
- Expresses desire to enhance comfort in one's faith
- Expresses desire to enhance connection with nature
- Expresses desire to enhance connection with power greater than self
- Expresses desire to enhance coping
- Expresses desire to enhance courage
- Expresses desire to enhance creative energy
- Expresses desire to enhance forgiveness from others
- Expresses desire to enhance harmony in the environment
- Expresses desire to enhance hope
- Expresses desire to enhance inner peace
- Expresses desire to enhance interaction with significant other
- Expresses desire to enhance joy
- Expresses desire to enhance love
- Expresses desire to enhance love of others
- Expresses desire to enhance meditative practice
- Expresses desire to enhance mystical experiences
- Expresses desire to enhance oneness with nature
- Expresses desire to enhance oneness with power greater than self
- Expresses desire to enhance participation in religious practices
- Expresses desire to enhance peace with power greater than self
- Expresses desire to enhance prayerfulness
- Expresses desire to enhance reverence
- Expresses desire to enhance satisfaction with life
- Expresses desire to enhance self-awareness
- Expresses desire to enhance self-forgiveness
- Expresses desire to enhance sense of awe
- Expresses desire to enhance sense of harmony within oneself
- Expresses desire to enhance sense of identity
- Expresses desire to enhance sense of magic in the environment
- Expresses desire to enhance serenity
- Expresses desire to enhance service to others

- Expresses desire to enhance strength in one's faith

- Expresses desire to enhance surrender

Domain 10 • Class 3 • Diagnosis Code 00184

Readiness for enhanced decision-making

Focus of the diagnosis: decision-making
Approved 2006 • Revised 2013 • Level of Evidence 2.1

Definition
A pattern of choosing a course of action for meeting short- and long-term health-related goals, which can be strengthened.

Defining characteristics

- Expresses desire to enhance congruency of decision with sociocultural goal
- Expresses desire to enhance congruency of decision with sociocultural values
- Expresses desire to enhance congruency of decisions with goal
- Expresses desire to enhance congruency of decisions with values
- Expresses desire to enhance decision-making
- Expresses desire to enhance risk-benefit analysis of decisions
- Expresses desire to enhance understanding of choices
- Expresses desire to enhance understanding of meaning of choices
- Expresses desire to enhance use of reliable evidence for decisions

Original literature support available at www.thieme.com/nanda-i.

Domain 10 • Class 3 • Diagnosis Code 00083

Decisional conflict

Focus of the diagnosis: decisional conflict
Approved 1988 • Revised 2006 • Level of Evidence 2.1

Definition

Uncertainty about course of action to be taken when choice among competing actions involves risk, loss, or challenge to values and beliefs.

Defining characteristics

- Delayed decision-making
- Expresses distress during decision-making
- Physical sign of distress
- Physical sign of tension
- Questions moral principle while attempting a decision
- Questions moral rule while attempting a decision
- Questions moral values while attempting a decision
- Questions personal beliefs while attempting a decision
- Questions personal values while attempting a decision
- Recognizes undesired consequences of potential actions
- Reports uncertainty about choices
- Self-focused
- Vacillating among choices

Related factors

- Conflict with moral obligation
- Conflicting information sources
- Inadequate information
- Inadequate social support
- Inexperience with decision-making
- Interference in decision-making
- Moral principle supports mutually inconsistent actions
- Moral rule supports mutually inconsistent actions
- Moral value supports mutually inconsistent actions
- Perceived danger to value system
- Unclear personal beliefs
- Unclear personal values

Domain 10 • Class 3 • Diagnosis Code 00242

Impaired emancipated decision-making

Focus of the diagnosis: emancipated decision-making
Approved 2013 • Revised 2017 • Level of Evidence 2.1

Definition

A process of choosing a health care decision that does not include personal knowledge and/or consideration of social norms, or does not occur in a flexible environment, resulting in decisional dissatisfaction.

Defining characteristics

- Delayed enactment of health care option
- Difficulty choosing a health care option that best fits current lifestyle
- Expresses constraint in describing own opinion
- Expresses distress about other's opinion
- Expresses excessive concern about others' opinions
- Expresses excessive fear of what others think about a decision
- Impaired ability to describe how option will fit into current lifestyle
- Limited verbalization about health care option in other's presence

Related factors

- Decreased understanding of available health care options
- Difficulty adequately verbalizing perceptions about health care options
- Inadequate confidence to openly discuss health care options
- Inadequate information regarding health care options
- Inadequate privacy to openly discuss health care options
- Inadequate self-confidence in decision-making
- Insufficient time to discuss health care options

At risk population

- Individuals with limited decision-making experience
- Women accessing health care from systems with patriarchal hierarchy
- Women living in families with patriarchal hierarchy

Original literature support available at www.thieme.com/nanda-i.

10. Life principles

Domain 10 • Class 3 • Diagnosis Code 00244

Risk for impaired emancipated decision-making

Focus of the diagnosis: emancipated decision-making
Approved 2013 • Revised 2017 • Level of Evidence 2.1

Definition
Susceptible to a process of choosing a health care decision that does not include personal knowledge and/or consideration of social norms, or does not occur in a flexible environment, resulting in decisional dissatisfaction.

Risk factors
- Decreased understanding of available health care options
- Difficulty adequately verbalizing perceptions about health care options
- Inadequate confidence to openly discuss health care options
- Inadequate information regarding health care options
- Inadequate privacy to openly discuss health care options
- Inadequate self-confidence in decision-making
- Insufficient time to discuss health care options

At risk population
- Individuals with limited decision-making experience
- Women accessing health care from systems with patriarchal hierarchy
- Women living in families with patriarchal hierarchy

Original literature support available at www.thieme.com/nanda-i.

Domain 10 • Class 3 • Diagnosis Code 00243

Readiness for enhanced emancipated decision-making

Focus of the diagnosis: emancipated decision-making
Approved 2013 • Level of Evidence 2.1

Definition

A process of choosing a health care decision that includes personal knowledge and/or consideration of social norms, which can be strengthened.

Defining characteristics

- Expresses desire to enhance ability to choose health care options that enhance current lifestyle
- Expresses desire to enhance ability to enact chosen health care option
- Expresses desire to enhance ability to understand all available health care options
- Expresses desire to enhance ability to verbalize own opinion without constraint
- Expresses desire to enhance comfort to verbalize health care options in the presence of others
- Expresses desire to enhance confidence in decision-making
- Expresses desire to enhance confidence to discuss health care options openly
- Expresses desire to enhance decision-making
- Expresses desire to enhance privacy to discuss health care options

Original literature support available at www.thieme.com/nanda-i.

455

Domain 10 • Class 3 • Diagnosis Code 00175

Moral distress

Focus of the diagnosis: moral distress
Approved 2006 • Level of Evidence 2.1

Definition
Response to the inability to carry out one's chosen ethical or moral decision and/or action.

Defining characteristics
- Reports anguish about acting on one's moral choice

Related factors
- Conflict among decision-makers
- Difficulty making end-of-life decisions
- Difficulty making treatment decision
- Information available for decision-making conflicts
- Time constraint for decision-making
- Values incongruent with cultural norms

At risk population
- Individuals experiencing loss of personal autonomy
- Individuals physically distant of decision-maker

Original literature support available at www.thieme.com/nanda-i.

Domain 10 • Class 3 • Diagnosis Code 00169

Impaired religiosity

Focus of the diagnosis: religiosity
Approved 2004 • Revised 2017 • Level of Evidence 2.1

Definition
Impaired ability to exercise reliance on beliefs and/or participate in rituals of a particular faith tradition.

Defining characteristics
- Desires to reconnect with belief pattern
- Desires to reconnect with customs
- Difficulty adhering to prescribed religious beliefs
- Difficulty adhering to prescribed religious rituals
- Expresses distress about separation from faith community
- Questions religious beliefs
- Questions religious customs

Related factors
- Anxiety
- Cultural barrier to practicing religion
- Depressive symptoms
- Environmental constraints
- Fear of death
- Inadequate social support
- Inadequate sociocultural interaction
- Inadequate transportation
- Ineffective caregiving
- Ineffective coping strategies
- Insecurity
- Pain
- Spiritual distress

At risk population
- Hospitalized individuals
- Individuals experiencing end of life crisis
- Individuals experiencing life transition
- Individuals experiencing personal crisis
- Individuals experiencing spiritual crisis
- Individuals with history of religious manipulation
- Older adults

Associated conditions
- Depression
- Impaired health status

Original literature support available at www.thieme.com/nanda-i.

Domain 10 • Class 3 • Diagnosis Code 00170

Risk for impaired religiosity

Focus of the diagnosis: religiosity
Approved 2004 • Revised 2013, 2017 • Level of Evidence 2.1

Definition

Susceptible to an impaired ability to exercise reliance on religious beliefs and/
or participate in rituals of a particular faith tradition, which may compromise
health.

Risk factors

- Anxiety
- Cultural barrier to practicing religion
- Depressive symptoms
- Environmental constraints
- Fear of death
- Inadequate social support
- Inadequate sociocultural interaction
- Inadequate transportation
- Ineffective caregiving
- Ineffective coping strategies
- Insecurity
- Pain
- Spiritual distress

At risk population

- Hospitalized individuals
- Individuals experiencing end of life crisis
- Individuals experiencing life transition
- Individuals experiencing personal crisis
- Individuals experiencing spiritual crisis
- Individuals with history of religious manipulation
- Older adults

Associated conditions

- Depression
- Impaired health status

Original literature support available at www.thieme.com/nanda-i.

Domain 10 · Class 3 · Diagnosis Code 00171

Readiness for enhanced religiosity

Focus of the diagnosis: religiosity
Approved 2004 · Revised 2013 · Level of Evidence 2.1

Definition
A pattern of reliance on religious beliefs and/or participation in rituals of a particular faith tradition, which can be strengthened.

Defining characteristics
- Expresses desire to enhance connection with a religious leader
- Expresses desire to enhance forgiveness
- Expresses desire to enhance participation in religious experiences
- Expresses desire to enhance participation in religious practices
- Expresses desire to enhance religious options
- Expresses desire to enhance use of religious material
- Expresses desire to reestablish belief patterns
- Expresses desire to reestablish religious customs

Original literature support available at www.thieme.com/nanda-i.

10. Life principles

Domain 10 • Class 3 • Diagnosis Code 00066

Spiritual distress

Focus of the diagnosis: spiritual distress
Approved 1978 • Revised 2002, 2013, 2017, 2020 • Level of Evidence 3.2

Definition

A state of suffering related to the impaired ability to integrate meaning and purpose in life through connections with self, others, the world, and/or a power greater than oneself.

Defining characteristics

- Anger behaviors
- Crying
- Decreased expression of creativity
- Disinterested in nature
- Dysomnias
- Excessive guilt
- Expresses alienation
- Expresses anger
- Expresses anger toward power greater than self
- Expresses concern about beliefs
- Expresses concern about the future
- Expresses concern about values system
- Expresses concerns about family
- Expresses feeling abandoned by power greater than self
- Expresses feeling of emptiness
- Expresses feeling unloved
- Expresses feeling worthless
- Expresses insufficient courage
- Expresses loss of confidence
- Expresses loss of control
- Expresses loss of hope
- Expresses loss of serenity
- Expresses need for forgiveness
- Expresses regret
- Expresses suffering
- Fatigue
- Fear
- Impaired ability for introspection
- Inability to experience transcendence
- Maladaptive grieving
- Perceived loss of meaning in life
- Questions identity
- Questions meaning of life
- Questions meaning of suffering
- Questions own dignity
- Refuses to interact with others

Related factors

- Altered religious ritual
- Altered spiritual practice
- Anxiety
- Barrier to experiencing love
- Cultural conflict
- Depressive symptoms
- Difficulty accepting the aging process
- Inadequate environmental control
- Inadequate interpersonal relations
- Loneliness
- Loss of independence
- Low self-esteem

- Pain
- Perception of having unfinished business
- Self-alienation
- Separation from support system
- Social alienation
- Sociocultural deprivation
- Stressors
- Substance misuse

At risk population

- Individuals experiencing birth of a child
- Individuals experiencing death of a significant other
- Individuals experiencing infertility
- Individuals experiencing life transition
- Individuals experiencing racial conflict
- Individuals experiencing unexpected life event
- Individuals exposed to death
- Individuals exposed to natural disaster
- Individuals exposed to traumatic events
- Individuals receiving bad news
- Individuals receiving terminal care
- Individuals with low educational level

Associated conditions

- Chronic disease
- Depression
- Loss of a body part
- Loss of function of a body part
- Treatment regimen

Original literature support available at www.thieme.com/nanda-i.

10. Life principles

Domain 10 • Class 3 • Diagnosis Code 00067

Risk for spiritual distress

Focus of the diagnosis: spiritual distress
Approved 1998 • Revised 2004, 2013, 2017, 2020 • Level of Evidence 3.2

Definition
Susceptible to a state of suffering related to the impaired ability to integrate meaning and purpose in life through connections with self, others, the world, and/or a power greater than oneself, which may compromise health.

Risk factors
- Altered religious ritual
- Altered spiritual practice
- Anxiety
- Barrier to experiencing love
- Cultural conflict
- Depressive symptoms
- Difficulty accepting the aging process
- Inadequate environmental control
- Inadequate interpersonal relations
- Loneliness
- Loss of independence
- Low self-esteem
- Pain
- Perception of having unfinished business
- Self-alienation
- Separation from support system
- Social alienation
- Sociocultural deprivation
- Stressors
- Substance misuse

At risk population
- Individuals experiencing birth of a child
- Individuals experiencing death of a significant other
- Individuals experiencing infertility
- Individuals experiencing life transition
- Individuals experiencing racial conflict
- Individuals experiencing unexpected life event
- Individuals exposed to death
- Individuals exposed to natural disaster
- Individuals exposed to traumatic events
- Individuals receiving bad news
- Individuals receiving terminal care
- Individuals with low educational level

Associated conditions
- Chronic disease
- Depression
- Loss of a body part
- Loss of function of a body part
- Treatment regimen

Original literature support available at www.thieme.com/nanda-i.

Domain 11. Safety/protection

Freedom from danger, physical injury, or immune system damage; preservation from loss; and protection of safety and security

Class 1. Infection
Host responses following pathogenic invasion

Code	Diagnosis	Page
00004	Risk for infection	466
00266	Risk for surgical site infection	467

Class 2. Physical injury
Bodily harm or hurt

Code	Diagnosis	Page
00031	Ineffective airway clearance	468
00039	Risk for aspiration	469
00206	Risk for bleeding	470
00048	Impaired dentition	471
00219	Risk for dry eye	472
00277	Ineffective dry eye self-management	473
00261	Risk for dry mouth	475
00303	Risk for adult falls	476
00306	Risk for child falls	478
00035	Risk for injury	480
00245	Risk for corneal injury	481
00320	Nipple-areolar complex injury	482
00321	Risk for nipple-areolar complex injury	484
00250	Risk for urinary tract injury	485
00087	Risk for perioperative positioning injury	486
00220	Risk for thermal injury	487
00045	Impaired oral mucous membrane integrity	488

Class 3. Violence

The exertion of excessive force or power to cause injury or abuse

Class 4. Environmental hazards

Sources of danger in the surroundings

Class 5. Defensive processes
The processes by which the self protects itself from the nonself

Code	Diagnosis	Page
00218	Risk for adverse reaction to iodinated contrast media	536
00217	Risk for allergy reaction	537
00042	Risk for latex allergy reaction	538

Class 6. Thermoregulation
The physiological process of regulating heat and energy within the body for purposes of protecting the organism

Code	Diagnosis	Page
00007	Hyperthermia	539
00006	Hypothermia	540
00253	Risk for hypothermia	541
00280	Neonatal hypothermia	542
00282	Risk for neonatal hypothermia	544
00254	Risk for perioperative hypothermia	545
00008	Ineffective thermoregulation	546
00274	Risk for ineffective thermoregulation	547

NANDA International, Inc. Nursing Diagnoses: Definitions and Classification 2021–2023, 12th Edition.
Edited by T. Heather Herdman, Shigemi Kamitsuru, and Camila Takáo Lopes.
© 2021 NANDA International, Inc. Published 2021 by Thieme Medical Publishers, Inc., New York.
Companion website: www.thieme.com/nanda-i.

Domain 11 • Class 1 • Diagnosis Code 00004

Risk for infection

Focus of the diagnosis: infection
Approved 1986 • Revised 2010, 2013, 2017, 2020 • Level of Evidence 3.1

Definition
Susceptible to invasion and multiplication of pathogenic organisms, which may compromise health.

Risk factors
- Difficulty managing long-term invasive devices
- Difficulty managing wound care
- Dysfunctional gastrointestinal motility
- Exclusive formula feeding
- Impaired skin integrity
- Inadequate access to individual protective equipment
- Inadequate adherence to public health recommendations
- Inadequate environmental hygiene
- Inadequate health literacy
- Inadequate hygiene
- Inadequate knowledge to avoid exposure to pathogens
- Inadequate oral hygiene habits
- Inadequate vaccination
- Malnutrition
- Mixed breastfeeding
- Obesity
- Smoking
- Stasis of body fluid

At risk population
- Economically disadvantaged individuals
- Individuals exposed to disease outbreak
- Individuals exposed to increased environmental pathogens
- Individuals with low level of education
- Infants who are not breastfed

Associated conditions
- Altered pH of secretion
- Anemia
- Chronic illness
- Decreased ciliary action
- Immunosuppression
- Invasive procedure
- Leukopenia
- Premature rupture of amniotic membrane
- Prolonged rupture of amniotic membrane
- Suppressed inflammatory response

Original literature support available at www.thieme.com/nanda-i.

Domain 11 • Class 1 • Diagnosis Code 00266

Risk for surgical site infection

Focus of the diagnosis: surgical site infection
Approved 2016 • Level of Evidence 2.1

Definition
Susceptible to invasion of pathogenic organisms at surgical site, which may compromise health.

Risk factors
- Alcoholism
- Obesity

- Smoking

At risk population
- Individuals exposed to cold operating room temperature
- Individuals exposed to excessive number of personnel during surgical procedure

- Individuals exposed to increased environmental pathogens
- Individuals with American Society of Anesthesiologists (ASA) Physical Status classification score ≥ 2

Associated conditions
- Diabetes mellitus
- Extensive surgical procedures
- General anesthesia
- Hypertension
- Immunosuppression
- Inadequate antibiotic prophylaxis
- Ineffective antibiotic prophylaxis
- Infections at other surgical sites
- Invasive procedure

- Post-traumatic osteoarthritis
- Prolonged duration of surgical procedure
- Prosthesis
- Rheumatoid arthritis
- Significant comorbidity
- Surgical implant
- Surgical wound contamination

Original literature support available at www.thieme.com/nanda-i.

11. Safety/protection

Domain 11 • Class 2 • Diagnosis Code 00031

Ineffective airway clearance

Focus of the diagnosis: airway clearance
Approved 1980 • Revised 1996, 1998, 2017, 2020 • Level of Evidence 3.3

> ### Definition
> Reduced ability to clear secretions or obstructions from the respiratory tract to maintain a clear airway.

Defining characteristics

- Absence of cough
- Adventitious breath sounds
- Altered respiratory rhythm
- Altered thoracic percussion
- Altered thoraco-vocal fremitus
- Bradypena
- Cyanosis
- Difficulty verbalizing
- Diminished breath sounds
- Excessive sputum
- Hypoxemia
- Ineffective cough
- Ineffective sputum elimination
- Nasal flaring
- Orthopnea
- Psychomotor agitation
- Subcostal retraction
- Tachypena
- Uses accessory muscles to breathe

Related factors

- Dehydration
- Excessive mucus
- Exposure to harmful substance
- Fear of pain
- Foreign body in airway
- Inattentive to second-hand smoke
- Mucus plug
- Retained secretions
- Smoking

At risk population

- Children
- Infants

Associated conditions

- Airway spasm
- Allergic airway
- Asthma
- Chronic obstructive pulmonary disease
- Congenital heart disease
- Critical illness
- Exudate in the alveoli
- General anesthesia
- Hyperplasia of the bronchial walls
- Neuromuscular diseases
- Respiratory tract infection

Domain 11 • Class 2 • Diagnosis Code 00039

Risk for aspiration

Focus of the diagnosis: aspiration
Approved 1988 • Revised 2013, 2017, 2020 • Level of Evidence 3.2

Definition

Susceptible to entry of gastrointestinal secretions, oropharyngeal secretions, solids, or fluids to the tracheobronchial passages, which may compromise health.

Risk factors

- Barrier to elevating upper body
- Decreased gastrointestinal motility
- Difficulty swallowing
- Enteral nutrition tube displacement
- Inadequate knowledge of modifiable factors
- Increased gastric residue
- Ineffective airway clearance

At risk population

- Older adults
- Premature infants

Associated conditions

- Chronic obstructive pulmonary disease
- Critical illness
- Decreased level of consciousness
- Delayed gastric emptying
- Depressed gag reflex
- Enteral nutrition
- Facial surgery
- Facial trauma
- Head and neck neoplasms
- Incompetent lower esophageal sphincter
- Increased intragastric pressure
- Jaw fixation techniques
- Medical devices
- Neck surgery
- Neck trauma
- Neurological diseases
- Oral surgical procedures
- Oral trauma
- Pharmaceutical preparations
- Pneumonia
- Stroke
- Treatment regimen

11. Safety/protection

Domain 11 • Class 2 • Diagnosis Code 00206

Risk for bleeding

Focus of the diagnosis: bleeding
Approved 2008 • Revised 2013, 2017 • Level of Evidence 2.1

Definition
Susceptible to a decrease in blood volume, which may compromise health.

Risk factors
- Inadequate knowledge of bleeding precautions

At risk population
- Individuals with history of falls

Associated conditions
- Aneurysm
- Circumcision
- Disseminated intravascular coagulopathy
- Gastrointestinal condition
- Impaired liver function
- Inherent coagulopathy
- Postpartum complication
- Pregnancy complication
- Trauma
- Treatment regimen

Additional risk factors to be developed.

Original literature support available at www.thieme.com/nanda-i.

Domain 11 • Class 2 • Diagnosis Code 00048

Impaired dentition

Focus of the diagnosis: dentition
Approved 1998 • Revised 2017

Definition
Disruption in tooth development/eruption pattern or structural integrity of individual teeth.

Defining characteristics
- Abraded teeth
- Absence of teeth
- Dental caries
- Enamel discoloration
- Eroded enamel
- Excessive oral calculus
- Excessive oral plaque
- Facial asymmetry
- Halitosis
- Incomplete tooth eruption for age
- Loose tooth
- Malocclusion
- Premature loss of primary teeth
- Root caries
- Tooth fracture
- Tooth misalignment
- Toothache

Related factors
- Difficulty accessing dental care
- Difficulty performing oral self-care
- Excessive intake of fluoride
- Excessive use of abrasive oral hygiene agents
- Habitual misuse of staining substance
- Inadequate dietary habits
- Inadequate knowledge of dental health
- Inadequate oral hygiene habits
- Malnutrition

At risk population
- Economically disadvantaged individuals
- Individuals with genetic predisposition to dental disorders

Associated conditions
- Bruxism
- Chronic vomiting
- Oral temperature sensitivity
- Pharmaceutical preparations

This diagnosis will retire from the NANDA-I Taxonomy in the 2024–2026 edition unless additional work is completed to bring it up to a level of evidence 2.1 or higher.

Domain 11 • Class 2 • Diagnosis Code 00219

Risk for dry eye

Focus of the diagnosis: dry eye
Approved 2010 • Revised 2013, 2017, 2020 • Level of Evidence 3.2

Definition
Susceptible to inadequate tear film, which may cause eye discomfort and/or damage ocular surface, which may compromise health.

Risk factors
- Air conditioning
- Air pollution
- Caffeine consumption
- Decreased blinking frequency
- Excessive wind
- Inadequate knowledge of modifiable factors
- Inappropriate use of contact lenses
- Inappropriate use of fans
- Inappropriate use of hairdryer
- Inattentive to second-hand smoke
- Insufficient fluid intake
- Low air humidity
- Omega-3 fatty acids deficiency
- Smoking
- Sunlight exposure
- Use of products with benzalkonium chloride preservatives
- Vitamin A deficiency

At risk population
- Contact lens wearer
- Individuals experiencing prolonged intensive care unit stay
- Individuals with history of allergy
- Older adults
- Women

Associated conditions
- Artificial respiration
- Autoimmune diseases
- Chemotherapy
- Decreased blinking
- Decreased level of consciousness
- Hormonal change
- Incomplete eyelid closure
- Leukocytosis
- Metabolic diseases
- Neurological injury with sensory or motor reflex loss
- Neuromuscular blockade
- Oxygen therapy
- Pharmaceutical preparations
- Proptosis
- Radiotherapy
- Reduced tear volume
- Surgical procedures

Original literature support available at www.thieme.com/nanda-i.

Domain 11 • Class 2 • Diagnosis Code 00277

Ineffective dry eye self-management

Focus of the diagnosis: dry eye self-management
Approved 2020 • Level of Evidence 2.1

Definition

Unsatisfactory management of symptoms, treatment regimen, physical, psychosocial, and spiritual consequences and lifestyle changes inherent in living with inadequate tear film.

Defining characteristics

Dry Eye Signs

- Chemosis
- Conjunctival hyperemia
- Epiphora
- Filamentary keratitis
- Keratoconjunctival staining with fluorescein
- Low aqueous tear production according to Schirmer I Test
- Mucous plaques

Dry Eye Symptoms

- Expresses dissatisfaction with quality of life
- Reports blurred vision
- Reports eye fatigue
- Reports feeling of burning eyes
- Reports feeling of ocular dryness
- Reports feeling of ocular foreign body
- Reports feeling of ocular itching
- Reports feeling of sand in eye

Behaviors

- Difficulty performing eyelid care
- Difficulty reducing caffeine consumption
- Inadequate maintenance of air humidity
- Inadequate use of eyelid closure device
- Inadequate use of prescribed medication
- Inappropriate use of contact lenses
- Inappropriate use of fans
- Inappropriate use of hairdryer
- Inappropriate use of moisture chamber goggles
- Inattentive to dry eye signs
- Inattentive to dry eye symptoms
- Inattentive to second-hand smoke
- Insufficient dietary intake of omega-3 fatty acids
- Insufficient dietary intake of vitamin A
- Insufficient fluid intake
- Nonadherence to recommended blinking exercises
- Nonadherence to recommended eye breaks
- Use of products with benzalkonium chloride preservatives

11. Safety/protection

Related factors

- Cognitive dysfunction
- Competing demands
- Competing lifestyle preferences
- Conflict between health behaviors and social norms
- Decreased perceived quality of life
- Difficulty accessing community resources
- Difficulty managing complex treatment regimen
- Difficulty navigating complex health care systems
- Difficulty with decision-making
- Inadequate commitment to a plan of action
- Inadequate health literacy
- Inadequate knowledge of treatment regimen
- Inadequate number of cues to action
- Inadequate role models
- Inadequate social support
- Limited ability to perform aspects of treatment regimen
- Low self efficacy
- Negative feelings toward treatment regimen
- Nonacceptance of condition
- Perceived barrier to treatment regimen
- Perceived social stigma associated with condition
- Unrealistic perception of seriousness of condition
- Unrealistic perception of susceptibility to sequelae
- Unrealistic perception of treatment benefit

At risk population

- Children
- Economically disadvantaged individuals
- Individuals experiencing prolonged hospitalization
- Individuals with history of ineffective health self-management
- Individuals with limited decision-making experience
- Individuals with low educational level
- Older adults
- Women experiencing menopause

Associated conditions

- Allergies
- Autoimmune diseases
- Chemotherapy
- Developmental disabilities
- Graft versus host disease
- Incomplete eyelid closure
- Leukocytosis
- Metabolic diseases
- Neurological injury with motor reflex loss
- Neurological injury with sensory reflex loss
- Oxygen therapy
- Pharmaceutical preparations
- Proptosis
- Radiotherapy
- Reduced tear volume
- Surgical procedures

Original literature support available at www.thieme.com/nanda-i.

Domain 11 • Class 2 • Diagnosis Code 00261

Risk for dry mouth

Focus of the diagnosis: dry mouth
Approved 2016 • Level of Evidence 2.1

Definition
Susceptible to discomfort or damage to the oral mucosa due to reduced quantity or quality of saliva to moisten the mucosa, which may compromise health.

Risk factors
- Dehydration
- Depressive symptoms
- Excessive stress
- Excitement
- Smoking

At risk population
- Pregnant women

Associated conditions
- Chemotherapy
- Depression
- Fluid restriction
- Inability to feed orally
- Oxygen therapy
- Pharmaceutical preparations
- Radiotherapy to the head and neck
- Systemic diseases

Original literature support available at www.thieme.com/nanda-i.

11. Safety/protection

Domain 11 • Class 2 • Diagnosis Code 00303

Risk for adult falls

Focus of the diagnosis: falls
Approved 2020 • Level of Evidence 3.4

> **Definition**
> Adult susceptible to experiencing an event resulting in coming to rest inadvertently on the ground, floor, or other lower level, which may compromise health.

Risk factors

Physiological Factors

- Chronic musculoskeletal pain
- Decreased lower extremity strength
- Dehydration
- Diarrhea
- Faintness when extending neck
- Faintness when turning neck
- Hypoglycemia
- Impaired physical mobility
- Impaired postural balance
- Incontinence
- Obesity
- Sleep disturbances
- Vitamin D deficiency

Psychoneurological Factors

- Agitated confusion
- Anxiety
- Cognitive dysfunction
- Depressive symptoms
- Fear of falling
- Persistent wandering
- Substance misuse

Unmodified Environmental Factors

- Cluttered environment
- Elevated bed surface
- Exposure to unsafe weather-related condition
- Inadequate anti-slip material in bathroom
- Inadequate anti-slip material on floors
- Inadequate lighting
- Inappropriate toilet seat height
- Inattentive to pets
- Lack of safety rails
- Objects out of reach
- Seats without arms
- Seats without backs
- Uneven floor
- Unfamiliar setting
- Use of throw rugs

Other Factors

- Factors identified by standardized, validated screening tool
- Getting up at night without help
- Inadequate knowledge of modifiable factors
- Inappropriate clothing for walking
- Inappropriate footwear

At risk population

- Economically disadvantaged individuals
- Individuals aged ≥ 60 years
- Individuals dependent for activities of daily living
- Individuals dependent for instrumental activities of daily living
- Individuals experiencing prolonged hospitalization
- Individuals in aged care settings
- Individuals in palliative care settings
- Individuals in rehabilitation settings
- Individuals in the early postoperative period
- Individuals living alone
- Individuals receiving home-based care
- Individuals with history of falls
- Individuals with low educational level
- Individuals with restraints

Associated conditions

- Anemia
- Assistive devices for walking
- Depression
- Endocrine system diseases
- Lower limb prosthetics
- Major injury
- Mental disorders
- Musculoskeletal diseases
- Neurocognitive disorders
- Orthostatic hypotension
- Pharmaceutical preparations
- Sensation disorders
- Vascular diseases

11. Safety/protection

Original literature support available at www.thieme.com/nanda-i.

Domain 11 • Class 2 • Diagnosis Code 00306

Risk for child falls

Focus of the diagnosis: falls
Approved 2020 • Level of Evidence 2.1

> **Definition**
> Child susceptible to experiencing an event resulting in coming to rest inadvertently on the ground, floor, or other lower level, which may compromise health.

Risk factors

Caregiver Factors

- Changes diapers on raised surfaces
- Exhaustion
- Fails to lock wheels of child equipment
- Inadequate knowledge of changes in developmental stages
- Inadequate supervision of child
- Inattentive to environmental safety
- Inattentive to safety devices during sports activities
- Places child in bouncer seat on raised surfaces
- Places child in infant walkers
- Places child in mobile seat on raised surfaces
- Places child in seats without a seat belt
- Places child in shopping cart basket
- Places child on play equipment unsuitable for age group
- Postpartum depressive symptoms
- Sleeps with child in arms without protective measures
- Sleeps with child on lap without protective measures

Physiological Factors

- Cognitive dysfunction
- Decreased lower extremity strength
- Dehydration
- Hypoglycemia
- Hypotension
- Impaired physical mobility
- Impaired postural balance
- Incontinence
- Malnutrition
- Neurobehavioral manifestations
- Obesity
- Sleep disturbances

Unmodified Environmental Factors

- Absence of stairway gate
- Absence of stairway handrail
- Absence of wheel locks on child equipment
- Absence of window guard
- Cluttered environment
- Furniture placement facilitates access to balconies

- Furniture placement facilitates access to windows
- High chairs positioned near tables or counters
- Inadequate anti-slip material on floors
- Inadequate automobile restraints
- Inadequate lighting
- Inadequate maintenance of play equipment
- Inadequate restraints on elevated surfaces
- Inattentive to pets
- Objects out of reach
- Seats without arms
- Seats without backs
- Uneven floor
- Unfamiliar setting
- Use of furniture without anti-tipping devices
- Use of non-age appropriate furniture
- Use of throw rugs

Other Factors

- Factors identified by standardized, validated screening tool
- Inappropriate clothing for walking
- Inappropriate footwear

At risk population

- Boys
- Children < 12 years of age
- Children born to economically disadvantaged families
- Children experiencing prolonged prescribed fasting period
- Children exposed to overcrowded environment
- Children in the labor force
- Children whose caregivers have low educational level
- Children whose caregivers have mental health issues
- Children with history of falls
- Children with stressed caregivers
- Children with young caregivers
- Children within the first week of hospitalization

Associated conditions

- Assistive devices for walking
- Feeding and eating disorders
- Musculoskeletal diseases
- Neurocognitive disorders
- Pharmaceutical preparations
- Sensation disorders

Original literature support available at www.thieme.com/nanda-i.

Domain 11 • Class 2 • Diagnosis Code 00035

Risk for injury

Focus of the diagnosis: injury
Approved 1978 • Revised 2013, 2017

Definition
Susceptible to physical damage due to environmental conditions interacting with the individual's adaptive and defensive resources, which may compromise health.

Risk factors
- Cognitive dysfunction
- Exposure to toxic chemicals
- Immunization level within community
- Inadequate knowledge of modifiable factors
- Malnutrition
- Neurobehavioral manifestations
- Nosocomial agent
- Pathogen exposure
- Physical barrier
- Tainted nutritional source
- Unsafe mode of transport

Associated conditions
- Abnormal blood profile
- Altered psychomotor performance
- Autoimmune diseases
- Biochemical dysfunction
- Effector dysfunction
- Hypoxia
- Immune system diseases
- Impaired primary defense mechanisms
- Sensation disorders
- Sensory integration dysfunction

This diagnosis will retire from the NANDA-I Taxonomy in the 2024–2026 edition unless additional work is completed to bring it up to a level of evidence 2.1 or higher.

11. Safety/protection

Domain 11 • Class 2 • Diagnosis Code 00245

Risk for corneal injury

Focus of the diagnosis: injury
Approved 2013 • Revised 2017 • Level of Evidence 2.1

Definition
Susceptible to infection or inflammatory lesion in the corneal tissue that can affect superficial or deep layers, which may compromise health.

Risk factors
- Exposure of the eyeball
- Inadequate knowledge of modifiable factors

At risk population
- Individuals experiencing prolonged hospitalization

Associated conditions
- Artificial respiration
- Blinking < 5 times per minute
- Glasgow Coma Scale score < 6
- Oxygen therapy
- Periorbital edema
- Pharmaceutical preparations
- Tracheostomy

Domain 11 • Class 2 • Diagnosis Code 00320

Nipple-areolar complex injury

Focus of the diagnosis: injury
Approved 2020 • Level of Evidence 2.1

Definition
Localized damage to nipple-areolar complex as a result of the breastfeeding process.

Defining characteristics
- Abraded skin
- Altered skin color
- Altered thickness of nipple-areolar complex
- Blistered skin
- Discolored skin patches
- Disrupted skin surface
- Ecchymosis
- Eroded skin
- Erythema
- Expresses pain
- Hematoma
- Macerated skin
- Scabbed skin
- Skin fissure
- Skin ulceration
- Skin vesicles
- Swelling
- Tissue exposure below the epidermis

Related factors
- Breast engorgement
- Hardened areola
- Improper use of milk pump
- Inadequate latching on
- Inappropriate maternal hand support of breast
- Inappropriate positioning of the infant during breastfeeding
- Inappropriate positioning of the mother during breastfeeding
- Ineffective infant sucking reflex
- Ineffective non-nutritive sucking
- Mastitis
- Maternal anxiety about breastfeeding
- Maternal impatience with the breastfeeding process
- Mother does not wait for the infant to spontaneously release the nipple
- Mother withdraws infant from breast without breaking the suction
- Nipple confusion due to use of artificial nipple
- Postprocedural pain
- Prolonged exposure to moisture
- Supplementary feeding
- Use of products that remove the natural protection of the nipple

At risk population
- Primiparous women
- Sole mother
- Women aged < 19 years

- Women breastfeeding for the first time
- Women with depigmented nipple-areolar complex
- Women with history of inadequate nipple-areolar preparation during prenatal care

- Women with history of nipple trauma in breastfeeding
- Women with non-protruding nipples
- Women with pink nipple-areolar complex

Associated conditions

- Ankylglossia

- Maxillofacial abnormalities

Original literature support available at www.thieme.com/nanda-i.

Domain 11 • Class 2 • Diagnosis Code 00321

Risk for nipple-areolar complex injury

Focus of the diagnosis: injury
Approved 2020 • Level of Evidence 2.1

Definition
Susceptible to localized damage to nipple-areolar complex as a result of the breastfeeding process.

Risk factors
- Breast engorgement
- Hardened areola
- Improper use of milk pump
- Inadequate latching on
- Inadequate nipple-areolar preparation during prenatal care
- Inappropriate maternal hand support of breast
- Inappropriate positioning of the infant during breastfeeding
- Inappropriate positioning of the mother during breastfeeding
- Ineffective infant sucking reflex
- Ineffective non-nutritive sucking
- Mastitis
- Maternal anxiety about breastfeeding
- Maternal impatience with the breastfeeding process
- Mother does not wait for the infant to spontaneously release the nipple
- Mother withdraws infant from breast without breaking the suction
- Nipple confusion due to use of artificial nipple
- Postprocedural pain
- Prolonged exposure to moisture
- Supplementary feeding
- Use of products that remove the natural protection of the nipple

At risk population
- Primiparous women
- Sole mother
- Women aged < 19 years
- Women breastfeeding for the first time
- Women with depigmented nipple-areolar complex
- Women with history of nipple trauma in breastfeeding
- Women with non-protruding nipples
- Women with pink nipple-areolar complex

Associated conditions
- Ankylglossia
- Maxillofacial abnormalities

Original literature support available at www.thieme.com/nanda-i.

Domain 11 • Class 2 • Diagnosis Code 00250

Risk for urinary tract injury

Focus of the diagnosis: injury
Approved 2013 • Revised 2017, 2020 • Level of Evidence 2.1

Definition
Susceptible to damage of the urinary tract structures from use of catheters, which may compromise health.

Risk factors
- Cognitive dysfunction
- Confusion
- Inadequate caregiver knowledge regarding urinary catheter care
- Inadequate knowledge regarding urinary catheter care
- Neurobehavioral manifestations
- Obesity

At risk population
- Individuals at extremes of age

Associated conditions
- Anatomical variation in the pelvic organs
- Condition preventing ability to secure catheter
- Detrusor sphincter dyssynergia
- Latex allergy
- Long term use of urinary catheter
- Medullary injury
- Prostatic hyperplasia
- Repetitive catheterizations
- Retention balloon inflated to ≥ 30 ml
- Use of large caliber urinary catheter

Original literature support available at www.thieme.com/nanda-i.

11. Safety/protection

Domain 11 • Class 2 • Diagnosis Code 00087

Risk for perioperative positioning injury

Focus of the diagnosis: perioperative positioning injury
Approved 1994 • Revised 2006, 2013, 2017, 2020 • Level of Evidence 2.1

Definition
Susceptible to inadvertent anatomical and physical changes as a result of posture or positioning equipment used during an invasive/surgical procedure, which may compromise health.

Risk factors
- Decreased muscle strength
- Dehydration
- Factors identified by standardized, validated screening tool
- Inadequate access to appropriate equipment
- Inadequate access to appropriate support surfaces
- Inadequate availability of equipment for individuals with obesity
- Malnutrition
- Obesity
- Prolonged non-anatomic positioning of limbs
- Rigid support surface

At risk population
- Individuals at extremes of age
- Individuals in lateral position
- Individuals in lithotomy position
- Individuals in prone position
- Individuals in Trendelenburg position
- Individuals undergoing surgical procedure > 1 hour

Associated conditions
- Diabetes mellitus
- Edema
- Emaciation
- General anesthesia
- Immobilization
- Neuropathy
- Sensoriperceptual disturbance from anesthesia
- Vascular diseases

Original literature support available at www.thieme.com/nanda-i.

Domain 11 • Class 2 • Diagnosis Code 00220

Risk for thermal injury

Focus of the diagnosis: thermal injury
Approved 2010 • Revised 2013, 2017 • Level of Evidence 2.1

Definition
Susceptible to extreme temperature damage to skin and mucous membranes, which may compromise health.

Risk factors
- Cognitive dysfunction
- Fatigue
- Inadequate caregiver knowledge of safety precautions
- Inadequate knowledge of safety precautions
- Inadequate protective clothing
- Inadequate supervision
- Inattentiveness
- Smoking
- Unsafe environment

At risk population
- Individuals exposed to environmental temperature extremes

Associated conditions
- Alcoholic intoxication
- Drug intoxication
- Neuromuscular diseases
- Neuropathy
- Treatment regimen

Original literature support available at www.thieme.com/nanda-i.

Domain 11 • Class 2 • Diagnosis Code 00045

Impaired oral mucous membrane integrity

Focus of the diagnosis: mucous membrane integrity
Approved 1982 • Revised 1998, 2013, 2017 • Level of Evidence 2.1

> **Definition**
> Injury to the lips, soft tissue, buccal cavity, and/or oropharynx.

Defining characteristics

- Bad taste in mouth
- Bleeding
- Cheilitis
- Coated tongue
- Decreased taste perception
- Desquamation
- Difficulty eating
- Difficulty swallowing
- Dysphonia
- Enlarged tonsils
- Geographic tongue
- Gingival hyperplasia
- Gingival pallor
- Gingival pocketing deeper than 4 mm
- Gingival recession
- Halitosis
- Hyperemia
- Macroplasia
- Mucosal denudation
- Oral discomfort
- Oral edema
- Oral fissure
- Oral lesion
- Oral mucosal pallor
- Oral nodule
- Oral pain
- Oral papule
- Oral ulcer
- Oral vesicles
- Pathogen exposure
- Presence of mass
- Purulent oral-nasal drainage
- Purulent oral-nasal exudates
- Smooth atrophic tongue
- Spongy patches in mouth
- Stomatitis
- White patches in mouth
- White plaque in mouth
- White, curd-like oral exudate
- Xerostomia

Related factors

- Alcohol consumption
- Cognitive dysfunction
- Decreased salivation
- Dehydration
- Depressive symptoms
- Difficulty performing oral self-care
- Inadequate access to dental care
- Inadequate knowledge of oral hygiene
- Inadequate oral hygiene habits
- Inappropriate use of chemical agent
- Malnutrition
- Mouth breathing
- Smoking
- Stressors

At risk population
- Economically disadvantaged individuals

Associated conditions
- Allergies
- Autosomal disorder
- Behavioral disorder
- Chemotherapy
- Decreased female hormone levels
- Decreased platelets
- Depression
- Immune system diseases
- Immunosuppression
- Infections
- Loss of oral support structure
- Mechanical factor
- Mouth abnormalities
- Nil per os (NPO) > 24 hours
- Oral trauma
- Radiotherapy
- Sjögren's Syndrome
- Surgical procedures
- Trauma
- Treatment regimen

Original literature support available at www.thieme.com/nanda-i.

11. Safety/protection

Domain 11 • Class 2 • Diagnosis Code 00247

Risk for impaired oral mucous membrane integrity

Focus of the diagnosis: mucous membrane integrity
Approved 2013 • Revised 2017 • Level of Evidence 2.1

Definition
Susceptible to injury to the lips, soft tissues, buccal cavity, and/or oropharynx, which may compromise health.

Risk factors
- Alcohol consumption
- Cognitive dysfunction
- Decreased salivation
- Dehydration
- Depressive symptoms
- Difficulty performing oral self-care
- Inadequate access to dental care
- Inadequate knowledge of oral hygiene
- Inadequate oral hygiene habits
- Inappropriate use of chemical agent
- Malnutrition
- Mouth breathing
- Smoking
- Stressors

At risk population
- Economically disadvantaged individuals

Associated conditions
- Allergies
- Autosomal disorder
- Behavioral disorder
- Chemotherapy
- Decreased female hormone levels
- Decreased platelets
- Depression
- Immune system diseases
- Immunosuppression
- Infections
- Loss of oral support structure
- Mechanical factor
- Mouth abnormalities
- Nil per os (NPO) > 24 hours
- Oral trauma
- Radiotherapy
- Sjögren's Syndrome
- Surgical procedures
- Trauma
- Treatment regimen

Original literature support available at www.thieme.com/nanda-i.

Domain 11 · Class 2 · Diagnosis Code 00086

Risk for peripheral neurovascular dysfunction

Focus of the diagnosis: neurovascular function
Approved 1992 · Revised 2013, 2017

Definition
Susceptible to disruption in the circulation, sensation, and motion of an extremity, which may compromise health.

Risk factors
- To be developed

Associated conditions
- Bone fractures
- Burns
- Immobilization
- Mechanical compression
- Orthopedic surgery
- Trauma
- Vascular obstruction

This diagnosis will retire from the NANDA-I Taxonomy in the 2024–2026 edition unless additional work is completed to bring it up to a level of evidence 2.1 or higher.

Original literature support available at www.thieme.com/nanda-i.

Domain 11 • Class 2 • Diagnosis Code 00038

Risk for physical trauma

Focus of the diagnosis: physical trauma
Approved 1980 • Revised 2013, 2017

> **Definition**
> Susceptible to physical injury of sudden onset and severity which require immediate attention.

Risk factors

External Factors

- Absence of call-for-aid device
- Absence of stairway gate
- Absence of window guard
- Bathing in very hot water
- Bed in high position
- Children riding in front seat of car
- Defective appliance
- Delay in ignition of gas appliance
- Dysfunctional call-for-aid device
- Easy access to weapon
- Electrical hazard
- Exposure to corrosive product
- Exposure to dangerous machinery
- Exposure to radiotherapy
- Exposure to toxic chemicals
- Flammable object
- Gas leak
- Grease on stove
- Icicles hanging from roof
- Inadequate anti-slip material on floors
- Inadequate lighting
- Inadequate protection from heat source
- Inadequate stair rails
- Inadequately stored combustible
- Inadequately stored corrosive
- Misuse of headgear
- Misuse of seat restraint
- Nonuse of seat restraints
- Obstructed passageway
- Playing with dangerous object
- Playing with explosive
- Pot handle facing front of stove
- Proximity to vehicle pathway
- Slippery floor
- Smoking in bed
- Smoking near oxygen
- Unanchored electric wires
- Unsafe operation of heavy equipment
- Unsafe road
- Unsafe walkway
- Use of cracked dishware
- Use of restraints
- Use of throw rugs
- Use of unstable chair
- Use of unstable ladder
- Wearing loose clothing around open flame

Internal Factors

- Cognitive dysfunction
- Excessive emotional disturbance
- Impaired postural balance
- Inadequate knowledge of safety precautions
- Neurobehavioral manifestations

- Unaddressed inadequate vision
- Weakness

At risk population

- Economically disadvantaged individuals
- Individuals exposed to high crime neighborhood
- Individuals with history of physical trauma

Associated conditions

- Decreased eye-hand coordination
- Decreased muscle coordination
- Sensation disorders

This diagnosis will retire from the NANDA-I Taxonomy in the 2024–2026 edition unless additional work is completed to bring it up to a level of evidence 2.1 or higher.

Domain 11 • Class 2 • Diagnosis Code 00213

Risk for vascular trauma

Focus of the diagnosis: trauma
Approved 2008 • Revised 2013, 2017 • Level of Evidence 2.1

Definition
Susceptible to damage to vein and its surrounding tissues related to the presence of a catheter and/or infused solutions, which may compromise health.

Risk factors
– Inadequate available insertion site
– Prolonged period of time catheter is in place

Associated conditions
– Irritating solution
– Rapid infusion rate

Original literature support available at www.thieme.com/nanda-i.

11. Safety/protection

Domain 11 • Class 2 • Diagnosis Code 00312

Adult pressure injury

Focus of the diagnosis: pressure injury
Approved 2020 • Level of Evidence 3.4

Definition
Localized damage to the skin and/or underlying tissue of an adult, as a result of pressure, or pressure in combination with shear (European Pressure Ulcer Advisory Panel, 2019).

Defining characteristics
- Blood-filled blister
- Erythema
- Full thickness tissue loss
- Full thickness tissue loss with exposed bone
- Full thickness tissue loss with exposed muscle
- Full thickness tissue loss with exposed tendon
- Localized heat in relation to surrounding tissue
- Pain at pressure points
- Partial thickness loss of dermis
- Purple localized area of discolored intact skin
- Ulcer is covered by eschar
- Ulcer is covered by slough

Related factors
External Factors

- Altered microclimate between skin and supporting surface
- Excessive moisture
- Inadequate access to appropriate equipment
- Inadequate access to appropriate health services
- Inadequate availability of equipment for individuals with obesity
- Inadequate caregiver knowledge of pressure injury prevention strategies
- Increased magnitude of mechanical load
- Pressure over bony prominence
- Shearing forces
- Surface friction
- Sustained mechanical load
- Use of linen with insufficient moisture wicking property

Internal Factors

- Decreased physical activity
- Decreased physical mobility
- Dehydration
- Dry skin
- Hyperthermia
- Inadequate adherence to incontinence treatment regimen

- Inadequate adherence to pressure injury prevention plan
- Inadequate knowledge of pressure injury prevention strategies

- Protein-energy malnutrition
- Smoking
- Substance misuse

Other Factors
- Factors identified by standardized, validated screening tool

At risk population
- Individuals in aged care settings
- Individuals in intensive care units
- Individuals in palliative care settings
- Individuals in rehabilitation settings
- Individuals in transit to or between clinical care settings
- Individuals receiving home-based care
- Individuals with American Society of Anesthesiologists (ASA) Physical Status classification score ≥ 3

- Individuals with body mass index above normal range for age and gender
- Individuals with body mass index below normal range for age and gender
- Individuals with history of pressure injury
- Individuals with physical disability
- Older adults

Associated conditions
- Anemia
- Cardiovascular diseases
- Central nervous system diseases
- Chronic neurological conditions
- Critical illness
- Decreased serum albumin level
- Decreased tissue oxygenation
- Decreased tissue perfusion
- Diabetes mellitus
- Edema
- Elevated C-reactive protein
- Hemodynamic instability

- Hip fracture
- Immobilization
- Impaired circulation
- Intellectual disability
- Medical devices
- Peripheral neuropathy
- Pharmaceutical preparations
- Physical trauma
- Prolonged duration of surgical procedure
- Sensation disorders
- Spinal cord injuries

Original literature support available at www.thieme.com/nanda-i.

Domain 11 • Class 2 • Diagnosis Code 00304

Risk for adult pressure injury

Focus of the diagnosis: pressure injury
Approved 2020 • Level of Evidence 3.4

Definition
Adult susceptible to localized damage to the skin and/or underlying tissue, as a result of pressure, or pressure in combination with shear, which may compromise health (European Pressure Ulcer Advisory Panel, 2019).

Risk factors

External Factors

- Altered microclimate between skin and supporting surface
- Excessive moisture
- Inadequate access to appropriate equipment
- Inadequate access to appropriate health services
- Inadequate availability of equipment for individuals with obesity
- Inadequate caregiver knowledge of pressure injury prevention strategies

- Increased magnitude of mechanical load
- Pressure over bony prominence
- Shearing forces
- Surface friction
- Sustained mechanical load
- Use of linen with insufficient moisture wicking property

Internal Factors

- Decreased physical activity
- Decreased physical mobility
- Dehydration
- Dry skin
- Hyperthermia
- Inadequate adherence to incontinence treatment regimen

- Inadequate adherence to pressure injury prevention plan
- Inadequate knowledge of pressure injury prevention strategies
- Protein-energy malnutrition
- Smoking
- Substance misuse

Other Factors

- Factors identified by standardized, validated screening tool

At risk population

- Individuals in aged care settings
- Individuals in intensive care units

- Individuals in palliative care settings

- Individuals in rehabilitation settings
- Individuals in transit to or between clinical care settings
- Individuals receiving home-based care
- Individuals with American Society of Anesthesiologists (ASA) Physical Status classification score ≥ 3
- Individuals with body mass index above normal range for age and gender
- Individuals with body mass index below normal range for age and gender
- Individuals with history of pressure injury
- Individuals with physical disability
- Older adults

Associated conditions

- Anemia
- Cardiovascular diseases
- Central nervous system diseases
- Chronic neurological conditions
- Critical illness
- Decreased serum albumin level
- Decreased tissue oxygenation
- Decreased tissue perfusion
- Diabetes mellitus
- Edema
- Elevated C-reactive protein
- Hemodynamic instability
- Hip fracture
- Immobilization
- Impaired circulation
- Intellectual disability
- Medical devices
- Peripheral neuropathy
- Pharmaceutical preparations
- Physical trauma
- Prolonged duration of surgical procedure
- Sensation disorders
- Spinal cord injuries

Original literature support available at www.thieme.com/nanda-i.

Domain 11 • Class 2 • Diagnosis Code 00313

Child pressure injury

Focus of the diagnosis: pressure injury
Approved 2020 • Level of Evidence 3.4

Definition
Localized damage to the skin and/or underlying tissue of a child or adolescent, as a result of pressure, or pressure in combination with shear (European Pressure Ulcer Advisory Panel, 2019).

Defining characteristics
- Blood-filled blister
- Erythema
- Full thickness tissue loss
- Full thickness tissue loss with exposed bone
- Full thickness tissue loss with exposed muscle
- Full thickness tissue loss with exposed tendon
- Localized heat in relation to surrounding tissue
- Pain at pressure points
- Partial thickness loss of dermis
- Purple localized area of discolored intact skin
- Ulcer is covered by eschar
- Ulcer is covered by slough

Related factors
External Factors

- Altered microclimate between skin and supporting surface
- Difficulty for caregiver to lift patient completely off bed
- Excessive moisture
- Inadequate access to appropriate equipment
- Inadequate access to appropriate health services
- Inadequate access to appropriate supplies
- Inadequate access to equipment for children with obesity
- Inadequate caregiver knowledge of appropriate methods for removing adhesive materials
- Inadequate caregiver knowledge of appropriate methods for stabilizing devices
- Inadequate caregiver knowledge of modifiable factors
- Inadequate caregiver knowledge of pressure injury prevention strategies
- Increased magnitude of mechanical load
- Pressure over bony prominence
- Shearing forces
- Surface friction
- Sustained mechanical load
- Use of linen with insufficient moisture wicking property

Internal Factors

- Decreased physical activity
- Decreased physical mobility
- Dehydration
- Difficulty assisting caregiver with moving self
- Difficulty maintaining position in bed
- Difficulty maintaining position in chair
- Dry skin
- Hyperthermia
- Inadequate adherence to incontinence treatment regimen
- Inadequate adherence to pressure injury prevention plan
- Inadequate knowledge of appropriate methods for removing adhesive materials
- Inadequate knowledge of appropriate methods for stabilizing devices
- Protein-energy malnutrition
- Water-electrolyte imbalance

Other Factors

- Factors identified by standardized, validated screening tool

At risk population

- Children in intensive care units
- Children in long-term care facilities
- Children in palliative care settings
- Children in rehabilitation settings
- Children in transit to or between clinical care settings
- Children receiving home-based care
- Children with body mass index above normal range for age and gender
- Children with body mass index below normal range for age and gender
- Children with developmental issues
- Children with growth issues
- Children with large head circumference
- Children with large skin surface area

Associated conditions

- Alkaline skin pH
- Altered cutaneous structure
- Anemia
- Cardiovascular diseases
- Decreased level of consciousness
- Decreased serum albumin level
- Decreased tissue oxygenation
- Decreased tissue perfusion
- Diabetes mellitus
- Edema
- Elevated C-reactive protein
- Frequent invasive procedures
- Hemodynamic instability
- Immobilization
- Impaired circulation
- Intellectual disability
- Medical devices
- Pharmaceutical preparations
- Physical trauma
- Prolonged duration of surgical procedure
- Sensation disorders
- Spinal cord injuries

Original literature support available at www.thieme.com/nanda-i.

11. Safety/protection

Domain 11 • Class 2 • Diagnosis Code 00286

Risk for child pressure injury

Focus of the diagnosis: pressure injury
Approved 2020 • Level of Evidence 3.4

Definition
Child or adolescent susceptible to localized damage to the skin and/or underlying tissue, as a result of pressure, or pressure in combination with shear, which may compromise health (European Pressure Ulcer Advisory Panel, 2019).

Risk factors

External Factors

- Altered microclimate between skin and supporting surface
- Difficulty for caregiver to lift patient completely off bed
- Excessive moisture
- Inadequate access to appropriate equipment
- Inadequate access to appropriate health services
- Inadequate access to appropriate supplies
- Inadequate access to equipment for children with obesity
- Inadequate caregiver knowledge of appropriate methods for removing adhesive materials
- Inadequate caregiver knowledge of appropriate methods for stabilizing devices
- Inadequate caregiver knowledge of modifiable factors
- Inadequate caregiver knowledge of pressure injury prevention strategies
- Increased magnitude of mechanical load
- Pressure over bony prominence
- Shearing forces
- Surface friction
- Sustained mechanical load
- Use of linen with insufficient moisture wicking property

Internal Factors

- Decreased physical activity
- Decreased physical mobility
- Dehydration
- Difficulty assisting caregiver with moving self
- Difficulty maintaining position in bed
- Difficulty maintaining position in chair
- Dry skin
- Hyperthermia
- Inadequate adherence to incontinence treatment regimen
- Inadequate adherence to pressure injury prevention plan
- Inadequate knowledge of appropriate methods for removing adhesive materials
- Inadequate knowledge of appropriate methods for stabilizing devices
- Protein-energy malnutrition
- Water-electrolyte imbalance

Other Factors
- Factors identified by standardized, validated screening tool

At risk population
- Children in intensive care units
- Children in long-term care facilities
- Children in palliative care settings
- Children in rehabilitation settings
- Children in transit to or between clinical care settings
- Children receiving home-based care
- Children with body mass index above normal range for age and gender
- Children with body mass index below normal range for age and gender
- Children with developmental issues
- Children with growth issues
- Children with large head circumference
- Children with large skin surface area

Associated conditions
- Alkaline skin pH
- Altered cutaneous structure
- Anemia
- Cardiovascular diseases
- Decreased level of consciousness
- Decreased serum albumin level
- Decreased tissue oxygenation
- Decreased tissue perfusion
- Diabetes mellitus
- Edema
- Elevated C-reactive protein
- Frequent invasive procedures
- Hemodynamic instability
- Immobilization
- Impaired circulation
- Intellectual disability
- Medical devices
- Pharmaceutical preparations
- Physical trauma
- Prolonged duration of surgical procedure
- Sensation disorders
- Spinal cord injuries

Use of a valid and reliable, standardized pressure injury risk screening tool is recommended.

Original literature support available at www.thieme.com/nanda-i.

Domain 11 • Class 2 • Diagnosis Code 00287

Neonatal pressure injury

Focus of the diagnosis: pressure injury
Approved 2020 • Level of Evidence 3.4

Definition
Localized damage to the skin and/or underlying tissue of a neonate, as a result of pressure, or pressure in combination with shear (European Pressure Ulcer Advisory Panel, 2019) .

Defining characteristics
– Blood-filled blister
– Erythema
– Full thickness tissue loss
– Full thickness tissue loss with exposed bone
– Full thickness tissue loss with exposed muscle
– Full thickness tissue loss with exposed tendon
– Localized heat in relation to surrounding tissue
– Maroon localized area of discolored intact skin
– Partial thickness loss of dermis
– Purple localized area of discolored intact skin
– Skin ulceration
– Ulcer is covered by eschar
– Ulcer is covered by slough

Related factors
External Factors

– Altered microclimate between skin and supporting surface
– Excessive moisture
– Inadequate access to appropriate equipment
– Inadequate access to appropriate health services
– Inadequate access to appropriate supplies
– Inadequate caregiver knowledge of appropriate methods for removing adhesive materials
– Inadequate caregiver knowledge of appropriate methods for stabilizing devices
– Inadequate caregiver knowledge of modifiable factors
– Inadequate caregiver knowledge of pressure injury prevention strategies
– Increased magnitude of mechanical load
– Pressure over bony prominence
– Shearing forces
– Surface friction
– Sustained mechanical load
– Use of linen with insufficient moisture wicking property

Internal Factors

- Decreased physical mobility
- Dehydration
- Dry skin
- Hyperthermia
- Water-electrolyte imbalance

Other Factors

- Factors identified by standardized, validated screening tool

At risk population

- Low birth weight neonates
- Neonates < 32 weeks gestation
- Neonates experiencing prolonged intensive care unit stay
- Neonates in intensive care units

Associated conditions

- Anemia
- Decreased serum albumin level
- Decreased tissue oxygenation
- Decreased tissue perfusion
- Edema
- Immature skin integrity
- Immature skin texture
- Immature stratum corneum
- Immobilization
- Medical devices
- Nutritional deficiencies related to prematurity
- Pharmaceutical preparations
- Prolonged duration of surgical procedure
- Significant comorbidity

Use of a valid and reliable, standardized pressure injury risk screening tool is recommended.

Original literature support available at www.thieme.com/nanda-i.

11. Safety/protection

Domain 11 • Class 2 • Diagnosis Code 00288

Risk for neonatal pressure injury

Focus of the diagnosis: pressure injury
Approved 2020 • Level of Evidence 3.4

> **Definition**
> Neonate susceptible to localized damage to the skin and/or underlying tissue, as a result of pressure, or pressure in combination with shear, which may compromise health (European Pressure Ulcer Advisory Panel, 2019).

Risk factors

External Factors

- Altered microclimate between skin and supporting surface
- Excessive moisture
- Inadequate access to appropriate equipment
- Inadequate access to appropriate health services
- Inadequate access to appropriate supplies
- Inadequate caregiver knowledge of appropriate methods for removing adhesive materials
- Inadequate caregiver knowledge of appropriate methods for stabilizing devices
- Inadequate caregiver knowledge of modifiable factors
- Inadequate caregiver knowledge of pressure injury prevention strategies
- Increased magnitude of mechanical load
- Pressure over bony prominence
- Shearing forces
- Surface friction
- Sustained mechanical load
- Use of linen with insufficient moisture wicking property

Internal Factors

- Decreased physical mobility
- Dehydration
- Dry skin
- Hyperthermia
- Water-electrolyte imbalance

Other Factors

- Factors identified by standardized, validated screening tool

At risk population

- Low birth weight neonates
- Neonates < 32 weeks gestation
- Neonates experiencing prolonged intensive care unit stay
- Neonates in intensive care units

Associated conditions

- Anemia
- Decreased serum albumin level
- Decreased tissue oxygenation
- Decreased tissue perfusion
- Edema
- Immature skin integrity
- Immature skin texture
- Immature stratum corneum
- Immobilization
- Medical devices
- Nutritional deficiencies related to prematurity
- Pharmaceutical preparations
- Prolonged duration of surgical procedure
- Significant comorbidity

Use of a valid and reliable, standardized pressure injury risk screening tool is recommended.

Original literature support available at www.thieme.com/nanda-i.

Domain 11 • Class 2 • Diagnosis Code 00205

Risk for shock

Focus of the diagnosis: shock
Approved 2008 • Revised 2013, 2017, 2020 • Level of Evidence 3.2

Definition
Susceptible to an inadequate blood flow to tissues that may lead to cellular dysfunction, which may compromise health.

Risk factors
- Bleeding
- Deficient fluid volume
- Factors identified by standardized, validated screening tool
- Hyperthermia
- Hypothermia
- Hypoxemia
- Hypoxia
- Inadequate knowledge of bleeding management strategies
- Inadequate knowledge of infection management strategies
- Inadequate knowledge of modifiable factors
- Ineffective medication self-management
- Nonhemorrhagic fluid losses
- Smoking
- Unstable blood pressure

At risk population
- Individuals admitted to the emergency care unit
- Individuals at extremes of age
- Individuals with history of myocardial infarction

Associated conditions
- Artificial respiration
- Burns
- Chemotherapy
- Diabetes mellitus
- Embolism
- Heart diseases
- Hypersensitivity
- Immunosuppression
- Infections
- Lactate levels ≥ 2 mmol/L
- Liver diseases
- Medical devices
- Neoplasms
- Nervous system diseases
- Pancreatitis
- Radiotherapy
- Sepsis
- Sequential Organ Failure Assessment (SOFA) Score ≥ 3
- Simplified Acute Physiology Score (SAPS) III > 70
- Spinal cord injuries
- Surgical procedures
- Systemic inflammatory response syndrome (SIRS)
- Trauma

Original literature support available at www.thieme.com/nanda-i.

Domain 11 • Class 2 • Diagnosis Code 00046

Impaired skin integrity

Focus of the diagnosis: skin integrity
Approved 1975 • Revised 1998, 2017, 2020 • Level of Evidence 3.2

Definition
Altered epidermis and/or dermis.

Defining characteristics

- Abscess
- Acute pain
- Altered skin color
- Altered turgor
- Bleeding
- Blister
- Desquamation
- Disrupted skin surface
- Dry skin
- Excoriation
- Foreign matter piercing skin
- Hematoma
- Localized area hot to touch
- Macerated skin
- Peeling
- Pruritus

Related factors

External Factors

- Excessive moisture
- Excretions
- Humidity
- Hyperthermia
- Hypothermia
- Inadequate caregiver knowledge about maintaining tissue integrity
- Inadequate caregiver knowledge about protecting tissue integrity
- Inadequate use of chemical agent
- Pressure over bony prominence
- Psychomotor agitation
- Secretions
- Shearing forces
- Surface friction
- Use of linen with insufficient moisture wicking property

Internal Factors

- Body mass index above normal range for age and gender
- Body mass index below normal range for age and gender
- Decreased physical activity
- Decreased physical mobility
- Edema
- Inadequate adherence to incontinence treatment regimen
- Inadequate knowledge about maintaining tissue integrity
- Inadequate knowledge about protecting tissue integrity
- Malnutrition
- Psychogenic factor
- Self mutilation
- Smoking
- Substance misuse
- Water-electrolyte imbalance

At risk population

- Individuals at extremes of age
- Individuals in intensive care units
- Individuals in long-term care facilities
- Individuals in palliative care settings
- Individuals receiving home-based care

Associated conditions

- Altered pigmentation
- Anemia
- Cardiovascular diseases
- Decreased level of consciousness
- Decreased tissue oxygenation
- Decreased tissue perfusion
- Diabetes mellitus
- Hormonal change
- Immobilization
- Immunodeficiency
- Impaired metabolism
- Infections
- Medical devices
- Neoplasms
- Peripheral neuropathy
- Pharmaceutical preparations
- Punctures
- Sensation disorders

Domain 11 • Class 2 • Diagnosis Code 00047

Risk for impaired skin integrity

Focus of the diagnosis: skin integrity
Approved 1975 • Revised 1998, 2010, 2013, 2017, 2020 • Level of Evidence 3.2

> **Definition**
> Susceptible to alteration in epidermis and/or dermis, which may compromise health.

Risk factors

External Factors

- Excessive moisture
- Excretions
- Humidity
- Hyperthermia
- Hypothermia
- Inadequate caregiver knowledge about maintaining tissue integrity
- Inadequate caregiver knowledge about protecting tissue integrity
- Inadequate use of chemical agent
- Pressure over bony prominence
- Psychomotor agitation
- Secretions
- Shearing forces
- Surface friction
- Use of linen with insufficient moisture wicking property

Internal Factors

- Body mass index above normal range for age and gender
- Body mass index below normal range for age and gender
- Decreased physical activity
- Decreased physical mobility
- Edema
- Inadequate adherence to incontinence treatment regimen
- Inadequate knowledge about maintaining skin integrity
- Inadequate knowledge about protecting skin integrity
- Malnutrition
- Psychogenic factor
- Self mutilation
- Smoking
- Substance misuse
- Water-electrolyte imbalance

At risk population

- Individuals at extremes of age
- Individuals in intensive care units
- Individuals in long-term care facilities
- Individuals in palliative care settings
- Individuals receiving home-based care

Associated conditions

- Altered pigmentation
- Anemia
- Cardiovascular diseases
- Decreased level of consciousness
- Decreased tissue oxygenation
- Decreased tissue perfusion
- Diabetes mellitus
- Hormonal change
- Immobilization

- Immunodeficiency
- Impaired metabolism
- Infections
- Medical devices
- Neoplasms
- Peripheral neuropathy
- Pharmaceutical preparations
- Punctures
- Sensation disorders

Domain 11 • Class 2 • Diagnosis Code 00156

Risk for sudden infant death

Focus of the diagnosis: sudden death
Approved 2002 • Revised 2013, 2017 • Level of Evidence 3.2

Definition
Infant susceptible to unpredicted death.

Risk factors

- Delayed prenatal care
- Inadequate prenatal care
- Inattentive to second-hand smoke
- Infant < 4 months placed in sitting devices for routine sleep
- Infant overheating
- Infant overwrapping
- Infant placed in prone position to sleep
- Infant placed in side-lying position to sleep
- Soft sleep surface
- Soft, loose objects placed near infant

At risk population

- Boys
- Infants aged 2-4 months
- Infants exposed to alcohol in utero
- Infants exposed to cold climates
- Infants exposed to illicit drug in utero
- Infants fed with expressed breast milk
- Infants not breastfed exclusively
- Infants of African descent
- Infants whose mothers smoked during pregnancy
- Infants with postnatal exposure to alcohol
- Infants with postnatal exposure to illicit drug
- Low birth weight infants
- Native American infants
- Premature infants

11. Safety/protection

Domain 11 • Class 2 • Diagnosis Code 00036

Risk for suffocation

Focus of the diagnosis: suffocation
Approved 1980 • Revised 2013, 2017

Definition
Susceptible to inadequate air availability for inhalation, which may compromise health.

Risk factors
- Access to empty refrigerator/ freezer
- Cognitive dysfunction
- Eating large mouthfuls of food
- Excessive emotional disturbance
- Gas leak
- Inadequate knowledge of safety precautions
- Low-strung clothesline
- Pacifier around infant's neck
- Playing with plastic bag
- Propped bottle in infant's crib
- Small object in airway
- Smoking in bed
- Soft sleep surface
- Unattended in water
- Unvented fuel-burning heater
- Vehicle running in closed garage

Associated conditions
- Altered olfactory function
- Face/neck disease
- Face/neck injury
- Impaired motor functioning

11. Safety/protection

Domain 11 • Class 2 • Diagnosis Code 00100

Delayed surgical recovery

Focus of the diagnosis: surgical recovery
Approved 1998 • Revised 2006, 2013, 2017, 2020 • Level of Evidence 3.3

Definition
Extension of the number of postoperative days required to initiate and perform activities that maintain life, health, and well-being.

Defining characteristics
- Anorexia
- Difficulty in moving about
- Difficulty resuming employment
- Excessive time required for recuperation
- Expresses discomfort
- Fatigue
- Interrupted surgical area healing
- Perceives need for more time to recover
- Postpones resumption of work
- Requires assistance for self-care

Related factors
- Delirium
- Impaired physical mobility
- Increased blood glucose level
- Malnutrition
- Negative emotional response to surgical outcome
- Obesity
- Persistent nausea
- Persistent pain
- Persistent vomiting
- Smoking

At risk population
- Individuals aged ≥ 80 years
- Individuals experiencing intraoperative hypothermia
- Individuals requiring emergency surgery
- Individuals requiring perioperative blood transfusion
- Individuals with American Society of Anesthesiologists (ASA) Physical Status classification score ≥ 3
- Individuals with history of myocardial infarction
- Individuals with low functional capacity
- Individuals with preoperative weight loss > 5%

Associated conditions

- Anemia
- Diabetes mellitus
- Extensive surgical procedures
- Pharmaceutical preparations
- Prolonged duration of perioperative surgical wound infection
- Psychological disorder in postoperative period
- Surgical wound infection

Original literature support available at www.thieme.com/nanda-i.

Domain 11 • Class 2 • Diagnosis Code 00246

Risk for delayed surgical recovery

Focus of the diagnosis: surgical recovery
Approved 2013 • Revised 2017, 2020 • Level of Evidence 3.3

Definition

Susceptible to an extension of the number of postoperative days required to initiate and perform activities that maintain life, health, and well-being, which may compromise health.

Risk factors

- Delirium
- Impaired physical mobility
- Increased blood glucose level
- Malnutrition
- Negative emotional response to surgical outcome

- Obesity
- Persistent nausea
- Persistent pain
- Persistent vomiting
- Smoking

At risk population

- Individuals aged ≥ 80 years
- Individuals experiencing intraoperative hypothermia
- Individuals requiring emergency surgery
- Individuals requiring perioperative blood transfusion

- Individuals with American Society of Anesthesiologists (ASA) Physical Status classification score ≥ 3
- Individuals with history of myocardial infarction
- Individuals with low functional capacity
- Individuals with preoperative weight loss > 5%

Associated conditions

- Anemia
- Diabetes mellitus
- Extensive surgical procedures
- Pharmaceutical preparations

- Prolonged duration of perioperative surgical wound infection
- Psychological disorder in postoperative period
- Surgical wound infection

Original literature support available at www.thieme.com/nanda-i.

Domain 11 • Class 2 • Diagnosis Code 00044

Impaired tissue integrity

Focus of the diagnosis: tissue integrity
Approved 1986 • Revised 1998, 2013, 2017, 2020 • Level of Evidence 3.2

Definition
Damage to the mucous membrane, cornea, integumentary system, muscular fascia, muscle, tendon, bone, cartilage, joint capsule, and/or ligament.

Defining characteristics
- Abscess
- Acute pain
- Bleeding
- Decreased muscle strength
- Decreased range of motion
- Difficulty bearing weight
- Dry eye
- Hematoma
- Impaired skin integrity
- Localized area hot to touch
- Localized deformity
- Localized loss of hair
- Localized numbness
- Localized swelling
- Muscle spasm
- Reports lack of balance
- Reports tingling sensation
- Stiffness
- Tissue exposure below the epidermis

Related factors
External Factors

- Excretions
- Humidity
- Hyperthermia
- Hypothermia
- Inadequate caregiver knowledge about maintaining tissue integrity
- Inadequate caregiver knowledge about protecting tissue integrity
- Inadequate use of chemical agent
- Pressure over bony prominence
- Psychomotor agitation
- Secretions
- Shearing forces
- Surface friction
- Use of linen with insufficient moisture wicking property

Internal Factors

- Body mass index above normal range for age and gender
- Body mass index below normal range for age and gender
- Decreased blinking frequency
- Decreased physical activity
- Fluid imbalance
- Impaired physical mobility
- Impaired postural balance
- Inadequate adherence to incontinence treatment regimen
- Inadequate blood glucose level management

- Inadequate knowledge about maintaining tissue integrity
- Inadequate knowledge about restoring tissue integrity
- Inadequate ostomy care
- Malnutrition

- Psychogenic factor
- Self mutilation
- Smoking
- Substance misuse

At risk population

- Homeless individuals
- Individuals at extremes of age
- Individuals exposed to environmental temperature extremes
- Individuals exposed to high-voltage power supply
- Individuals participating in contact sports

- Individuals participating in winter sports
- Individuals with family history of bone fracture
- Individuals with history of bone fracture

Associated conditions

- Anemia
- Autism spectrum disorder
- Cardiovascular diseases
- Chronic neurological conditions
- Critical illness
- Decreased level of consciousness
- Decreased serum albumin level
- Decreased tissue oxygenation
- Decreased tissue perfusion

- Hemodynamic instability
- Immobilization
- Intellectual disability
- Medical devices
- Metabolic diseases
- Peripheral neuropathy
- Pharmaceutical preparations
- Sensation disorders
- Surgical procedures

Original literature support available at www.thieme.com/nanda-i.

Domain 11 • Class 2 • Diagnosis Code 00248

Risk for impaired tissue integrity

Focus of the diagnosis: tissue integrity
Approved 2013 • Revised 2017, 2020 • Level of Evidence 3.2

Definition
Susceptible to damage to the mucous membrane, cornea, integumentary system, muscular fascia, muscle, tendon, bone, cartilage, joint capsule, and/or ligament, which may compromise health.

Risk factors

External Factors

- Excretions
- Humidity
- Hyperthermia
- Hypothermia
- Inadequate caregiver knowledge about maintaining tissue integrity
- Inadequate caregiver knowledge about protecting tissue integrity
- Inadequate use of chemical agent
- Pressure over bony prominence
- Psychomotor agitation
- Secretions
- Shearing forces
- Surface friction
- Use of linen with insufficient moisture wicking property

Internal Factors

- Body mass index above normal range for age and gender
- Body mass index below normal range for age and gender
- Decreased blinking frequency
- Decreased physical activity
- Fluid imbalance
- Impaired physical mobility
- Impaired postural balance
- Inadequate adherence to incontinence treatment regimen
- Inadequate blood glucose level management
- Inadequate knowledge about maintaining tissue integrity
- Inadequate knowledge about restoring tissue integrity
- Inadequate ostomy care
- Malnutrition
- Psychogenic factor
- Self mutilation
- Smoking
- Substance misuse

At risk population

- Homeless individuals
- Individuals at extremes of age
- Individuals exposed to environmental temperature extremes
- Individuals exposed to high-voltage power supply
- Individuals participating in contact sports

11. Safety/protection

- Individuals participating in winter sports
- Individuals with family history of bone fracture

- Individuals with history of bone fracture

Associated conditions

- Anemia
- Autism spectrum disorder
- Cardiovascular diseases
- Chronic neurological conditions
- Critical illness
- Decreased level of consciousness
- Decreased serum albumin level
- Decreased tissue oxygenation
- Decreased tissue perfusion

- Hemodynamic instability
- Immobilization
- Intellectual disability
- Medical devices
- Metabolic diseases
- Peripheral neuropathy
- Pharmaceutical preparations
- Sensation disorders
- Surgical procedures

Original literature support available at www.thieme.com/nanda-i.

Domain 11 • Class 3 • Diagnosis Code 00272

Risk for female genital mutilation

Focus of the diagnosis: female genital mutilation
Approved 2016 • Level of Evidence 2.1

Definition
Susceptible to full or partial ablation of the female external genitalia and other lesions of the genitalia, whether for cultural, religious or any other non-therapeutic reasons, which may compromise health.

Risk factors
- Lack of family knowledge about impact of practice on physical health
- Lack of family knowledge about impact of practice on psychosocial health
- Lack of family knowledge about impact of practice on reproductive health

At risk population
- Women belonging to ethnic group in which practice is accepted
- Women belonging to family in which any female member has been subjected to practice
- Women from families with favorable attitude towards practice
- Women planning to visit family's country of origin in which practice is accepted
- Women residing in country where practice is accepted
- Women whose family leaders belong to ethnic group in which practice is accepted

Original literature support available at www.thieme.com/nanda-i.

11. Safety/protection

Domain 11 • Class 3 • Diagnosis Code 00138

Risk for other-directed violence

Focus of the diagnosis: other-directed violence
Approved 1980 • Revised 1996, 2013, 2017

Definition
Susceptible to behaviors in which an individual demonstrates that he or she can be physically, emotionally, and/or sexually harmful to others.

Risk factors

- Cognitive dysfunction
- Easy access to weapon
- Ineffective impulse control
- Negative body language
- Pattern of aggressive anti-social behavior
- Pattern of indirect violence
- Pattern of other-directed violence
- Pattern of threatening violence
- Suicidal behavior

At risk population

- Individuals with history of childhood abuse
- Individuals with history of cruelty to animals
- Individuals with history of firesetting
- Individuals with history of motor vehicle offense
- Individuals with history of substance misuse
- Individuals with history of witnessing family violence

Associated conditions

- Neurological impairment
- Pathological intoxication
- Perinatal complications
- Prenatal complications
- Psychotic disorders

11. Safety/protection

Domain 11 • Class 3 • Diagnosis Code 00140

Risk for self-directed violence

Focus of the diagnosis: self-directed violence
Approved 1994 • Revised 2013, 2017

Definition
Susceptible to behaviors in which an individual demonstrates that he or she can be physically, emotionally, and/or sexually harmful to self.

Risk factors
- Behavioral cues of suicidal intent
- Conflict about sexual orientation
- Conflict in interpersonal relations
- Employment concern
- Engagement in autoerotic sexual acts
- Inadequate personal resources
- Social isolation
- Suicidal ideation
- Suicidal plan
- Verbal cues of suicidal intent

At risk population
- Individuals aged 15-19 years
- Individuals aged ≥ 45 years
- Individuals in occupations with high suicide risk
- Individuals with history of multiple suicide attempts
- Individuals with pattern of difficulties in family background

Associated conditions
- Mental health issues
- Physical health issues
- Psychological disorder

This diagnosis will retire from the NANDA-I Taxonomy in the 2024–2026 edition unless additional work is completed to bring it up to a level of evidence 2.1 or higher.

Domain 11 • Class 3 • Diagnosis Code 00151

Self-mutilation

Focus of the diagnosis: self-mutilation
Approved 2000 • Revised 2017

Definition
Deliberate self-injurious behavior causing tissue damage with the intent of causing nonfatal injury to attain relief of tension.

Defining characteristics
- Abrading skin
- Biting
- Constricting a body part
- Cuts on body
- Hitting
- Ingested harmful substance
- Inhaled harmful substance
- Insertion of object into body orifice
- Picking at wound
- Scratches on body
- Self-inflicted burn
- Severing of a body part

Related factors
- Absence of family confidant
- Altered body image
- Dissociation
- Disturbed interpersonal relations
- Eating disorder
- Excessive emotional disturbance
- Feeling threatened with loss of significant interpersonal relations
- Impaired self-esteem
- Inability to express tension verbally
- Ineffective communication between parent and adolescent
- Ineffective coping strategies
- Ineffective impulse control
- Irresistible urge for self-directed violence
- Irresistible urge to cut self
- Labile behavior
- Loss of control over problem-solving situation
- Low self-esteem
- Mounting tension that is intolerable
- Negative feelings
- Pattern of inability to plan solutions
- Pattern of inability to see long-term consequences
- Perfectionism
- Requires rapid stress reduction
- Social isolation
- Substance misuse
- Use of manipulation to obtain nurturing interpersonal relations with others

At risk population
- Adolescents
- Battered children
- Incarcerated individuals

- Individuals experiencing family divorce
- Individuals experiencing family substance misuse
- Individuals experiencing loss of significant interpersonal relations
- Individuals experiencing sexual identity crisis
- Individuals living in nontraditional setting
- Individuals whose peers self-mutilate
- Individuals with family history of self-destructive behavior
- Individuals with history of childhood abuse
- Individuals with history of childhood illness
- Individuals with history of childhood surgery
- Individuals with history of self-directed violence
- Individuals witnessing violence between parental figures

Associated conditions

- Autism
- Borderline personality disorder
- Character disorder
- Depersonalization
- Developmental disabilities
- Psychotic disorders

This diagnosis will retire from the NANDA-I Taxonomy in the 2024–2026 edition unless additional work is completed to bring it up to a level of evidence 2.1 or higher.

Domain 11 • Class 3 • Diagnosis Code 00139

Risk for self-mutilation

Focus of the diagnosis: self-mutilation
Approved 1992 • Revised 2000, 2013, 2017

Definition
Susceptible to deliberate self-injurious behavior causing tissue damage with the intent of causing nonfatal injury to attain relief of tension.

Risk factors

- Absence of family confidant
- Altered body image
- Dissociation
- Disturbed interpersonal relations
- Eating disorder
- Excessive emotional disturbance
- Feeling threatened with loss of significant interpersonal relations
- Impaired self-esteem
- Inability to express tension verbally
- Ineffective communication between parent and adolescent
- Ineffective coping strategies
- Ineffective impulse control
- Irresistible urge for self-directed violence
- Irresistible urge to cut self
- Labile behavior
- Loss of control over problem-solving situation
- Low self-esteem
- Mounting tension that is intolerable
- Negative feelings
- Pattern of inability to plan solutions
- Pattern of inability to see long-term consequences
- Perfectionism
- Requires rapid stress reduction
- Social isolation
- Substance misuse
- Use of manipulation to obtain nurturing interpersonal relations with others

At risk population

- Adolescents
- Battered children
- Incarcerated individuals
- Individuals experiencing family divorce
- Individuals experiencing family substance misuse
- Individuals experiencing loss of significant interpersonal relations
- Individuals experiencing sexual identity crisis
- Individuals living in nontraditional setting
- Individuals whose peers self-mutilate
- Individuals with family history of self-destructive behavior
- Individuals with history of childhood abuse
- Individuals with history of childhood illness
- Individuals with history of childhood surgery

- Individuals with history of self-directed violence
- Individuals witnessing violence between parental figures

Associated conditions

- Autism
- Borderline personality disorder
- Character disorder
- Depersonalization
- Developmental disabilities
- Psychotic disorders

This diagnosis will retire from the NANDA-I Taxonomy in the 2024–2026 edition unless additional work is completed to bring it up to a level of evidence 2.1 or higher.

Domain 11 • Class 3 • Diagnosis Code 00289

Risk for suicidal behavior

Focus of the diagnosis: suicidal behavior
Approved 2020 • Level of Evidence 3.2

> **Definition**
> Susceptible to self-injurious acts associated with some intent to die.

Risk factors

Behavioral Factors

- Apathy
- Difficulty asking for help
- Difficulty coping with unsatisfactory performance
- Difficulty expressing feelings
- Ineffective chronic pain self-management
- Ineffective impulse control
- Self-injurious behavior
- Self-negligence
- Stockpiling of medication
- Substance misuse

Psychological

- Anxiety
- Depressive symptoms
- Hostility
- Expresses deep sadness
- Expresses frustration
- Expresses loneliness
- Low self-esteem
- Maladaptive grieving
- Perceived dishonor
- Perceived failure
- Reports excessive guilt
- Reports helplessness
- Reports hopelessness
- Reports unhappiness
- Suicidal ideation

Situational

- Easy access to weapon
- Loss of independence
- Loss of personal autonomy

Social Factors

- Dysfunctional family processes
- Inadequate social support
- Inappropriate peer pressure
- Legal difficulty
- Social deprivation
- Social devaluation
- Social isolation
- Unaddressed violence by others

At risk population

- Adolescents
- Adolescents living in foster care

- Economically disadvantaged individuals
- Individuals changing a will
- Individuals experiencing situational crisis
- Individuals facing discrimination
- Individuals giving away possessions
- Individuals living alone
- Individuals obtaining potentially lethal materials
- Individuals preparing a will
- Individuals who frequently seek care for vague symptomatology
- Individuals with disciplinary problems
- Individuals with family history of suicide
- Individuals with history of suicide attempt
- Individuals with history of violence
- Individuals with sudden euphoric recovery from major depression
- Institutionalized individuals
- Men
- Native American individuals
- Older adults

Associated conditions

- Depression
- Mental disorders
- Physical illness
- Terminal illness

Original literature support available at www.thieme.com/nanda-i.

11. Safety/protection

Domain 11 • Class 4 • Diagnosis Code 00181

Contamination

Focus of the diagnosis: contamination
Approved 2006 • Revised 2017 • Level of Evidence 2.1

> **Definition**
> Exposure to environmental contaminants in doses sufficient to cause adverse health effects.

Defining characteristics

Pesticides

- Dermatological effects of pesticide exposure
- Gastrointestinal effects of pesticide exposure
- Neurological effects of pesticide exposure
- Pulmonary effects of pesticide exposure
- Renal effects of pesticide exposure

Chemicals

- Dermatological effects of chemical exposure
- Gastrointestinal effects of chemical exposure
- Immunological effects of chemical exposure
- Neurological effects of chemical exposure
- Pulmonary effects of chemical exposure
- Renal effects of chemical exposure

Biologics

- Dermatological effects of biologic exposure
- Gastrointestinal effects of biologic exposure
- Neurological effects of biologic exposure
- Pulmonary effects of biologic exposure
- Renal effects of biologic exposure

Pollution

- Neurological effects of pollution exposure
- Pulmonary effects of pollution exposure

Waste

- Dermatological effects of waste exposure
- Gastrointestinal effects of waste exposure
- Hepatic effects of waste exposure
- Pulmonary effects of waste exposure

Radiation
- Genetic effects of radiotherapy exposure
- Immunological effects of radiotherapy exposure
- Neurological effects of radiotherapy exposure
- Oncological effects of radiotherapy exposure

Related factors
External Factors
- Carpeted flooring
- Chemical contamination of food
- Chemical contamination of water
- Flaking, peeling surface in presence of young children
- Inadequate breakdown of contaminant
- Inadequate household hygiene practices
- Inadequate municipal services
- Inadequate personal hygiene practices
- Inadequate protective clothing
- Inappropriate use of protective clothing
- Individuals who ingested contaminated material
- Playing where environmental contaminants are used
- Unprotected exposure to chemical
- Unprotected exposure to heavy metal
- Unprotected exposure to radioactive material
- Use of environmental contaminant in the home
- Use of noxious material in inadequately ventilated area
- Use of noxious material without effective protection

Internal Factors
- Concomitant exposure
- Malnutrition
- Smoking

At risk population
- Children aged < 5 years
- Economically disadvantaged individuals
- Individuals exposed perinatally
- Individuals exposed to areas with high contaminant level
- Individuals exposed to atmospheric pollutants
- Individuals exposed to bioterrorism
- Individuals exposed to disaster
- Individuals with history of exposure to contaminant
- Older adults
- Pregnant women
- Women

Associated conditions
- Pre-existing disease
- Radiotherapy

Original literature support available at www.thieme.com/nanda-i.

11. Safety/protection

Domain 11 • Class 4 • Diagnosis Code 00180

Risk for contamination

Focus of the diagnosis: contamination
Approved 2006 • Revised 2013, 2017 • Level of Evidence 2.1

Definition
Susceptible to exposure to environmental contaminants, which may compromise health.

Risk factors

External Factors

- Carpeted flooring
- Chemical contamination of food
- Chemical contamination of water
- Flaking, peeling surface in presence of young children
- Inadequate breakdown of contaminant
- Inadequate household hygiene practices
- Inadequate municipal services
- Inadequate personal hygiene practices
- Inadequate protective clothing
- Inappropriate use of protective clothing
- Individuals who ingested contaminated material
- Playing where environmental contaminants are used
- Unprotected exposure to chemical
- Unprotected exposure to heavy metal
- Unprotected exposure to radioactive material
- Use of environmental contaminant in the home
- Use of noxious material in inadequately ventilated area
- Use of noxious material without effective protection

Internal Factors

- Concomitant exposure
- Malnutrition
- Smoking

At risk population

- Children aged < 5 years
- Economically disadvantaged individuals
- Individuals exposed perinatally
- Individuals exposed to areas with high contaminant level
- Individuals exposed to atmospheric pollutants
- Individuals exposed to bioterrorism
- Individuals exposed to disaster
- Individuals with history of exposure to contaminant
- Older adults
- Pregnant women
- Women

Associated conditions
- Pre-existing disease
- Radiotherapy

Original literature support available at www.thieme.com/nanda-i.

Domain 11 • Class 4 • Diagnosis Code 00265

Risk for occupational injury

Focus of the diagnosis: occupational injury
Approved 2016 • Level of Evidence 2.1

Definition
Susceptible to a work-related accident or illness, which may compromise health.

Risk factors
Individual

- Distraction from interpersonal relations
- Excessive stress
- Improper use of personal protective equipment
- Inadequate knowledge
- Inadequate time management skills
- Ineffective coping strategies
- Misinterpretation of information
- Overconfident behaviors
- Psychological distress
- Unhealthy habits
- Unsafe work behaviors

Unmodified Environmental Factors

- Environmental constraints
- Exposure to biological agents
- Exposure to chemical agents
- Exposure to noise
- Exposure to radiotherapy
- Exposure to teratogenic agents
- Exposure to vibration
- Inadequate access to individual protective equipment
- Inadequate physical environment
- Labor relationships
- Night shift work rotating to day shift work
- Occupational burnout
- Physical workload
- Shift work

At risk population
- Individuals exposed to environmental temperature extremes

Original literature support available at www.thieme.com/nanda-i.

Domain 11 • Class 4 • Diagnosis Code 00037

Risk for poisoning

Focus of the diagnosis: poisoning
Approved 1980 • Revised 2006, 2013, 2017 • Level of Evidence 2.1

Definition
Susceptible to accidental exposure to, or ingestion of, drugs or dangerous products in sufficient doses, which may compromise health.

Risk factors

External Factors

- Access to dangerous product
- Access to illicit drugs potentially contaminated by poisonous additives
- Access to pharmaceutical preparations
- Occupational setting without adequate safeguards

Internal Factors

- Cognitive dysfunction
- Excessive emotional disturbance
- Inadequate knowledge of pharmaceutical preparations
- Inadequate knowledge of poisoning prevention
- Inadequate precautions against poisoning
- Neurobehavioral manifestations
- Unaddressed inadequate vision

Original literature support available at www.thieme.com/nanda-i.

11. Safety/protection

Domain 11 • Class 5 • Diagnosis Code 00218

Risk for adverse reaction to iodinated contrast media

Focus of the diagnosis: adverse reaction to iodinated contrast media
Approved 2010 • Revised 2013, 2017 • Level of Evidence 2.1

Definition
Susceptible to noxious or unintended reaction that can occur within seven days after contrast agent injection, which may compromise health.

Risk factors
– Dehydration

– Generalized weakness

At risk population
– Individuals at extremes of age
– Individuals with history of adverse effect from iodinated contrast media

– Individuals with history of allergy

Associated conditions
– Chronic disease
– Concurrent use of pharmaceutical preparations

– Decreased level of consciousness
– Individuals with fragile veins

Original literature support available at www.thieme.com/nanda-i.

Domain 11 • Class 5 • Diagnosis Code 00217

Risk for allergy reaction

Focus of the diagnosis: allergy reaction
Approved 2010 • Revised 2013, 2017 • Level of Evidence 2.1

Definition
Susceptible to an exaggerated immune response or reaction to substances, which may compromise health.

Risk factors
- Exposure to allergen
- Exposure to environmental allergen
- Exposure to toxic chemicals
- Inadequate knowledge about avoidance of relevant allergens
- Inattentive to potential allergen exposure

At risk population
- Individuals with history of food allergy
- Individuals with history of insect sting allergy
- Individuals with repeated exposure to allergen-producing environmental substance

Original literature support available at www.thieme.com/nanda-i.

11. Safety/protection

Domain 11 • Class 5 • Diagnosis Code 00042

Risk for latex allergy reaction

Focus of the diagnosis: latex allergy reaction
Approved 1998 • Revised 2006, 2013, 2017, 2020 • Level of Evidence 2.1

Definition
Susceptible to a hypersensitive reaction to natural latex rubber products or latex reactive foods, which may compromise health.

Risk factors
- Inadequate knowledge about avoidance of relevant allergens
- Inattentive to potential environmental latex exposure
- Inattentive to potential exposure to latex reactive foods

At risk population
- Individuals frequently exposed to latex product
- Individuals receiving repetitive injections from rubber topped bottles
- Individuals with family history of atopic dermatitis
- Individuals with history of latex reaction
- Infants undergoing numerous operations beginning soon after birth

Associated conditions
- Asthma
- Atopy
- Food allergy
- Hypersensitivity to natural latex rubber protein
- Multiple surgical procedures
- Poinsettia plant allergy
- Urinary bladder diseases

Original literature support available at www.thieme.com/nanda-i.

Domain 11 • Class 6 • Diagnosis Code 00007

Hyperthermia

Focus of the diagnosis: hyperthermia
Approved 1986 • Revised 2013, 2017 • Level of Evidence 2.2

Definition
Core body temperature above the normal diurnal range due to failure of thermoregulation.

Defining characteristics
- Abnormal posturing
- Apnea
- Coma
- Flushed skin
- Hypotension
- Infant does not maintain suck
- Irritable mood
- Lethargy
- Seizure
- Skin warm to touch
- Stupor
- Tachycardia
- Tachypnea
- Vasodilation

Related factors
- Dehydration
- Inappropriate clothing
- Vigorous activity

At risk population
- Individuals exposed to high environmental temperature

Associated conditions
- Decreased sweat response
- Impaired health status
- Increased metabolic rate
- Ischemia
- Pharmaceutical preparations
- Sepsis
- Trauma

Refer to staging criteria.

Original literature support available at www.thieme.com/nanda-i.

11. Safety/protection

Domain 11 • Class 6 • Diagnosis Code 00006

Hypothermia

Focus of the diagnosis: hypothermia
Approved 1986 • Revised 1988, 2013, 2017, 2020 • Level of Evidence 2.2

> **Definition**
> Core body temperature below the normal diurnal range in individuals > 28 days of life.

Defining characteristics

- Acrocyanosis
- Bradycardia
- Cyanotic nail beds
- Decreased blood glucose level
- Decreased ventilation
- Hypertension
- Hypoglycemia
- Hypoxia
- Increased metabolic rate
- Increased oxygen consumption
- Peripheral vasoconstriction
- Piloerection
- Shivering
- Skin cool to touch
- Slow capillary refill
- Tachycardia

Related factors

- Alcohol consumption
- Excessive conductive heat transfer
- Excessive convective heat transfer
- Excessive evaporative heat transfer
- Excessive radiative heat transfer
- Inactivity
- Inadequate caregiver knowledge of hypothermia prevention
- Inadequate clothing
- Low environmental temperature
- Malnutrition

At risk population

- Economically disadvantaged individuals
- Individuals at extremes of age
- Individuals at extremes of weight

Associated conditions

- Damage to hypothalamus
- Decreased metabolic rate
- Pharmaceutical preparations
- Radiotherapy
- Trauma

Refer to appropriate and validated staging criteria.
Original literature support available at www.thieme.com/nanda-i.

Domain 11 • Class 6 • Diagnosis Code 00253

Risk for hypothermia

Focus of the diagnosis: hypothermia
Approved 2013 • Revised 2017, 2020 • Level of Evidence 2.2

Definition
Susceptible to a failure of thermoregulation that may result in a core body temperature below the normal diurnal range in individuals > 28 days of life, which may compromise health.

Risk factors
- Alcohol consumption
- Excessive conductive heat transfer
- Excessive convective heat transfer
- Excessive evaporative heat transfer
- Excessive radiative heat transfer
- Inactivity
- Inadequate caregiver knowledge of hypothermia prevention
- Inadequate clothing
- Low environmental temperature
- Malnutrition

At risk population
- Economically disadvantaged individuals
- Individuals at extremes of age
- Individuals at extremes of weight

Associated conditions
- Damage to hypothalamus
- Decreased metabolic rate
- Pharmaceutical preparations
- Radiotherapy
- Trauma

Refer to appropriate and validated staging criteria.

Original literature support available at www.thieme.com/nanda-i.

11. Safety/protection

Domain 11 • Class 6 • Diagnosis Code 00280

Neonatal hypothermia

Focus of the diagnosis: hypothermia
Approved 2020 • Level of Evidence 3.1

Definition
Core body temperature of an infant below the normal diurnal range.

Defining characteristics
- Acrocyanosis
- Bradycardia
- Decreased blood glucose level
- Decreased metabolic rate
- Decreased peripheral perfusion
- Decreased ventilation
- Hypertension
- Hypoglycemia
- Hypoxia
- Increased oxygen demand
- Insufficient energy to maintain sucking
- Irritability
- Metabolic acidosis
- Pallor
- Peripheral vasoconstriction
- Respiratory distress
- Skin cool to touch
- Slow capillary refill
- Tachycardia
- Weight gain < 30 g/day

Related factors
- Delayed breastfeeding
- Early bathing of newborn
- Excessive conductive heat transfer
- Excessive convective heat transfer
- Excessive evaporative heat transfer
- Excessive radiative heat transfer
- Inadequate caregiver knowledge of hypothermia prevention
- Inadequate clothing
- Malnutrition

At risk population
- Low birth weight neonates
- Neonates aged 0-28 days
- Neonates born by cesarean delivery
- Neonates born to an adolescent mother
- Neonates born to economically disadvantaged families
- Neonates exposed to low environmental temperatures
- Neonates with high-risk out of hospital birth
- Neonates with inadequate subcutaneous fat
- Neonates with increased body surface area to weight ratio
- Neonates with unplanned out-of-hospital birth
- Premature neonates

Associated conditions

- Damage to hypothalamus
- Immature stratum corneum
- Increased pulmonary vascular resistance
- Ineffective vascular control
- Inefficient nonshivering thermogenesis
- Low Appearance, Pulse, Grimace, Activity, & Respiration (APGAR) scores
- Pharmaceutical preparations

Refer to appropriate and validated hypothermia staging criteria.

Original literature support available at www.thieme.com/nanda-i.

Domain 11 • Class 6 • Diagnosis Code 00282

Risk for neonatal hypothermia

Focus of the diagnosis: hypothermia
Approved 2020 • Level of Evidence 3.1

Definition
Susceptibility of an infant to a core body temperature below the normal diurnal range, which may compromise health.

Risk factors
- Delayed breastfeeding
- Early bathing of newborn
- Excessive conductive heat transfer
- Excessive convective heat transfer
- Excessive evaporative heat transfer
- Excessive radiative heat transfer
- Inadequate caregiver knowledge of hypothermia prevention
- Inadequate clothing
- Malnutrition

At risk population
- Low birth weight neonates
- Neonates aged 0-28 days
- Neonates born by cesarean delivery
- Neonates born to an adolescent mother
- Neonates born to economically disadvantaged families
- Neonates exposed to low environmental temperatures
- Neonates with high-risk out of hospital birth
- Neonates with inadequate subcutaneous fat
- Neonates with increased body surface area to weight ratio
- Neonates with unplanned out-of-hospital birth
- Premature neonates

Associated conditions
- Damage to hypothalamus
- Immature stratum corneum
- Increased pulmonary vascular resistance
- Ineffective vascular control
- Inefficient nonshivering thermogenesis
- Low Appearance, Pulse, Grimace, Activity, & Respiration (APGAR) scores
- Pharmaceutical preparations

Refer to appropriate and validated hypothermia staging criteria.

Original literature support available at www.thieme.com/nanda-i.

Domain 11 • Class 6 • Diagnosis Code 00254

Risk for perioperative hypothermia

Focus of the diagnosis: perioperative hypothermia
Approved 2013 • Revised 2017, 2020 • Level of Evidence 2.2

Definition
Susceptible to an inadvertent drop in core body temperature below 36 °C / 96.8 °F occurring one hour before to 24 hours after surgery, which may compromise health.

Risk factors
- Anxiety
- Body mass index below normal range for age and gender
- Environmental temperature < 21 °C / 69.8 °F
- Inadequate availability of appropriate warming equipment
- Wound area uncovered

At risk population
- Individuals aged ≥ 60 years
- Individuals in environment with laminar air flow
- Individuals receiving anesthesia for a period > 2 hours
- Individuals undergoing long induction time
- Individuals undergoing open surgery
- Individuals undergoing surgical procedure > 2 hours
- Individuals with American Society of Anesthesiologists (ASA) Physical Status classification score > 1
- Individuals with high Model for End-Stage Liver Disease (MELD) score
- Individuals with increased intra-operative blood loss
- Individuals with intraoperative diastolic arterial blood pressure < 60 mmHg
- Individuals with intraoperative systolic blood pressure < 140 mmHg
- Individuals with low body surface area
- Neonates < 37 weeks gestational age
- Women

Associated conditions
- Acute hepatic failure
- Anemia
- Burns
- Cardiovascular complications
- Chronic renal impairment
- Combined regional and general anesthesia
- Neurological disorder
- Pharmaceutical preparations
- Trauma

11. Safety/protection

Original literature support available at www.thieme.com/nanda-i.

Domain 11 • Class 6 • Diagnosis Code 00008

Ineffective thermoregulation

Focus of the diagnosis: thermoregulation
Approved 1986 • Revised 2017 • Level of Evidence 2.1

Definition
Temperature fluctuation between hypothermia and hyperthermia.

Defining characteristics

- Cyanotic nail beds
- Flushed skin
- Hypertension
- Increased body temperature above normal range
- Increased respiratory rate
- Mild shivering
- Moderate pallor
- Piloerection
- Reduction in body temperature below normal range
- Seizure
- Skin cool to touch
- Skin warm to touch
- Slow capillary refill
- Tachycardia

Related factors

- Dehydration
- Environmental temperature fluctuations
- Inactivity
- Inappropriate clothing for environmental temperature
- Increased oxygen demand
- Vigorous activity

At risk population

- Individuals at extremes of weight
- Individuals exposed to environmental temperature extremes
- Individuals with inadequate supply of subcutaneous fat
- Individuals with increased body surface area to weight ratio

Associated conditions

- Altered metabolic rate
- Brain injuries
- Condition affecting temperature regulation
- Decreased sweat response
- Impaired health status
- Inefficient nonshivering thermogenesis
- Pharmaceutical preparations
- Sedation
- Sepsis
- Trauma

Domain 11 • Class 6 • Diagnosis Code 00274

Risk for ineffective thermoregulation

Focus of the diagnosis: thermoregulation
Approved 2016 • Level of Evidence 2.1

Definition
Susceptible to temperature fluctuation between hypothermia and hyperthermia, which may compromise health.

Risk factors
- Dehydration
- Environmental temperature fluctuations
- Inactivity
- Inappropriate clothing for environmental temperature
- Increased oxygen demand
- Vigorous activity

At risk population
- Individuals at extremes of weight
- Individuals exposed to environmental temperature extremes
- Individuals with inadequate supply of subcutaneous fat
- Individuals with increased body surface area to weight ratio

Associated conditions
- Altered metabolic rate
- Brain injuries
- Condition affecting temperature regulation
- Decreased sweat response
- Impaired health status
- Inefficient nonshivering thermogenesis
- Pharmaceutical preparations
- Sedation
- Sepsis
- Trauma

11. Safety/protection

Domain 12. Comfort

Sense of mental, physical, or social well-being or ease

Class 3.   Social comfort
Sense of well-being or ease with one's social situation

Code	Diagnosis	Page
00214	Impaired comfort	562
00183	Readiness for enhanced comfort	563
00054	Risk for loneliness	564
00053	Social isolation	565

NANDA International, Inc. Nursing Diagnoses: Definitions and Classification 2021–2023, 12th Edition.
Edited by T. Heather Herdman, Shigemi Kamitsuru, and Camila Takáo Lopes.
© 2021 NANDA International, Inc. Published 2021 by Thieme Medical Publishers, Inc., New York.
Companion website: www.thieme.com/nanda-i.

Domain 12 • Class 1 • Diagnosis Code 00214

Impaired comfort

Focus of the diagnosis: comfort
Approved 2008 • Revised 2010, 2017 • Level of Evidence 2.1

Definition
Perceived lack of ease, relief, and transcendence in physical, psychospiritual, environmental, cultural, and/or social dimensions.

Defining characteristics

- Anxiety
- Crying
- Difficulty relaxing
- Expresses discomfort
- Expresses discontentment with situation
- Expresses fear
- Expresses feeling cold
- Expresses feeling warm
- Expresses itching
- Expresses psychological distress
- Irritable mood
- Moaning
- Psychomotor agitation
- Reports altered sleep-wake cycle
- Reports hunger
- Sighing
- Uneasy in situation

Related factors

- Inadequate control over environment
- Inadequate health resources
- Inadequate situational control
- Insufficient privacy
- Unpleasant environmental stimuli

Associated conditions

- Illness-related symptoms
- Treatment regimen

This diagnosis is classified under Class 1 (Physical comfort), Class 2 (Environmental comfort), and Class 3 (Social comfort).

Original literature support available at www.thieme.com/nanda-i.

12. Comfort

Domain 12 · Class 1 · Diagnosis Code 00183

Readiness for enhanced comfort

Focus of the diagnosis: comfort
Approved 2006 · Revised 2013 · Level of Evidence 2.1

Definition
A pattern of ease, relief, and transcendence in physical, psychospiritual, environmental, and/or social dimensions, which can be strengthened.

Defining characteristics
- Expresses desire to enhance comfort
- Expresses desire to enhance feeling of contentment
- Expresses desire to enhance relaxation
- Expresses desire to enhance resolution of complaints

This diagnosis is classified under Class 1 (Physical comfort), Class 2 (Environmental comfort), and Class 3 (Social comfort).

Original literature support available at www.thieme.com/nanda-i.

Domain 12 • Class 1 • Diagnosis Code 00134

Nausea

Focus of the diagnosis: nausea
Approved 1998 • Revised 2002, 2010, 2017 • Level of Evidence 2.1

Definition
A subjective phenomenon of an unpleasant feeling in the back of the throat and stomach, which may or may not result in vomiting.

Defining characteristics
- Food aversion
- Gagging sensation
- Increased salivation
- Increased swallowing
- Sour taste

Related factors
- Anxiety
- Exposure to toxin
- Fear
- Noxious taste
- Unpleasant sensory stimuli

At risk population
- Pregnant women

Associated conditions
- Abdominal neoplasms
- Altered biochemical phenomenon
- Esophageal disease
- Gastric distention
- Gastrointestinal irritation
- Intracranial hypertension
- Labyrinthitis
- Liver capsule stretch
- Localized tumor
- Meniere's disease
- Meningitis
- Motion sickness
- Pancreatic diseases
- Pharmaceutical preparations
- Psychological disorder
- Splenic capsule stretch
- Treatment regimen

12. Comfort

Original literature support available at www.thieme.com/nanda-i.

Domain 12 • Class 1 • Diagnosis Code 00132

Acute pain

Focus of the diagnosis: pain
Approved 1996 • Revised 2013 • Level of Evidence 2.1

Definition

Unpleasant sensory and emotional experience associated with actual or potential tissue damage, or described in terms of such damage (International Association for the Study of Pain); sudden or slow onset of any intensity from mild to severe with an anticipated or predictable end, and with a duration of less than 3 months.

Defining characteristics

- Altered physiological parameter
- Appetite change
- Diaphoresis
- Distraction behavior
- Evidence of pain using standardized pain behavior checklist for those unable to communicate verbally
- Expressive behavior
- Facial expression of pain
- Guarding behavior
- Hopelessness

- Narrow focus
- Positioning to ease pain
- Protective behavior
- Proxy report of activity changes
- Proxy report of pain behavior
- Pupil dilation
- Reports intensity using standardized pain scale
- Reports pain characteristics using standardized pain instrument
- Self-focused

Related factors

- Biological injury agent
- Inappropriate use of chemical agent

- Physical injury agent

Original literature support available at www.thieme.com/nanda-i.

Domain 12 • Class 1 • Diagnosis Code 00133

Chronic pain

Focus of the diagnosis: pain
Approved 1986 • Revised 1996, 2013, 2017 • Level of Evidence 2.1

Definition
Unpleasant sensory and emotional experience associated with actual or potential tissue damage, or described in terms of such damage (International Association for the Study of Pain); sudden or slow onset of any intensity from mild to severe, constant or recurring without an anticipated or predictable end, and with a duration of greater than 3 months.

Defining characteristics
- Altered ability to continue activities
- Anorexia
- Evidence of pain using standardized pain behavior checklist for those unable to communicate verbally
- Expresses fatigue
- Facial expression of pain
- Proxy report of activity changes
- Proxy report of pain behavior
- Reports altered sleep-wake cycle
- Reports intensity using standardized pain scale
- Reports pain characteristics using standardized pain instrument
- Self-focused

Related factors
- Body mass index above normal range for age and gender
- Fatigue
- Ineffective sexuality pattern
- Injury agent
- Malnutrition
- Prolonged computer use
- Psychological distress
- Repeated handling of heavy loads
- Social isolation
- Whole-body vibration

At risk population
- Individuals aged > 50 years
- Individuals with history of being abused
- Individuals with history of genital mutilation
- Individuals with history of over indebtedness
- Individuals with history of static work postures
- Individuals with history of substance misuse
- Individuals with history of vigorous exercise
- Women

12. Comfort

Associated conditions

- Bone fractures
- Central nervous system sensitization
- Chronic musculoskeletal diseases
- Contusion
- Crush syndrome
- Imbalance of neurotransmitters, neuromodulators and receptors
- Immune system diseases
- Impaired metabolism
- Inborn genetic diseases
- Ischemia
- Neoplasms
- Nerve compression syndromes
- Nervous system diseases
- Post-trauma related condition
- Prolonged increase in cortisol level
- Soft tissue injuries
- Spinal cord injuries

Original literature support available at www.thieme.com/nanda-i.

Domain 12 • Class 1 • Diagnosis Code 00255

Chronic pain syndrome

Focus of the diagnosis: chronic pain syndrome
Approved 2013 • Revised 2020 • Level of Evidence 2.2

Definition
Recurrent or persistent pain that has lasted at least 3 months, and that significantly affects daily functioning or well-being.

Defining characteristics

- Anxiety (00146)
- Constipation (00011)
- Disturbed sleep pattern (00198)
- Fatigue (00093)
- Fear (00148)

- Impaired mood regulation (00241)
- Impaired physical mobility (00085)
- Insomnia (00095)
- Social isolation (00053)
- Stress overload (00177)

Related factors

- Body mass index above normal range for age and gender
- Fear of pain
- Fear-avoidance beliefs

- Inadequate knowledge of pain management behaviors
- Negative affect
- Sleep disturbances

12. Comfort

Original literature support available at www.thieme.com/nanda-i.

Domain 12 • Class 1 • Diagnosis Code 00256

Labor pain

Focus of the diagnosis: labor pain
Approved 2013 • Revised 2017, 2020 • Level of Evidence 2.2

Definition
Sensory and emotional experience that varies from pleasant to unpleasant, associated with labor and childbirth.

Defining characteristics
- Altered blood pressure
- Altered heart rate
- Altered muscle tension
- Altered neuroendocrine functioning
- Altered respiratory rate
- Altered urinary functioning
- Anxiety
- Appetite change
- Diaphoresis
- Distraction behavior
- Expressive behavior
- Facial expression of pain
- Narrow focus
- Nausea
- Perineal pressure
- Positioning to ease pain
- Protective behavior
- Pupil dilation
- Reports altered sleep-wake cycle
- Self-focused
- Uterine contraction
- Vomiting

Related factors
Behavioral Factors
- Insufficient fluid intake
- Supine position

Cognitive Factors
- Fear of childbirth
- Inadequate knowledge about childbirth
- Inadequate preparation to deal with labor pain
- Low self efficacy
- Perception of labor pain as nonproductive
- Perception of labor pain as negative
- Perception of labor pain as threatening
- Perception of labor pain as unnatural
- Perception of pain as meaningful

Social Factors
- Interference in decision-making
- Unsupportive companionship

Unmodified Environmental Factors

- Noisy delivery room
- Overcrowded delivery room

- Turbulent environment

At risk population

- Women experiencing emergency situation during labor
- Women from cultures with negative perspective of labor pain
- Women giving birth in a disease-based health care system
- Women whose mothers have a high level of education

- Women with history of pre-pregnancy dysmenorrhea
- Women with history of sexual abuse during childhood
- Women without supportive companion

Associated conditions

- Cervical dilation
- Depression
- Fetal expulsion

- High maternal trait anxiety
- Prescribed mobility restriction
- Prolonged duration of labor

12. Comfort

Original literature support available at www.thieme.com/nanda-i.

Domain 12 • Class 2 • Diagnosis Code 00214

Impaired comfort

Focus of the diagnosis: comfort
Approved 2008 • Revised 2010, 2017 • Level of Evidence 2.1

Definition
Perceived lack of ease, relief, and transcendence in physical, psychospiritual, environmental, cultural, and/or social dimensions.

Defining characteristics
- Anxiety
- Crying
- Difficulty relaxing
- Expresses discomfort
- Expresses discontentment with situation
- Expresses fear
- Expresses feeling cold
- Expresses feeling warm
- Expresses itching
- Expresses psychological distress
- Irritable mood
- Moaning
- Psychomotor agitation
- Reports altered sleep-wake cycle
- Reports hunger
- Sighing
- Uneasy in situation

Related factors
- Inadequate control over environment
- Inadequate health resources
- Inadequate situational control
- Insufficient privacy
- Unpleasant environmental stimuli

Associated conditions
- Illness-related symptoms
- Treatment regimen

This diagnosis is classified under Class 1 (Physical comfort), Class 2 (Environmental comfort), and Class 3 (Social comfort).

Original literature support available at www.thieme.com/nanda-i.

12. Comfort

Domain 12 • Class 2 • Diagnosis Code 00183

Readiness for enhanced comfort

Focus of the diagnosis: comfort
Approved 2006 • Revised 2013 • Level of Evidence 2.1

Definition
A pattern of ease, relief, and transcendence in physical, psychospiritual, environmental, and/or social dimensions, which can be strengthened.

Defining characteristics
- Expresses desire to enhance comfort
- Expresses desire to enhance feeling of contentment
- Expresses desire to enhance relaxation
- Expresses desire to enhance resolution of complaints

This diagnosis is classified under Class 1 (Physical comfort), Class 2 (Environmental comfort), and Class 3 (Social comfort).

Original literature support available at www.thieme.com/nanda-i.

12. Comfort

Domain 12 • Class 3 • Diagnosis Code 00214

Impaired comfort

Focus of the diagnosis: comfort
Approved 2008 • Revised 2010, 2017 • Level of Evidence 2.1

Definition
Perceived lack of ease, relief, and transcendence in physical, psychospiritual, environmental, cultural, and/or social dimensions.

Defining characteristics

- Anxiety
- Crying
- Difficulty relaxing
- Expresses discomfort
- Expresses discontentment with situation
- Expresses fear
- Expresses feeling cold
- Expresses feeling warm
- Expresses itching

- Expresses psychological distress
- Irritable mood
- Moaning
- Psychomotor agitation
- Reports altered sleep-wake cycle
- Reports hunger
- Sighing
- Uneasy in situation

Related factors

- Inadequate control over environment
- Inadequate health resources
- Inadequate situational control

- Insufficient privacy
- Unpleasant environmental stimuli

Associated conditions

- Illness-related symptoms

- Treatment regimen

This diagnosis is classified under Class 1 (Physical comfort), Class 2 (Environmental comfort), and Class 3 (Social comfort).

Original literature support available at www.thieme.com/nanda-i.

Domain 12 • Class 3 • Diagnosis Code 00183

Readiness for enhanced comfort

Focus of the diagnosis: comfort
Approved 2006 • Revised 2013 • Level of Evidence 2.1

Definition
A pattern of ease, relief, and transcendence in physical, psychospiritual, environmental, and/or social dimensions, which can be strengthened.

Defining characteristics

- Expresses desire to enhance comfort
- Expresses desire to enhance feeling of contentment
- Expresses desire to enhance relaxation
- Expresses desire to enhance resolution of complaints

This diagnosis is classified under Class 1 (Physical comfort), Class 2 (Environmental comfort), and Class 3 (Social comfort).

Original literature support available at www.thieme.com/nanda-i.

12. Comfort

Domain 12 • Class 3 • Diagnosis Code 00054

Risk for loneliness

Focus of the diagnosis: loneliness
Approved 1994 • Revised 2006, 2013 • Level of Evidence 2.1

Definition
Susceptible to experiencing discomfort associated with a desire or need for more contact with others, which may compromise health.

Risk factors
- Affectional deprivation
- Emotional deprivation
- Physical isolation
- Social isolation

Original literature support available at www.thieme.com/nanda-i.

Domain 12 • Class 3 • Diagnosis Code 00053

Social isolation

Focus of the diagnosis: social isolation
Approved 1982 • Revised 2017, 2020 • Level of Evidence 3.1

Definition
A state in which the individual lacks a sense of relatedness connected to positive, lasting, and significant interpersonal relationships.

Defining characteristics

- Altered physical appearance
- Expresses dissatisfaction with respect from others
- Expresses dissatisfaction with social connection
- Expresses dissatisfaction with social support
- Expresses loneliness
- Flat affect
- Hostility
- Impaired ability to meet expectations of others
- Low levels of social activities
- Minimal interaction with others
- Preoccupation with own thoughts
- Purposelessness
- Reduced eye contact
- Reports feeling different from others
- Reports feeling insecure in public
- Sad affect
- Seclusion imposed by others
- Sense of alienation
- Social behavior incongruent with cultural norms
- Social withdrawal

Related factors

- Cognitive dysfunction
- Difficulty establishing satisfactory reciprocal interpersonal relations
- Difficulty performing activities of daily living
- Difficulty sharing personal life expectations
- Fear of crime
- Fear of traffic
- Impaired physical mobility
- Inadequate psychosocial support system
- Inadequate social skills
- Inadequate social support
- Inadequate transportation
- Low self-esteem
- Negative perception of support system
- Neurobehavioral manifestations
- Values incongruent with cultural norms

At risk population

- Economically disadvantaged individuals
- Immigrants
- Individuals experiencing altered social role

12. Comfort

- Individuals experiencing loss of significant other
- Individuals living alone
- Individuals living far from significant others
- Individuals moving to unfamiliar locations
- Individuals with history of rejection

- Individuals with history of traumatic event
- Individuals with ill family member
- Individuals with no children
- Institutionalized individuals
- Older adults
- Widowed individuals

Associated conditions

- Chronic disease

- Cognitive disorders

Domain 13.
Growth/development

Age-appropriate increases in physical dimensions, maturation of organ systems, and/or progression through the developmental milestones

Class 1. Growth
Increase in physical dimensions or maturity of organ systems

Code	Diagnosis	Page
This class does not currently contain any diagnoses		

Class 2. Development
Progress or regression through a sequence of recognized milestones in life

Code	Diagnosis	Page
00314	Delayed child development	568
00305	Risk for delayed child development	570
00315	Delayed infant motor development	571
00316	Risk for delayed infant motor development	573

Domain 13 • Class 2 • Diagnosis Code 00314

Delayed child development

Focus of the diagnosis: development
Approved 2020 • Level of Evidence 2.3

Definition
Child who continually fails to achieve developmental milestones within the expected timeframe.

Defining characteristics

- Consistent difficulty performing cognitive skills typical of age group
- Consistent difficulty performing language skills typical of age group
- Consistent difficulty performing motor skills typical of age group
- Consistent difficulty performing psychosocial skills typical of age group

Related factors

Infant or Child Factors

- Inadequate access to health care provider
- Inadequate attachment behavior
- Inadequate stimulation
- Unaddressed abuse
- Unaddressed psychological neglect

Caregiver Factors

- Anxiety
- Decreased emotional support availability
- Depressive symptoms
- Excessive stress
- Unaddressed domestic violence

At risk population

- Children aged 0-9 years
- Children born to economically disadvantaged families
- Children exposed to community violence
- Children exposed to environmental pollutants
- Children whose caregivers have developmental disabilities
- Children whose mothers had inadequate prenatal care
- Children with below normal growth standards for age and gender
- Institutionalized children
- Low birth weight infants
- Premature infants

Associated conditions

- Antenatal pharmaceutical preparations
- Congenital disorders
- Depression
- Inborn genetic diseases

- Maternal mental disorders
- Maternal physical illnesses
- Prenatal substance misuse
- Sensation disorders

Use of a valid and reliable, standardized development assessment scale is recommended.

Original literature support available at www.thieme.com/nanda-i.

Domain 13 • Class 2 • Diagnosis Code 00305

Risk for delayed child development

Focus of the diagnosis: development
Approved 2020 • Level of Evidence 2.3

Definition
Child who is susceptible to failure to achieve developmental milestones within the expected timeframe.

Risk factors

Infant or Child Factors

- Inadequate access to health care provider
- Inadequate attachment behavior

- Inadequate stimulation
- Unaddressed psychological neglect

Caregiver Factors

- Anxiety
- Decreased emotional support availability
- Depressive symptoms

- Excessive stress
- Unaddressed domestic violence

At risk population

- Children aged 0-9 years
- Children born to economically disadvantaged families
- Children exposed to community violence
- Children exposed to environmental pollutants
- Children whose caregivers have developmental disabilities

- Children whose mothers had inadequate prenatal care
- Children with below normal growth standards for age and gender
- Institutionalized children
- Low birth weight infants
- Premature infants

Associated conditions

- Antenatal pharmaceutical preparations
- Congenital disorders
- Depression
- Inborn genetic diseases

- Maternal mental disorders
- Maternal physical illnesses
- Prenatal substance misuse
- Sensation disorders

Original literature support available at www.thieme.com/nanda-i.

Domain 13 • Class 2 • Diagnosis Code 00315

Delayed infant motor development

Focus of the diagnosis: motor development
Approved 2020 • Level of Evidence 3.1

Definition
Individual who consistently fails to achieve developmental milestones related to the normal strengthening of bones, muscles and ability to move and touch one's surroundings.

Defining characteristics
- Difficulty lifting head
- Difficulty maintaining head position
- Difficulty picking up blocks
- Difficulty pulling self to stand
- Difficulty rolling over
- Difficulty sitting with support
- Difficulty sitting without support
- Difficulty standing with assistance
- Difficulty transferring objects
- Difficulty with hand-and-knee crawling
- Does not engage in activities
- Does not initiate activities

Related factors
Infant Factors
- Difficulty with sensory processing
- Insufficient curiosity
- Insufficient initiative
- Insufficient persistence

Caregiver Factors
- Anxiety about infant care
- Carries infant in arms for excessive time
- Does not allow infant to choose physical activities
- Does not allow infant to choose toys
- Does not encourage infant to grasp
- Does not encourage infant to reach
- Does not encourage sufficient infant play with other children
- Does not engage infant in games about body parts
- Does not teach movement words
- Insufficient fine motor toys for infant
- Insufficient gross motor toys for infant
- Insufficient time between periods of infant stimulation
- Limits infant experiences in the prone position
- Maternal postpartum depressive symptoms
- Negative perception of infant temperament
- Overstimulation of infant
- Perceived infant care incompetence

13. Growth/development

At risk population

- Boys
- Infants aged 0-12 months
- Infants born to economically disadvantaged families
- Infants born to large families
- Infants born to parents with low educational levels
- Infants in intensive care units
- Infants living in home with inadequate physical space
- Infants whose mothers had inadequate antenatal diet
- Infants with below normal growth standards for age and gender
- Low birth weight infants
- Premature infants
- Premature infants who do not receive physiotherapy during hospitalization

Associated conditions

- 5 minute Appearance, Pulse, Grimace, Activity, & Respiration (APGAR) score < 7
- Antenatal pharmaceutical preparations
- Complex medical conditions
- Failure to thrive
- Maternal anemia in late pregnancy
- Maternal mental health disorders in early pregnancy
- Maternal prepregnancy obesity
- Neonatal abstinence syndrome
- Neurodevelopmental disorders
- Postnatal infection of preterm infant
- Sensation disorders

Original literature support available at www.thieme.com/nanda-i.

Domain 13 • Class 2 • Diagnosis Code 00316

Risk for delayed infant motor development

Focus of the diagnosis: motor development
Approved 2020 • Level of Evidence 3.1

Definition
Individual susceptible to fails to achieve developmental milestones related to the normal strengthening of bones, muscles and ability to move and touch one's surroundings.

Risk factors

Infant Factors

- Difficulty with sensory processing
- Insufficient curiosity
- Insufficient initiative
- Insufficient persistence

Caregiver Factors

- Anxiety about infant care
- Carries infant in arms for excessive time
- Does not allow infant to choose toys
- Does not encourage infant to grasp
- Does not encourage infant to reach
- Does not encourage sufficient infant play with other children
- Does not engage infant in games about body parts
- Does not teach movement words
- Insufficient fine motor toys for infant
- Insufficient gross motor toys for infant
- Insufficient time between periods of infant stimulation
- Limits infant experiences in the prone position
- Maternal postpartum depressive symptoms
- Negative perception of infant temperament
- Overstimulation of infant
- Perceived infant care incompetence

At risk population

- Boys
- Infants aged 0-12 months
- Infants born to economically disadvantaged families
- Infants born to large families
- Infants born to parents with low educational levels
- Infants in intensive care units
- Infants living in home with inadequate physical space
- Infants whose mothers had inadequate antenatal diet
- Infants with below normal growth standards for age and gender
- Low birth weight infants
- Premature infants

- Premature infants who do not receive physiotherapy during hospitalization

Associated conditions

- 5 minute Appearance, Pulse, Grimace, Activity, & Respiration (APGAR) score < 7
- Antenatal pharmaceutical preparations
- Complex medical conditions
- Failure to thrive
- Maternal anemia in late pregnancy

- Maternal mental health disorders in early pregnancy
- Maternal prepregnancy obesity
- Neonatal abstinence syndrome
- Neurodevelopmental disorders
- Postnatal infection of preterm infant
- Sensation disorders

Original literature support available at www.thieme.com/nanda-i.

Index

The foci of the nursing diagnoses in NANDA-I Taxonomy II and their associated diagnoses start on the following pages: